The Paleo
Answer

Also by Loren Cordain

The Paleo Diet
The Paleo Diet Cookbook (with Lorrie Cordain
    and Nell Stephenson)
The Paleo Diet for Athletes (with Joe Friel)
The Dietary Cure for Acne

The Paleo Answer

7 Days to Lose Weight, Feel Great, Stay Young

Loren Cordain, Ph.D.

WILEY

John Wiley & Sons, Inc.

For Lorrie and the Boys

Contents

Preface

I think it's important to give you a history of the Paleo Diet concept. The Paleo Diet and Paleo in general have recently become very hot topics. These ideas have become household words in the last few years; however, it hasn't always been this way. On the next page is a graph from Google Trends for the words "Paleo Diet."

It's clear from this graph that the Paleo Diet was unknown to all but dedicated fans until three years ago. Fortunately, I've been in the middle of this worldwide movement nearly from its beginnings.

Last October, I approached my sixtieth birthday with some trepidation. I was part of the 1960s generation whose mantra was not to trust anyone over thirty, and now I'm twice that age. As I look back over my life, I can pinpoint a few key events that led me to discover and appreciate the Paleo Diet.

I came of age as a track and field athlete at the University of Nevada, Reno, in the late 1960s and the early 1970s, and I was always interested in diet, fitness, and athletic performance. Later as lifeguards at Lake Tahoe, my friends and I read all of the now-classic vegetarian diet and health books such as Francis Moore Lappé's *Diet for a Small Planet*, Paivo Airola's *Are You Confused?* and Dick Gregory's *Natural Diet for Folks Who Eat*, among others. I attended a Dick Gregory lecture in Seattle and got to shake the famous comedian's hand. My lifeguard friends

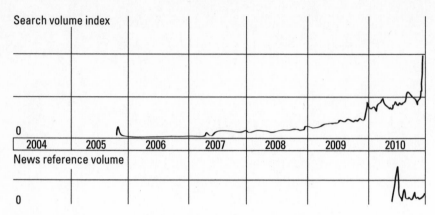

Google Trends Search for "Paleo Diet"

and I experimented with vegan diets, fasting, and all kinds of vitamins and supplements. Almost everyone seemed to own a juicer.

Each summer, instead of shying away from the sun and using sunscreens, we all tried to get the deepest tans possible. We swam in Tahoe's icy, invigorating, nonchlorinated waters, and decades before Vibram Five Fingers and Nike Frees (shoes that mimic bare feet) were the rage, we ran barefoot in the sand along Sand Harbor's pristine shoreline. Those twenty memorable summers as a lifeguard at Tahoe heightened my awareness of the outdoor, natural world, sunshine, health, fitness, and diet.

I completed my Ph.D. in exercise physiology at the University of Utah in the spring of 1981 and was promptly hired as an assistant professor in the Department of Health and Exercise Science at Colorado State University. For the first five to ten years of my career, my research focused mainly on how diet and exercise affected fitness and athletic performance. I still hadn't encountered Paleo, but I read widely and had a considerable interest in anthropology.

In the spring of 1987, I happened upon Boyd Eaton, M.D.'s now-classic scientific paper "Paleolithic Nutrition: A Consideration of Its Nature and Current Implications," which had been published two years earlier in the prestigious *New England Journal of Medicine*. This article made a lasting impression on me; it was the single factor that caused me to focus my research interests on ancestral human diets from that point forward.

One of the surprising points that Dr. Eaton made in a subsequent paper was that cereal grains were rarely or never consumed by pre-agricultural hunter-gatherers.

In the days and months after reading Boyd's groundbreaking paper, I became engrossed in studying ancestral human diets, and I voraciously read everything I could about the topic. At first, I simply filed all of the scientific papers and documents into a single file folder I labeled "Paleolithic Nutrition." Early on, I realized that this strategy wouldn't work because of the enormous volume and diversity of topics that materialized.

As I read more and more, patterns began to emerge. Stone Age people did not drink milk or consume dairy products. So I created a file folder labeled "Dairy." They also didn't eat cereal grains, as Dr. Eaton pointed out, so I created a single file folder called "Cereal Grains." Just like the single folder I had originally created for "Paleolithic Nutrition," it soon became apparent that the topic of cereal grains and their potential for adversely affecting health was an enormous topic that ultimately would require a huge number of file folders.

Eating Paleo

As my lifeguarding days drew to a close in 1991, my wife, Lorrie, and I began to eat Paleo. During the course of the next seven or eight years, I collected more than twenty-five thousand scientific papers and filled five large filing cabinets—each with hundreds of categories dealing with all aspects of the Paleo Diet and the Paleo lifestyle. In 1994, I mustered enough courage to telephone (no one used e-mail then) the man who was responsible for my collection of articles on anything and everything related to Paleo. Dr. Eaton is a true gentleman and a scholar in every sense of the word. We spoke for almost an hour on that first telephone call. He gave me one of the greatest compliments of my life at the end of the conversation when he said, "It sounds to me like you know more about this than I do."

Boyd and I eventually met in 1995, and two years later he invited me to speak with him at an international conference on fitness and diet organized by Dr. Artemis Simopoulos in Athens, Greece. Artemis was a wonderful hostess for the conference, and during my two-week stay in Greece, we had many conversations about diet and health. I mentioned that I had written a partially completed manuscript on the nutritional shortcomings of cereal grains. About a year later, she asked me if I could complete the paper and submit it for publication in a scientific journal she edited. I did, and the paper "Cereal Grains: Humanity's Double Edged Sword," published in 1999, launched my academic career in Paleo nutrition.

The Paleo Diet concept is now taken seriously in the scientific world, thanks in part to Boyd Eaton's pioneering work. There is no doubt in my mind that without Dr. Eaton's influential 1985 *New England Journal of Medicine* paper, Paleo would continue to be an obscure word known mainly to anthropologists and would not have become a household term now recognized by millions. The Paleo Diet and the Paleo lifestyle are clearly much larger than either my writings or Boyd Eaton's. Hundreds, if not thousands, of scientists, physicians, and people from all walks of life are responsible for creating this incredibly powerful idea, full of the wisdom of the ages, that can be used to bring order to your dietary, health, and lifestyle questions and issues.

Some of the key players who came before Dr. Eaton in the Paleo Diet and lifestyle world bear mention. Charles Darwin's *Origins of the Species* was published in 1859 and started it all. It still amazes me that the most powerful idea in biology—evolution via natural selection—generally had not been applied to nutritional thought until 126 years later, with Dr. Eaton's classic paper. Theodosius Dobzhansky, a well-known Russian evolutionary biologist, said, "Nothing in biology makes sense, except under the light of evolution." Indeed, his statement could easily be reworked to *"Nothing in nutrition makes sense except under the light of evolution."* This quote could be applied to a multitude of lifestyle issues, which I discuss later in this book.

One way that we can look at how and where the Paleo Diet and Paleo lifestyle concepts arose would be to examine the contributions of a few of the key players who came both before and after Dr. Eaton's landmark paper. Charles Darwin started it all, but a number of other noteworthy people recognized the value of ancestral dietary patterns decades before the publication of Boyd's article.

Perhaps the first book about non-Western diets and disease to receive attention was Weston Price's *Nutrition and Physical Degeneration, A Comparison of Primitive and Modern Diets and Their Effects*, published in 1939. Dr. Price, an American dentist, extensively traveled the world in the 1920s and the 1930s and made detailed observations about diet and health in numerous non-Westernized populations, including Amazon Indians, Alaskan Eskimos, Australian Aborigines, Canadian Indians, Polynesians, and African tribal populations, among many others. His book is a treasure and contains hundreds of photographs of non-Westernized people in excellent health taken in an era when modern processed foods were not universally available. Dr. Price noted that wherever and whenever modern diets were adopted by non-Westernized cultures, their health declined. His statement was just as true then as it is today.

An intriguing aspect of early books such as Dr. Price's is that frequently the diet/health observations were correct, but the underlying mechanisms about how diet and lifestyle specifically affected health were either unknown or poorly understood. In the early part of the twentieth century, before population-wide vaccination programs existed, tuberculosis remained a major public health problem responsible for millions of deaths worldwide. In his book, Dr. Price noted that in Europe, sunbathing was being effectively used to treat tuberculosis. At the time and even decades later, these kinds of observations were commonly ridiculed by the "best medical minds" because they seemed ludicrous and had no known physiological basis.

Let's fast-forward sixty-five years and look at this 1930s observation from a modern perspective. Discoveries made in the last four or five years show that sunlight exposure might be one of the best strategies to prevent or cure tuberculosis infections. When you sunbathe, ultraviolet radiation from the sun causes vitamin D to be produced in your skin. The more sun you get, the more vitamin D is produced. Blood concentrations of vitamin D regulate the synthesis of a recently identified substance called cathelicidin, which turns out to be one of the most potent bacteria-killing peptides that our bodies produce. Cathelicidin shows specific killing activity against bacteria that cause tuberculosis, and indeed studies confirm that vitamin D insufficiency is a risk factor for tuberculosis. Most of us have been vaccinated against tuberculosis, so we really don't need to worry about it, but, as I show you in this book, sunlight and vitamin D are good medicine for all of us.

Although Dr. Price's book was advanced for its time, the evolutionary basis for optimal nutrition and a healthy lifestyle still lay decades in the future. Other early popular books touching on ancestral diets and health include Arnold DeVries's *Primitive Man and His Food* (1952), Walter Voegtlin's *The Stone Age Diet* (1975), Leon Chaitow's *Stone Age Diet* (1987), and Boyd Eaton's *The Paleolithic Prescription* (1988). All of these books are out of print, and, except for Boyd's, the books faded into obscurity because they didn't have the bigger picture right—without the evolutionary template correctly in place, they were incomplete and inconclusive.

Prior to the publication of Boyd's 1985 paper, a few scientists had independently recognized the evolutionary underpinnings for healthful diets and lifestyles, but their work was published in obscure scientific journals that received little or no attention. I list most of these articles in the extensive reference section at the end of the book.

After publication of Boyd Eaton's influential paper in the *New England Journal of Medicine*, a number of events ultimately set the stage for the worldwide recognition of the Paleo Diet, as well as the evolutionary basis for modern-day Paleo lifestyles.

The Paleo Diet and Darwinian Medicine

The foundation of the Paleo Diet concept is a recently recognized discipline called Darwinian medicine. Following in the footsteps of Boyd's landmark paper came the revolutionary 1991 scientific publication in the *Quarterly Review of Biology* by Drs. George Williams and Randy Neese, "The Dawn of Darwinian Medicine." This was the first scientific publication addressing how our ancestral evolutionary experience affects the manner in which we view and treat modern diseases. Although this paper is almost twenty years old, its message is finally being filtered down to many physicians, their patients, and the public.

Here's a quote: "Human biology is designed for Stone Age conditions. Modern environments may cause many diseases . . . [and evolutionary medicine] provides new insights into the causes of medical disorders." Cough, fever, vomiting, diarrhea, fatigue, pain, nausea, and anxiety, for instance, are widespread medical problems. Many orthodox physicians focus on relieving short-term distress by prescribing drugs to block these responses. Darwinian medicine would say these responses are not necessarily harmful but rather signify the body's effort to remedy a problem. In most situations, coughing when you are sick is a natural and healthy response because it helps purge disease-causing microbes from your throat and lungs. Similarly, fever increases your body temperature, which helps destroy pathogens that have infected your body. Medications that suppress coughs and block fever may relieve symptoms but actually prolong the illness.

Obviously, certain extreme situations necessitate a balanced approach between our bodies' evolutionary responses to disease and modern medicine. For example, blocking fever can prevent febrile seizures, and stopping vomiting can prevent severe dehydration.

The bottom line: We need to balance our hunter-gatherer genetic legacy with the best technology of our modern world. In *The Paleo Answer*, I show you how the majority of chronic health problems we suffer from today can be traced to our modern world and its discordance with the ancient world for which our bodies are genetically adapted.

Having been a faculty member at a major research university for the past thirty years, I can tell you that your personal experience with the Paleo Diet and a dollar will buy you no more than one cup of coffee in the scientific community. No matter how much weight you have dropped on the Paleo Diet, no matter how much your blood chemistry has improved or how much better you feel, the medical and scientific community will, by and large, not listen to you. What the academic community of science and medicine require is not your personal anecdotal evidence, but rather experimental evidence based upon one of the following four scientific methods: animal studies, tissue or organ studies, epidemiological (population) studies, or randomized, controlled human trials.

When *The Paleo Diet* came out in 2002, thousands of indirect experimental studies had already supported its general principles in promoting weight loss, improving overall health, and curing disease:

- A multitude of well-controlled experimental studies had already confirmed that low-glycemic-load diets improved health and promoted weight loss. The Paleo Diet is a low-glycemic-load diet.
- High-protein diets were shown to be the most effective strategy to improve blood chemistry and help you lose weight. The Paleo Diet is a high-protein diet.
- Even in 2002, you would have been hard-pressed to find a single nutritionist who would disagree with the notion that omega 3 fats improve health and well-being in almost every conceivable way. The Paleo Diet is a diet rich in omega 3 fats.

By 2002, thousands of scientific papers had independently verified that certain individual aspects of the Paleo Diet normalized body weight and improved health and well-being. But at that time, not a single study had yet examined all of the combined nutritional characteristics of the Paleo Diet. Was a diet high in animal protein, omega 3 fats, monounsaturated fats, vitamins, minerals, phytochemicals, and fiber and low in salt, refined sugars, cereal grains, dairy products, vegetable oils, and processed foods healthy? Was it more healthful than the officially sanctioned USDA MyPyramid, which was renamed MyPlate in June of 2011 (both MyPyramid and MyPlate base their recommendations upon the 2010 Dietary Guidelines for Americans), or even the highly touted Mediterranean diet? The direct scientific answers to these questions had yet to be answered.

Fortunately, in the past five years a number of scientists have dared to test contemporary versions of humanity's original diet against supposedly "healthful diets." One of the key figures behind this groundbreaking research is my friend and colleague Dr. Staffan Lindeberg, M.D., Ph.D., from Lund University in Sweden.

Staffan became interested in the Paleo Diet almost twenty years ago through his medical studies of the Kitavans, a non-Westernized group of 2,250 people living on remote islands near Papua New Guinea. The Kitavans obtain virtually all of their food from either the land or the sea and have little contact with the modern world. Common Western foods such as cereals, dairy, refined sugars, vegetable oils, and processed foods are nearly absent from their diets. These people represent the epitome of health compared to the average citizen living in the Western world. No one is over-weight, and heart disease and stroke are extremely rare. High blood pressure and type 2 diabetes are nonexistent, and acne is not present among their children or teenagers. I doubt that you could round up a random group of two thousand Western people anywhere on the planet without encountering high rates of all of these diseases.

In the late 1990s, I first began to correspond with Dr. Lindeberg. We soon discovered that we had read almost all of the same scientific papers and were interested in most of the same diet/health topics.

Paleo Clues from the Outback

One study that stood out to both of us was an extraordinary experiment performed by Dr. Kerin O'Dea and published in the journal *Diabetes* in 1984. In this study, Dr. O'Dea gathered together

ten middle-aged Australian Aborigines who had been born in the
Outback. They had lived their early days primarily as hunter-
gatherers until they had no choice but to finally settle into a rural
community with access to Western goods. All ten subjects eventually
became overweight and developed type 2 diabetes as they adopted
Western sedentary lifestyles in the community of Mowwanjum in
the northern Kimberley region of western Australia. Inherent in their
upbringing, however, was the knowledge to live and survive in
this seemingly desolate land without any of the trappings of the
modern world.

Dr. O'Dea requested that these ten middle-aged subjects revert
to their former lives as hunter-gatherers for a seven-week period.
All agreed and traveled back into the isolated land from which they
originated. Their daily sustenance came only from native foods that
could be foraged, hunted, or gathered. Instead of white bread,
corn, sugar, powdered milk, and canned foods, they began to eat
the traditional fresh foods of their ancestral past: kangaroos, birds,
crocodiles, turtles, shellfish, yams, figs, yabbies (freshwater cray-
fish), freshwater bream, and bush honey. At the experiment's conclusion, the results were spectacular: the average weight loss in the
group was 16.5 pounds; blood cholesterol dropped by 12 percent,
and triglycerides were reduced by a whopping 72 percent. Insulin
and glucose metabolism became normal, and their diabetes effectively disappeared.

Dr. Lindeberg and I both realized that this type of experiment
would probably never be repeated, simply because the hunter-
gather lifestyle is nearly extinct and because very few contemporary
people have the knowledge or skills to live entirely off the land. Yet
we both had the same vision. This experiment should be conducted
in a slightly different manner but not with Westernized, former
hunter-gatherers. Why not take a group of typically unhealthy
Westerners and put them on commonly available contemporary
foods that mimic the nutritional characteristics of hunter-gatherer
diets? We knew that this experiment was precisely what Dr. Eaton
had in mind with his inspirational paper.

It took nearly twenty-two years for Dr. Eaton's dream of an experimental modern-day Paleo Diet to come true, but it finally happened with the publication of a paper by Dr. Lindeberg's research group in 2007. Staffan followed this publication with two additional papers in 2009 and 2010. Good ideas catch on, and two other independent research groups around the world followed suit with similar results—the first in 2008 by Dr. Osterdahl in Sweden and the next in 2009 by my colleague Lynda Frassetto, M.D., from the University of California San Francisco School of Medicine. Although science may move slowly, it eventually does move forward as old ideas are replaced with new and better thoughts and information.

I can assure you that the Paleo Diet, a fundamental diet and lifestyle concept based on evolutionary biology and scientific research, is not a fad and will not fade away.

PART ONE

The Paleo Way

If man made it, don't eat it.
—Jack LaLanne

1

Paleo 2.0

The reason I wrote this book is quite simple. Paleo Dieters, as well as newbies to the concept, want to learn more about the Paleo Diet and how it can help them lose weight and improve their health. Although the term "Paleo" has become a household word since the publication of my first book, *The Paleo Diet*, many people simply don't know where the term originated or what it means.

"Paleo" means "old" and is short for the Paleolithic Era or the Old Stone Age. The Paleolithic period began 2.6 million years ago with the invention of primitive stone tools and ended with the beginning of the agricultural revolution about ten thousand years ago. During the Paleolithic Era, all of our ancestors lived as hunter-gatherers until the arrival of farming, animal husbandry, and permanent villages. Although ten thousand years ago seems to be historically far away, on an evolutionary time scale only 333 human generations have come and gone since the advent of agriculture. Research confirms that our Paleolithic genomes have barely changed in the last ten thousand years. We are literally Stone Agers living in the Space Age. The Paleo Way means the Old Way, and this is a book about adopting a modern healthy diet and lifestyle consistent with our genetic heritage as hunter-gatherers.

I am not suggesting that we abandon electricity, central heating, public sanitation, or clean water. We need to recognize our humble roots as hunter-gatherers and adopt the best of their world, while leaving the worst behind. Many aspects of hunter-gatherer lifestyles are unpleasant, detrimental, and life threatening. Think about camping out for your entire life, and you can begin to comprehend some of the shortcomings of hunter-gatherer lives. Our foraging ancestors were at the constant mercy of the elements and risked life and limb on a daily basis in a treacherous environment. I am thankful for the skilled physicians and surgeons whose application of modern medicine can intervene to save our lives in the case of trauma, serious injury, or severe disease. I think very few of us would consider trading the comforts and securities of our twenty-first-century world with the stark reality of hunter-gatherer existence.

Perhaps the most important lifestyle change we can make to improve our health and well-being is to put our twenty-first-century diet in sync with the Stone Age by mimicking our ancestors in the food groups they ate. Improving our diet is far and away the most important lifestyle modification we can make to increase the quality and length of our lives. By following the evolutionary template, we can gain insight into complex diet/health issues in our modern world that will allow us to live longer, more healthful, fuller lives.

In this book, I focus on a variety of nutritional issues about the Paleo Diet concept that require more detail or have become contentious since the publication of my first book. For instance, the saturated fat question has become huge in recent years. What is the evolutionary perspective? Should we eat or avoid saturated fats? How about whey protein powders as nutritional supplements? Should we use them or not? How can vegetarian diets influence fertility? What about soy products and concentrated soy proteins—thumbs-up or thumbs-down? What is the evolutionary approach to meal patterns? Should we eat three meals a day or small frequent daily meals? How about snacking between meals? Fasting and intermittent fasting have become contested matters. What about the new governmental recommendations for vitamin D? Should we take supplements? How about the water we drink?

In *The Paleo Diet*, I spoke of the 85/15 rule—meaning that if you are 85 percent compliant with the diet most of the time, significant improvements in your health can occur. The other 15 percent—normally, three meals a week—are open meals, meaning you can choose to eat a normal amount of foods that fall outside the diet plan.

There are actually many ways you can individualize and customize your own Paleo Diet, as you'll see in *The Paleo Answer*. I refer to this variety as "Paleo diets."

Jack LaLanne's Story

In January 2011, I had the pleasure of meeting Chris LaLanne, the grandnephew of fitness legend Jack LaLanne. Chris invited me to speak at his CrossFit Gym in San Francisco. As I walked into Chris's fitness center, there before me on the entry wall was a larger-than-life poster of Jack LaLanne in his signature jump suit, flexing his muscles. Sadly, Jack passed away a few weeks later, and I never got to meet this inspirational man. But what a life he led—the epitome of health and fitness throughout his effervescent ninety-six years. My favorite Jack LaLanne quote is, "If man made it, don't eat it." Jack clearly got it right and was eating Paleo about eighty years before this lifelong nutritional plan became mainstream.

We should all be so lucky to live a long and vibrant life as Jack LaLanne did. As I'm sure Jack would have concurred, his longevity and health had less to do with luck and more to do with proper diet and exercise. Jack got a head start on us all by not eating man-made foods for most of his life.

What better time than now to start the Paleo Diet? I believe that many aspects of ill health caused by decades of improper diet can be reversed within weeks or months of adopting humanity's original nutritional plan. People with serious health issues or who are grossly overweight will require considerably more time to restore their health and vigor, but your body is a wonderful biological instrument, and when you provide it with the foods nature intended, you will be amazed at its restorative powers, regardless of your age.

Recent Paleo Research

As of December 2010, only four human experiments involving Paleo diets have been published in the scientific literature. All four studies show good success in ameliorating disease symptoms and/ or promoting weight loss.

In his first study in 2007, Dr. Lindeberg and associates placed twenty-nine patients with type 2 diabetes and heart disease on either a Paleo diet or a Mediterranean diet based on whole grains, low-fat dairy products, vegetables, fruits, fish, oils, and margarines. Note that the Paleo diet excludes grains, dairy products, and margarines, while encouraging a greater consumption of meat and fish. After twelve weeks on either diet, blood glucose tolerance—a risk factor for heart disease—improved in both groups but was better in the Paleo dieters. In a 2010 follow-up publication of this same experiment, the Paleo diet was shown to be more satiating on a calorie-by-calorie basis than the Mediterranean diet because it caused greater changes in leptin, a hormone that regulates appetite and body weight.

In a second study of Paleo diets in 2008, Dr. Osterdahl and coworkers put fourteen healthy subjects on a Paleo diet. After only three weeks, the subjects lost weight, reduced their waist size, and experienced significant reductions in blood pressure and plasmino-gen activator inhibitor, a substance in blood that promotes clotting and accelerates artery clogging. Because no control group was employed in this study, some scientists would argue that the benefi-cial changes might not necessarily be due to the Paleo diet.

In 2009, Dr. Frasetto and coworkers put nine inactive subjects on a Paleo diet for just ten days. In this experiment, the Paleo diet was exactly matched in calories with the subjects' usual diet. Almost any time people observe diets that are calorically reduced, no matter what foods are involved, they exhibit beneficial health effects. The beauty of this experiment was that any therapeutic changes in the subjects' health could not be credited to a reduction in calories, but rather to changes in the types of food eaten. While on the Paleo diet, participants experienced improvements in blood pres-sure, arterial function, insulin, total cholesterol, LDL cholesterol, and triglycerides. What is most amazing about this experiment is how rapidly so many markers of health improved—and that they occurred in every single patient.

In an even more convincing experiment in 2009, Dr. Lindeberg and colleagues compared the effects of a Paleo diet to a diabetes diet generally recommended for patients with type 2 diabetes. The diabetes diet was intended to reduce total fat by increasing whole-grain bread and cereals, low-fat dairy products, fruits, and vegetables, while restricting animal foods. By contrast, the Paleo diet was lower in cereals, dairy products, potatoes, beans, and baked goods but higher in fruits, vegetables, meat, and eggs compared to the diabetes diet. The strength of this experiment was its crossover design, in which all thirteen diabetes patients first followed one diet for three months and then crossed over and followed the other diet for three months. Compared to the diabetes diet, the Paleo diet resulted in improved weight loss, waist size, blood pressure, HDL cholesterol, triglycerides, blood glucose, and hemoglobin A1c (a marker for long-term blood glucose control). This experiment represents the most powerful example to date of the Paleo Diet's effectiveness in treating people with serious health problems. Yet you don't have to have serious health problems to enjoy the advantages of the Paleo Diet and the Paleo lifestyle.

Paleo Success: Ross Werland's Story

I was stunned a year ago when my doctor mentioned that I should lose some weight. Compared with most Americans, I thought I rated on the thin side, except for a gut that refused to melt after I quit smoking for the first time about fifteen years ago.

I probably wouldn't have tried to lose weight, except that the idea of the Paleo-type dietary regimen seemed to make sense, gut or no.

For me, it wasn't as though I had been a slouch physically. After quitting smoking the second time, about eight years ago, I started to cultivate a healthier lifestyle. I cut back on red meat; began to limit fast foods, added more vegetables, legumes, and lots more fish to my diet; and started a moderate weight-lifting routine. With in-line skating, bicycling, canoeing, kayaking, and lots of walking, I figured I already did enough cardio.

Then I read *The Paleo Diet*. Following it strictly on weekdays and more loosely on weekends, I cut back dramatically on grain and dairy products and quit adding salt or sugar to anything. As with my religion, I simply tried to get it mostly right but forgave myself easily.

The hardest thing to give up was wheat grain. It had never dawned on me how often most of us eat wheat, especially refined grain such as pasta, pastries, and white bread. I still allowed myself whole-wheat toast and jam on weekends.

My diet primarily became three heaping bowls of fresh vegetables daily; lots of fresh and frozen fruits, especially berries; plus sardines, salmon, and low-sodium turkey. Sparkling water became my beverage of choice, but I also had plain water, coffee, and unsweetened tea. Sugary soft drinks didn't pass my lips. Wine and the occasional martini did.

Within two weeks, I was down 9 pounds. Within six weeks, I was down 15, to 150 pounds. During the next couple of months, I drifted even further down to 145 and plateaued there. At a height of 5 foot 7, that still—unbelievably—puts me on the high end of my ideal body mass index, at 22.7, according to the Centers for Disease Control and Prevention.

Nevertheless, my gut vanished, leaving me with a waistline I haven't seen since college: 30 inches, down from 34 when I first went mostly Paleo four months ago. All obvious fat under the skin is gone.

My cholesterol after three months on the diet was a total of 153, with HDL at 60 and LDL at 76. By most measures, that's fantastic. My highest reading in total cholesterol was about 220 right before I quit smoking the second time.

Now my energy level seems boundless. My weight-lifting goals in repetitions are much easier to reach than before. Even running, which I never really cared for, is fun.

Maintaining the diet has become easier, once I figured I could find all of the vegetables and the fruits I wanted at nearly any salad bar. Trips to the grocery store still tend to feel like an alien experience, but I've learned to ignore all of my previous loves, especially Lucky Charms.

In fact, now I burn excess calories simply by rolling my eyes at all of the processed foods that are offered to us as sustenance.

Oh, yeah, I've also gotten a little preachy.

So—welcome to *The Paleo Answer!*

2

The Truth about Saturated Fat

Wonderful Results with Paleo: Marilyn's Story

I started following this diet five weeks ago after it was recommended by an osteopath I was seeing. I am about to turn sixty-five and have been struggling with high blood pressure for about four years and elevated cholesterol for about fifteen years. Until very recently, I was taking 25 mg of a diuretic and 40 mg of lisinopril (a blood pressure drug).

The first two weeks on the diet were not easy, because I was especially weak until I adjusted my blood pressure medication, first cutting out my diuretic and then lowering the dosage of my lisinopril. I monitor my blood pressure daily, and with my doctor's supervision I am now keeping it within a normal range, usually about 110/75, with only 10 mg of lisinopril daily.

As to my lipids, the change is remarkable. On March 7, 2006, my total cholesterol was 263, HDL was 48, and LDL was 158, with a ratio of 5.4. My triglycerides were 284. My results today: total cholesterol is 163 (in my entire life I have never been this low), with an HDL of 53, an LDL of 94, and a ratio of 3.1. My triglycerides are 76.

Prior to following this eating program, I was a fairly health-conscious person who exercised regularly, yet was never able to control my weight or other health issues. I tried for twenty years to lose my last ten pounds and was never successful. I have already lost at least eight pounds and hope to drop five more. Most important, I am very excited to finally find a program that keeps me off medication.

Blood Miracles: Sam's Story

Dr. Cordain spoke last semester at the USAF Academy. I listened to his lecture, bought and read *The Paleo Diet*, and decided to try the diet myself, due to concerns about coronary artery disease. I had my lipid profile checked the day before starting the diet and again after two and a half weeks—I had dropped my total cholesterol by 66 points, and my total cholesterol was lower than my LDL had been when I started. (Total cholesterol 141, down from 207; LDL 86, down from 145; HDL 42, down from 44; risk factor 3.4, down from 4.7.)
Phenomenal!

If you are a Paleo Dieter or follow a low-carb diet, you know a storm has been brewing for some time about saturated fats. This question of saturated fats and disease has been hotly debated in recent years and has created a rift in both the Paleo and the scientific communities. My perspective on dietary saturated fat has changed substantially in the last decade as new data has arisen and as we gain a better understanding of atherosclerosis, the process that clogs arteries and promotes heart disease.

The correct answer to the saturated fat issue lies in the wisdom of our evolutionary past. By examining the dietary and lifestyle patterns of our hunter-gatherer ancestors, we can gain insight into this difficult problem. The evolutionary template allows us to peer into the future and provides us with the proper solution to complex dietary/health questions before any laboratory experiments are ever conducted. This powerful tool gives us a huge advantage. The Paleo evolutionary template allows us to connect the dots, piecing together and making sense of the scientific evidence so that we can truly understand how to eat for optimal health the way nature intended. To find an answer to the saturated fat problem, I examined the saturated fat intake of the world's 229 hunter-gather societies and published the results of my analysis in 2006; the outcome changed the way I now view saturated fats.

Saturated Fat, Blood Cholesterol Levels, and Heart Disease

Let us critically evaluate both sides of the saturated fat argument. The traditional viewpoint is that dietary saturated fats raise blood cholesterol levels and increase our risk for heart disease. On the opposite side of the argument, a growing number of scientists, physicians, and writers now believe that dietary saturated fats have little or nothing to do with atherosclerosis and heart disease. Both factions strongly rely on epidemiological (population) studies to support their opposing viewpoints. Who's right and who's wrong? You may ask yourself how in the world could two seemingly well-informed and well-educated groups of scientists interpret similar studies in such different ways? And does it matter?

One of the reasons why epidemiological studies frequently yield conflicting results for identical topics is because of variables that cause confusion in the interpretation of the results. For example, although some studies have shown a link between animal protein consumption and symptoms of heart disease, it is entirely possible that this association was false because the measurement of animal protein was confounded by another variable also linked to heart disease symptoms: meat is a major source of animal protein in the

U.S. diet, but it is also a major source of saturated fat. Because meat often comes as an inseparable package of protein plus saturated fat, animal protein is highly related to saturated fat, thereby making it difficult to separate the effects of saturated fat from those of animal protein.

Given the shortcomings of epidemiological studies, human experimental studies are more helpful because they can separate factors and determine which specific variable may be causing certain effects. So is it the protein or the saturated fat that elicits heart disease symptoms? To answer this question, an experiment was conducted by Dr. Andy Sinclair and coworkers at Deakin University in Australia in 1990. Ten adults were fed a low-fat, lean beef–based diet for five weeks. Caloric intake was kept constant during the entire experiment. Total blood cholesterol concentrations fell significantly within one week of beginning the high-protein diet but rose as beef fat drippings were added back into the diet during weeks four and five. The authors concluded, "[I]t is the beef fat, not lean beef itself, that is associated with elevations in cholesterol concentrations."

More research conducted during the last five years has confirmed that increases in dietary protein have a beneficial effect on our blood cholesterol and blood lipid profiles.

Saturated Fats Defined

When most people align themselves with the saturated fat issue one way or another, they are frequently unaware that the term "saturated fat" is not a single item. Although most people know that saturated fats are concentrated in foods such as butter, eggs, lard, cheese, shortening, cream, fatty meats, and baked goods, few realize that not all saturated fats affect our blood cholesterol equally. There are four dietary saturated fats (actually, fatty acids) we need to concern ourselves with:

1. Lauric acid
2. Myristic acid

3. Palmitic acid
4. Stearic acid

Each of these dietary saturated fatty acids has slightly different effects on our blood.

Early studies supported the viewpoint that myristic acid and palmitic acid generally raised total blood cholesterol levels, whereas lauric acid did so slightly, and stearic acid didn't increase it at all. In those days, it was routine to carry out nutritional experiments under meticulous "metabolic ward" conditions—meaning that the subjects could eat only the food provided to them and nothing else. All meals were designed to precisely control the types of fats consumed. Subjects who didn't faithfully comply with the experimental diets were eliminated from the study.

The precision and accuracy of these early experiments are unquestionable, and the conclusion that saturated fats increase blood cholesterol is indisputable. As you will soon see, however, there are important limitations to these experiments that were unrecognized in their day. The most important shortcoming was that the endpoint variable that was measured—total blood cholesterol—was misleading and incomplete. We now realize that additional blood chemistry measurements are required to more accurately predict the risk of heart disease.

Total blood cholesterol levels are a crude marker for heart disease, as they don't reflect the dynamics of cholesterol entering or leaving the bloodstream. Some cholesterol is taken out of our bodies by HDL (good) particles, while other cholesterol is deposited in our arteries by LDL (bad) particles and forms part of the plaque that clogs our arteries. Because total cholesterol represents a summation of both good (HDL) and bad (LDL) cholesterol, by itself it is a poor measure of heart disease risk. The total cholesterol/HDL cholesterol ratio is a much better index for heart disease risk—and it is even more predictive if we know our general state of inflammation, which I cover in later chapters.

Putting It All Together

Lower values for the total cholesterol/HDL cholesterol ratio reduce our risk for heart disease, whereas higher values increase it. Let's go back and reevaluate Dr. Sinclair's experiment, in which he fed subjects a low-fat, beef-based diet for five weeks and then added beef fat back into the subjects' diets during weeks four and five—all the while keeping the calories constant. Remember that total blood cholesterol increased during weeks four and five after the beef fat drippings were added back in, leading the authors of the study to conclude that saturated fats raise total blood cholesterol. Dr. Sinclair didn't report the total cholesterol/HDL cholesterol ratio in his experiment, but it is easy to calculate these numbers, as I have done in the table below. As you can see, the addition of high-saturated-fat beef drippings worsened total blood cholesterol values but actually improved the total cholesterol/HDL cholesterol ratio. If you were to look only at the total blood cholesterol values, it would appear as if saturated fats increased the risk for heart disease. And herein lies the problem with much of the human experimental studies conducted from the 1960s until the late 1980s—the single measurement of total cholesterol was an inappropriate and misleading endpoint.

Don't get too excited about my reanalysis of Dr. Sinclair's study. Remember, it is only a single experiment and, by itself, can't overturn the dogma of thirty or more years of studies examining only total blood cholesterol as the endpoint risk factor for heart disease. What

How Dietary Changes Affect Your Cholesterol

	Week 1	Week 2	Week 3	Week 4	Week 5
Calories	2,264	2,164	2,175	2,234	2,213
% Carbohydrate	43.8	62.6	62.5	53.3	43.6
% Fat	38.2	8.8	9.3	19.2	29.1
% Protein	16.1	25.6	26.9	25.4	25.4
Total Blood Cholesterol	5.84	4.69	4.84	4.94	5.39
HDL Cholesterol	1.71	1.41	1.60	1.64	1.76
Total Cholesterol/HDL	3.42	3.33	3.03	3.01	3.06

we really need to look at are analyses combining all experiments that have examined how saturated fats affect the total cholesterol/HDL cholesterol ratio. Studies that combine the results from many experiments are called meta analyses. In addition, we can check out what meta analyses tell us about how the four different types of saturated fatty acids—lauric acid, myristic acid, palmitic acid, and stearic acid—affect the total cholesterol/HDL cholesterol ratio, as well as other blood markers that increase heart disease risk.

Amazingly, these types of comprehensive meta analyses of human dietary interventions are few and far between. A recent meta analysis involving saturated fats and blood chemistry was published in 2010 by Drs. Micha and Mozaffarian of the Harvard School of Public Health. Let's examine an important issue these authors have stirred up. If national nutritional policy dictates that dietary saturated fats should be slashed across the board for every man, woman, and child in the country, what should they be replaced with: carbohydrates, polyunsaturated fats, monounsaturated fats, or what? The default nutrient that the government decided on to replace saturated fats became carbohydrates—this official governmental dictate occurred with very little discussion or debate on the issue. Incredibly, this recommendation was never rigorously tested using human dietary interventions or meta analyses. It simply became the unquestioned national policy that was spoon-fed to our entire medical/health-care system for decades. The simplistic thinking of the day was that if carbs contained no saturated fats, how could they possibly be dangerous?

Now let's take a look at the facts about saturated fats that should have been considered before national policy unilaterally rejected them. Drs. Micha and Mozaffarian's 2010 meta analysis showed that when carbs were used to replace saturated fats, carbs *increased the risk for heart disease* by increasing blood triglycerides and lowering HDL cholesterol levels. More important, this comprehensive meta analysis showed that the substitution of carbs for saturated fats neither raised nor lowered the total cholesterol/HDL cholesterol ratio. In effect, when compared to carbs, saturated fats were shown to be neutral and neither increased nor decreased the risk for heart disease. In addition, when individual saturated fatty acids were compared to carbs, it was demonstrated that lauric acid, myristic acid, and stearic acid actually lowered the total cholesterol/HDL cholesterol ratio. The authors concluded the most wide-ranging meta analysis on saturated fats and heart disease ever with this statement:

> These meta-analyses suggest no overall effect of saturated fatty acid consumption on coronary heart disease events.

What a turn of events! The best science of 2010 with the most comprehensive database ever assembled flew in the face of more than forty to fifty years of public and private recommendations that we should severely reduce dietary saturated fats to diminish our risk for heart disease. From the time I was twenty until very recently, I grew up with dietary recommendations that were flawed. Fortunately for me, during the last twenty years I have not followed the USDA MyPyramid Guidelines, which were in effect until mid-2011, but rather have followed humanity's original diet as my road map for optimal health and well-being.

So, should you go out and eat bacon, hot dogs, salami, and fatty processed meats until you can't eat any more? Absolutely not. Processed meats are synthetic mixtures of meat and fat combined artificially at the meatpacker's or the butcher's whim with no regard for the true fatty acid profile of the wild animal carcasses our hunter-gatherer ancestors ate. In addition to their unnatural fatty acid profiles—high in omega 6 fatty acids, low in omega 3 fatty acids, and high in saturated fatty acids—processed fatty meats are chock full of the preservatives nitrites and nitrates, which are converted into potent cancer-causing nitrosamines in our guts. To make a bad situation worse, these unnatural meats are typically laced full of salt, high-fructose corn syrup, wheat, grains, and other additives that have multiple adverse health effects. In a 2010 meta analysis, scientists from the Harvard School of Public Health reported that red meat consumption was not associated with either heart disease or type 2 diabetes, whereas eating processed meats resulted in a 42 percent greater risk for heart disease and a 19 percent greater risk for type 2 diabetes.

Saturated Fats in Hunter-Gatherer Diets

In 2006, I published a chapter in a scientific book that essentially overturned my prior convictions about saturated fat and health. The correct science behind the saturated fat issue and heart disease did not happen overnight, and had I used the evolutionary template as my guide quite a bit earlier, I would have known that population-wide recommendations to reduce saturated fats were flawed. The U.S. Dietary Guidelines and the World Health Organization both recommend consuming less than 10 percent of our calories as saturated fats. The American Heart Association's recommendations are lower still, advising us to get less than 7 percent of our daily calories as saturated fat. Let's take a look at the evolutionary evidence and see how it compares to these official recommendations.

In 2001, I published a paper in the *American Journal of Clinical Nutrition*, in which my colleagues and I examined the dietary macronutrient (protein, fat, and carbohydrate) content in 229 hunter-gatherer societies. We showed that animal fare almost always made up the greater part of hunter-gatherers' daily food intake. In fact, most (73 percent) of the world's hunter-gatherers obtained more than 50 percent of their subsistence from hunted and fished animal foods. In contrast, only 14 percent of worldwide hunter-gatherers obtained more than 50 percent of their daily subsistence from plant foods. You can see from these numbers that our ancestors ate a lot of meat. It is possible to look at any nutrient, including saturated fats, using the same mathematical model I developed for this study.

The results of this study are compiled in the following table. Notice that in my model I varied two factors: (1) the percentage of plant and animal foods in the diet and (2) the percentage of fat for the animal foods. These procedures allowed me to calculate the saturated fat in a wide range of hunter-gatherer diets. Finally, any combination of values that exceeded 35 percent protein was excluded, as protein is toxic above 35 percent of a person's daily calories.

Saturated Fat Intake for Different Levels
of Dietary Meats and Plant Foods

Ratio of Plant to Animal Foods in Diet	% Animal Fat	% Protein	% Carb	% Fat	% Saturated Fat
35/65	20	21	22	58	17.6
35/65	15	28	22	50	16.3
35/65	10	35	22	43	14.1
45/55	20	20	28	52	15.8
45/55	15	26	28	46	14.5
45/55	10	32	28	40	12.3
50/50	20	20	31	49	15.1
50/50	15	25	31	44	13.8
50/50	10	31	31	38	11.6
55/45	20	19	34	47	14.5
55/45	15	24	34	42	13.1
55/45	10	29	34	37	11.0
65/35	20	19	40	41	13.1
65/35	15	22	40	37	11.8
65/35	10	26	40	34	9.6
65/35	5	32	40	28	6.1

A few key points jump out from this table. First and foremost is the average dietary saturated fat intake, which comes in at 13.1 percent of the total calories. If we look at the typical hunter-gatherer diet, in which animal food consumption falls between 55 and 65 percent of the total calories, the dietary saturated fat intake is higher still at 15.1 percent. Even in plant-dominated hunter-gatherer diets, the dietary saturated fat (11.3 percent) is considerably higher than the American Heart Association's recommended healthful values of less than 7 percent.

You can see that the normal dietary intake of saturated fats for historically studied hunter-gatherers likely accounted for 10 to 15 percent of their total energy. Values lower than 10 percent or higher than 15 percent would have been the exception, rather than the rule.

I cannot lend my support to population-wide recommendations to lower dietary saturated fat below 10 percent to reduce our risk for heart disease. This advice has little or no support from an evolutionary basis. Just as the replacement of saturated fat with carbohydrate was a poor idea that had not been adequately tested, studies of sufficient duration examining how low-saturated-fat diets may affect our health and well-being have never been carried out. They certainly don't protect us from heart disease, and recommendations to reduce dietary saturated fats may potentially have adverse health consequences.

So my new advice for you is this: *If you are faithful to the basic principles of the Paleo Diet, consumption of saturated fats within the range of 10 to15 percent of your daily calories will not increase your risk for heart disease.* In fact, the opposite may be true, as new information suggests that elevations in LDL cholesterol may actually reduce systemic inflammation, a potent risk factor for heart disease. Consumption of fatty meats and organs had survival value in an earlier time, because fat provided a lot of energy and organs were rich in nutrients including iron, vitamin A, and the B-vitamins.

In Paleolithic times, humans didn't eat grains, legumes, dairy products, refined sugars, and salty processed foods, the modern foods that produce chronic low-level inflammation in our bodies. Some medical studies now attribute many diseases, including heart disease, to chronic inflammation. Perhaps inflammation will prove to be more of a risk factor than high total cholesterol was thought to be.

Good and Bad Saturated Fats

Saturated fats have always been part of the ancestral human diet, and you should not avoid them when they are found in "real," non-processed foods. The following table shows the sources of most of the saturated fats in the typical American diet. Notice that two-thirds of all of the saturated fats that Americans consume come from processed foods and dairy products. These are the foods you want to eliminate or restrict when you adopt the Paleo Diet. Remarkably, computerized dietary analyses from our laboratory show that despite their high meat content, modern-day Paleo diets actually contain lower quantities of saturated fats than are found in the typical U.S. diet.

Sources of Saturated Fats	% of Total Saturated Fats
Non-Paleo Foods	
Milk, cheese, butter, and dairy	20.0
Processed foods with grains and beef (burritos, tacos, spaghetti)	9.8
Bread, cereals, rice, pasta, tortilla chips, potato chips	9.5
Desserts (ice cream, cakes)	8.6
Processed foods with grains and cheese (pizza, macaroni and cheese)	6.9
Beverages, miscellaneous	3.7
French fries, hash browns	3.3
Salad dressings	3.0
Margarine	1.2
Total	**66.0**
Paleo Foods	
Beef	13.2
Pork	8.8
Poultry	6.0
Eggs	3.2
Seafood	1.8
Total	**33.0**

Stay away from saturated fats in processed foods. These artificial concoctions carry the baggage of refined grains, sugars, vegetable oils, trans fats, dairy, salt, preservatives, and additives that are definitely not good for our bodies. The saturated fats you consume from grass-fed beef, poultry, pork, eggs, fish, and seafood will not promote heart disease, cancer, or any chronic health problem. In fact, these foods can ensure your birthright—a long, healthy, and happy life.

Paleo Bottom Line

Not all saturated fats are created equal. Enjoy the right kinds and live a healthy, long life.

3

Your Own Paleo Diet

Beating Metabolic Syndrome:
Barbara's Story

I have had high blood pressure, high cholesterol, and high
triglycerides for years and was recently diagnosed with type
2 diabetes. Just a few days later, I began the Paleo Diet,
and within a week, my blood sugar dropped from the 200–300
range down into the 130–180 range. I am noticeably losing
body fat, and I feel 100 percent better.

During the last three or four years since Paleo has become a household word, I have been interviewed a lot by the media and the popular
press. The first question I often get asked is how the "caveman diet"
works. Before I launch into my explanations, I correct the interviewer
and make sure they know the Paleo Diet is also a nutritional plan for
cavewomen and cave children. Then I say that the Paleo Diet is not
really a "diet" at all, but rather a lifetime way of eating to maximize
health and well-being to prevent and cure illnesses and diseases that

run rampant in Westernized countries. I call the Paleo approach to nutrition Paleo diets (the foundation of the Paleo Diet).

With Paleo diets, we try to replicate the nutritional qualities in our ancestral hunter-gatherer diets by consuming the food groups they ate, chosen from common foods found in our local supermarkets, farmer's markets, and grocery stores. What many people don't completely understand is that Paleo diets are mimicking Stone Age diets but not exactly duplicating them. By reducing or eliminating refined sugars, processed foods, dairy products, cereal grains, and legumes (except occasionally, per the 85/15 rule), we can go a long way toward getting close to the nutrient characteristics of hunter-gatherer diets. Modern-day Paleo diets are composed of meats (grass-produced, preferably), fish, seafood, fresh fruits, veggies, nuts and seeds, and healthful oils. By replacing processed, feedlot-produced meats with grass-fed meats and free-range, organically fed poultry, we can get closer still to the original Stone Age diet.

The incredible cornucopia of fresh fruits, vegetables, meats, fish, seafood, and nuts that are routinely available year round in most major food stores in the Western world would be mind-boggling to any hunter-gatherer. On a daily basis, we can eat a luxuriously rich and diversified diet that most hunter-gatherers could only dream about. Modern-day Paleo diets could not have existed fifty to seventy-five years ago in most parts of the world. These diets are only possible now due to the advent of industrialization, refrigeration, modern agricultural practices, worldwide air transportation, and current technology. Let's consider ourselves fortunate to live in these times.

Yet contemporary Paleo Dieters face a number of dietary issues that we need to consider as we adopt this lifetime nutritional plan. Here are a few:

- Hunter-gatherers typically did not eat three meals a day. Should we follow lockstep in their example?
- Hunter-gatherers ate only wild plant foods that were available seasonally from their local environment, whereas we can eat

fresh fruits and vegetables all year round because of worldwide air transportation and various food-processing and agricultural practices.

- Hunter-gatherers certainly did not ingest pesticides, synthetic hormones, artificial sweeteners, or plastic compounds, but these items frequently find their way into present-day Paleo diets.
- Are there potential problems with our chemically treated water supply?
- We have the luxury to bake, broil, barbecue, microwave, fry, sauté, or cook our foods any way that we please—are there nutritional issues or concerns here?

The worldwide adoption of modern-day Paleo diets has been with us now for less than a decade, and clearly all of the answers to these questions have not been completely worked out. Let's once again let the data speak for itself, however, and examine each of these topics from an evolutionary perspective.

Meal Timing the Paleo Way

The evolutionary template is an excellent way to answer complex questions of diet and health. The timing and the number of meals we should eat are controversial issues and not well understood. Many health-care professionals, as well as the lay press, state that consumption of smaller and more frequent meals is healthier than eating larger and less frequent meals. This advice is offered despite the lack of scientific evidence to justify it.

Studies examining the effects of meal frequency on health and body weight are inconclusive and have produced mixed results. Some studies show that skipping breakfast is unhealthy and may promote weight gain; other studies have shown that daily caloric intake was higher among women who ate breakfast compared to those who didn't. Similarly, children who reported that they never ate breakfast had lower daily caloric intakes than regular breakfast eaters did. Furthermore, children who skipped breakfast lost more weight during a one-year period compared to daily breakfast eaters.

These kinds of controversies typify the chaos and disarray that are endemic in nutritional science. By placing the evolutionary template over the meal controversy fiasco, we can gain instant insight into the dietary patterns for which our species is genetically adapted. Yet before we get into the dietary patterns of hunter-gatherers, let's see why the number of daily meals we eat can affect our health.

Caloric Restriction, Longevity, and Health

Numerous review papers from diverse research groups around the world are unanimous in their conclusion: caloric restriction increases life span and improves health. Caloric restriction by as little as 30 percent can increase life span by up to 40 percent in short-lived mammals such as rodents. To date, caloric restriction is the only intervention known to slow the rate of aging and increase life span in a variety of smaller animal species. Studies of caloric restriction in longer-lived primates such as the rhesus monkey were started in 1987. These ongoing experiments, though not yet complete, parallel the results of rodent studies and are predictive of an increased life span.

Perhaps more important than longevity are the beneficial health effects that caloric restriction has to offer. Caloric restriction improves virtually all indices of cardiovascular health—not only in lab animals but also in humans. In animal models, caloric restriction delays or prevents all types of cancers, kidney disease, diabetes, and autoimmune diseases and delays the age-related decline in wound healing, while improving immune function. Virtually all mechanisms that protect the body's cells from injury remain at youthful levels longer during caloric restriction, including antioxidants, DNA repair mechanisms, protein turnover, corticosteroids, and heat shock proteins.

It is still not clear whether caloric restriction can extend life span in human beings, but some of the world's longest-lived and healthiest people, the Okinawans, consume 20 percent fewer calories than adults on the Japanese mainland. Death rates for stroke, cancer, and heart disease were only 59 percent, 69 percent, and 59 percent, respectively, of those for the rest of Japan.

Intermittent Fasting

Does how many meals we eat influence our total caloric intake? During the fasting month of Ramadan, Muslims abstain from food and drink from dawn until sunset. Numerous studies demonstrate that this dietary pattern causes a spontaneous reduction in caloric intake and a slight weight loss. To date, no clinical studies have examined how a single large evening meal influences weight during the long term—six months or longer. The consumption of a single daily meal is a form of intermittent fasting, which in animals causes them to spontaneously reduce their caloric intake by 30 percent. In human studies, intermittent fasting reduces blood pressure, improves insulin sensitivity, improves kidney function, and increases resistance to disease and cancer.

Hunter-Gatherer Patterns

I am currently in the process of compiling meal times and patterns in the world's historically studied hunter-gatherers. If any single picture is beginning to surface, it clearly is not three meals per day plus snacking as per the typical U.S. grazing pattern. Here are a few examples:

1. The Ingalik hunter-gatherers of interior Alaska: The only meal of the day is eaten in the evening.
2. The Guayaki (Ache) hunter-gatherers of Paraguay: The evening meal is the most consistent of the day. This is understandable, because the day is generally spent hunting for food that will be eaten in the evening.

3. The !Kung hunter-gatherers of Botswana: Members move out of camp each day individually or in small groups to work through the surrounding range and return in the evening to pool the collected resources for the evening meal.
4. Hawaiians, Tahitians, Fijians, and other Oceanic peoples (pre-Westernization): Typically, meals, as defined by Westerners, were consumed once or twice a day. The main meal, usually freshly cooked, was generally eaten in the late afternoon after the day's work was over.

From my ongoing analysis of hunter-gatherers, the most consistent daily eating pattern appears to be a single large meal consumed in the late afternoon or evening. A midday meal or lunch was rarely or never taken, and a small breakfast (consisting of the remainders of the previous evening meal) was sometimes eaten. Some snacking may have occurred during gathering; however, the bulk of the day's food was consumed in the late afternoon or the evening. The hunter-gatherer pattern of eating could be described as intermittent fasting, compared to our Western customs, particularly when daily gathering or hunting was unsuccessful or marginal. There is wisdom in the ways of our hunter-gatherer ancestors, and perhaps it is time to rethink three squares a day.

Fruit Guidelines

Fresh produce is an absolutely essential component of modern-day Paleo diets, and my previous recommendations were for you to eat as much of these delicious foods as you like. This advice still holds true. The only banned vegetables are potatoes, cassava root, sweet corn, and legumes (beans, peas, soy, green beans, peanuts, etc.). Fruits are Mother Nature's natural sweets, and the only fruits you should completely avoid are canned fruits packed in syrups. Dried fruits should be consumed in limited quantities, as they can contain as much concentrated sugar as a candy bar. See the following table for a comparison of the sugar content in fresh and dried fruits. If you are overweight or have one or more diseases of the metabolic syndrome (hypertension, type 2 diabetes, heart disease, or abnormal blood lipids), you should avoid dried fruit altogether and eat sparingly of "very high" and "high" sugar fruits.

Sugar Content in Dried and Fresh Fruits

Dried Fruits	Total Sugars per 100 Grams
Extremely High in Total Sugars	
Dried mango	73.0
Raisins, golden	70.6
Zante currants	70.6
Raisins	65.0
Dates	64.2
Dried figs	62.3
Dried papaya	53.5
Dried pears	49.0
Dried peaches	44.6
Dried prunes	44.0
Dried apricots	38.9
Fresh Fruits	
Very High in Total Sugars	
Grapes	18.1
Banana	15.6
Mango	14.8
Cherries, sweet	14.6
High in Total Sugars	
Apple	13.3
Pineapple	11.9
Purple passion fruit	11.2

Once your weight normalizes and your disease symptoms wane, feel free to eat as much fresh fruit as you like.

Domesticated versus Wild Produce

Of the many fruits and veggies that are available in the produce sections of our supermarkets, specialty food stores, and ethnic markets, most bear little resemblance to their wild ancestors. For instance, when you visualize a carrot, what do you see? Most likely, a large, bright-orange, tapering root. The wild version is tiny, thin, and perhaps not much bigger than your little finger. It is either black or dark or light purple, and frequently splits into multiple roots. Similarly, modern varieties of apples are big, sweet, and luscious, whereas the wild versions are more like crabapples—small, fibrous, and definitely not sweet. Almost all domesticated fruits and vegetables have been bred over thousands of years since the agricultural revolution to produce foods that are bigger, sweeter, and less fibrous. See the table below to compare the fiber content in wild versus cultivated plants.

Is domesticated produce nutritionally inferior to wild plant foods? The table at the top of the next page contrasts the vitamin and mineral content of wild plant foods and their domesticated counterparts.

The B vitamins and iron and zinc concentrations are similar between the two, whereas wild plants have more calcium and magnesium. Cultured plants win out when it comes to vitamin C. Unless you are lucky enough to live in a part of the country where you can pick wild berries or gather wild asparagus, most of us will rarely eat wild plant foods. It really doesn't matter, however, as the differences between wild and cultured plants are generally inconsequential.

Comparison of the Fiber Content of Wild and Cultivated Plants (100-gram samples)

	Wild	Cultivated
Fruit	8 grams	3 grams
Roots	8 grams	2 grams
Bulbs	8 grams	3 grams
Legumes	32 grams	13 grams
Seeds/grains	14 grams	10 grams
Nuts	11 grams	7 grams
Leaves	5 grams	5 grams

**Comparison of the Vitamin and Mineral
Content of Wild and Domesticated Plants**

	Wild	Domesticated
Vitamin B$_1$	0.19 mg	0.15 mg
Vitamin B$_2$	0.11 mg	0.10 mg
Vitamin C	8.1 mg	22.5 mg
Magnesium	98 mg	67 mg
Calcium	117 mg	49 mg
Iron	7.6 mg	7.4 mg
Zinc	3.5 mg	1.5 mg

Organic versus Conventional Produce

Are there any advantages to organic produce? Should you pay the higher price? The table below shows the results of a study by Dr. Worthington that tabulated thirty-four scientific papers contrasting the nutrient content of organic versus conventionally grown produce.

The research has generally concluded that except for somewhat more vitamin C in organic vegetables (but not in fruit), no differences existed for any nutrient. So, if you're considering buying organic produce for its superior vitamin and mineral qualities, it's really not worth it.

Notice, though, that the concentration of nitrate in organic produce is consistently lower than in conventionally grown fruits and veggies. In addition, many studies have demonstrated reduced amounts of pesticides and toxic chemicals in organic produce.

Nutrient	Higher	No Difference	Lower
Protein	3	0	0
Nitrate	5	10	25
Vitamin C	21	12	3
Beta carotene	5	5	3
B vitamins	2	12	2
Calcium	21	20	6
Magnesium	17	24	4
Iron	15	14	6
Zinc	4	9	3

Higher environmental and dietary exposure to both pesticides and nitrates are associated with a greater risk for developing certain cancers. If this issue is of concern to you, then definitely go with organic produce, if you can afford it.

Waxed Foods

When you visit the produce section of your local supermarket, I'm sure you have noticed the glossy wax that is frequently present on cucumbers and apples and sometimes on bell peppers and other fruits and veggies. Have you wondered why these waxes were applied and whether they are safe? The purpose of fruit and vegetable waxes is to reduce shrinkage from water loss; to provide a barrier to gas exchange, which prolongs shelf life by simultaneously reducing the oxygen content and increasing the carbon dioxide content of the fruit or the vegetable; to improve appearance by adding a shiny film; and/or to provide a carrier for fungicides or other chemical agents to prevent microbial decay.

The waxes applied to fruits and vegetables can take on many different formulations. Listed below are five common waxing formulas:

1. 18.6% oxidized polyethylene, 3.4% oleic acid, 2.8% morpholine, 0.01% polydimethylsiloxane antifoam
2. 18.3% candelilla wax, 2.1% oleic acid, 2.4% morpholine, 0.02% polydimethylsiloxane antifoam
3. 9.5% shellac, 8.3% carnauba wax, 3.3% morpholine, 1.7% oleic acid, 0.17% ammonia, 0.01% polydimethylsiloxane antifoam
4. 19% shellac, 1.0% oleic acid, 4.4% morpholine, 0.3% ammonia, and 0.01% polydimethylsiloxane antifoam
5. 13.3% shellac, 3.0% whey protein isolate, 3.1% morpholine, 0.7% oleic acid, 0.2% ammonia, 0.01% polydimethylsiloxane antifoam

Not very appetizing, is it? It's important that we take a closer look so that you can see the risks involved in consuming these waxes. Note that morpholine is a common element in most waxing formulas. This chemical is permitted for use in the United States, Australia, Canada, and other countries but not in Germany. The function of morpholine is to serve as a fungicide and as a solvent to help liquefy the wax.

By itself, in the low doses present in fruits and vegetables, this chemical probably does not constitute a health risk. During the digestive process, however, if there are nitrites (compounds found in processed meats and most vegetables) simultaneously present, morpholine is chemically changed into N-nitrosomorpholine (NMOR), a potent cancer-causing agent in rats and mice. The safe lower limit for NMOR is 4.3 ng (nanograms) per kg of body weight a day. It has been estimated that for adults, consuming waxed apples and a mixed diet, NMOR ingestion can approach 3.6 ng per kg of body weight a day, which represents the lower limit of safety.

These estimates did not actually measure NMOR formation in humans, though. Additionally, nitrite ingestion is quite variable, depending on your intake of vegetables and processed meats. It is entirely possible that regular consumption of waxed fruit and vegetables containing morpholine, along with the rest of your diet, could represent a significant cancer risk.

Notice that shellac is a major ingredient in three of the five most common formulas that are used to wax produce. Shellac comes from the hardened secretion of the female lac insect, which is native to India and Thailand and can be a potent allergen in some people, as can carnauba wax, which is also an ingredient in wax formulas.

Waxes cannot be removed by regular washing. If you prefer not to consume waxes, you must buy unwaxed produce or peel the fruit or the vegetable. Fruits and vegetables that are waxed include:

- Apples
- Avocados
- Bell peppers
- Cantaloupes
- Cucumbers
- Eggplants
- Grapefruits
- Lemons
- Limes
- Melons
- Oranges
- Parsnips
- Passion fruit
- Peaches
- Pineapples
- Pumpkins
- Rutabagas
- Squash
- Sweet potatoes
- Tomatoes
- Turnips
- Yucca

Because many of these fruits and vegetables are typically peeled and the peel is not consumed, only a few common fruits and vegetables present a problem.

Until recent times, fruits and vegetables were generally harvested when ripe and brought to market without wax coatings. Even today, fruit and vegetables can be harvested, packed, and stored without the use of waxes, and storage life can be extended through careful handling. The relative cancer risk of not eating fresh fruits and vegetables is much greater than the small risk posed by consuming waxed fruits and vegetables, but personally, I prefer my produce wax-free and as fresh as possible.

Artificial Sweeteners

It's pretty clear that if we follow the example of our hunter-gatherer ancestors, artificial sweeteners should not be part of contemporary Paleo diets. In my first book, I mentioned that beverages made with these substances were an acceptable replacement for high-fructose corn syrup sweetened sodas. I no longer can make this recommendation, based on some intriguing new population and animal studies that have been conducted recently.

Don't forget the 85/15 rule, which allows you to occasionally consume food or drink that is normally off limits. I would never recommend that you drink these artificially sweetened beverages on a daily basis, though, and as I will soon show you, it is definitely not a good idea for pregnant women to ingest artificial sweeteners at all.

The table on page 34 lists the five artificial sweeteners that the U.S. Food and Drug Administration (FDA) has approved for consumption.

In addition, the FDA has sanctioned a sugar substitute, stevia, as a dietary supplement since 1995. Stevia is a crystalline substance made from the leaves of a plant native to Central and South America and is 100 to 300 times sweeter than table sugar. A new concentrated derivative of stevia leaves called rebaudioside A was

Sweetener	Trade Name	Sweetness Comparison to Table Sugar	Acceptable Daily Intake
Saccharin	Sweet 'N' Low	300 times sweeter	5 mg/kg body weight
Aspartame	NutraSweet, Equal	160–220 times sweeter	50 mg/kg body weight
Acesulfame	Sunett, Sweet & Safe, Sweet One	200 times sweeter	15 mg/kg body weight
Sucralose	Splenda	600 times sweeter	5 mg/kg body weight
Neotame	Made by NutraSweet	7,000–13,000 times sweeter	0.10 mg/ kg body weight

authorized by the FDA in 2008 and goes by the trade names of Only Sweet, PureVia, Reb-A, Rebiana, SweetLeaf, and Truvia.

Since 1980, the number of people consuming artificially sweetened products in the United States has more than doubled. Today, at least forty-six million Americans regularly ingest foods and drinks sweetened by these chemicals—mainly in the form of soft drinks but also in a large number of other products, including baby food.

Most people know that soft drinks sweetened with sugar promote obesity, type 2 diabetes, and the metabolic syndrome (high blood pressure, high blood cholesterol, and heart disease). And most people also believe that if we removed refined sugars from our diets and replaced them with artificial sweeteners, we would all be a lot healthier. A number of recent epidemiological and animal studies suggest that they are not part of the solution to the U.S. obesity epidemic but rather may be part of the problem. Unexpectedly, a series of large population-based studies, including the National Health and Nutrition Examination Survey, have clearly demonstrated strong associations between the increased intake of artificial sweeteners and obesity and the metabolic syndrome, a cluster of health problems that includes high cholesterol, high blood pressure, and high blood glucose. Alarmingly, these effects have been observed in children, as well as in adults, and were utterly unanticipated because most artificial sweeteners were previously thought to be inert and not to react with our metabolism in an unsafe manner. Recent animal experiments conducted by Dr. Susan Swithers at Purdue have reversed these erroneous assumptions. Rats that were allowed to eat their normal chow consumed more food and gained more weight when artificial sweeteners were added to their diet. We do not currently know precisely how artificial sweeteners cause us to gain weight, but the most likely explanation is that they somehow interfere with our normal appetites and how our bodies handle both glucose and insulin.

Who would have thought that a mass-marketed product that was designed to help us lose weight may have actually caused exactly the opposite result? In 1958, the federal government deemed both saccharin and cyclamate "generally recognized as safe artificial sweeteners." Eleven years later, the FDA banned cyclamate and announced its intention to ban saccharin in 1977 because of worries over increased cancer risks from both of these chemicals. Consumer protests eventually led to a congressional moratorium on the ban for saccharin, and it is still with us today. Aspartame was sanctioned for use as a sweetener by the FDA in 1982 for food and in 1983 for drinks, followed by sucralose in 1999, neotame in 2002, and acesulfame in 2003. You may think that any time chemical additives such as artificial sweeteners were permitted into our food supply, they would have been thoroughly tested and conclusively shown to be safe. Unfortunately, this is not always the case, and the potential toxicity of some of these sweetening compounds is widely disputed in the scientific community, particularly in the light of newer, more carefully controlled animal studies.

A series of experiments by Dr. Soffritti has shown that even low doses of aspartame given to rats during the course of their lives leads to increased cancer rates. This study is important, because many people may consume much higher concentrations of this chemical by drinking artificially sweetened beverages on a daily basis for years and years. Aspartame has also been shown to trigger migraine headaches in certain people because it breaks down into methanol—wood alcohol—in our bodies.

It's not only aspartame that may prove dangerous to our health when we ingest these synthetic concoctions on a regular basis. Animal experiments by Dr. Bandyopadhyay have revealed that sac- charin, acesulfame, and aspartame caused DNA damage in mice bone marrow. Frequently, it is difficult to translate results from animal experiments into meaningful recommendations for humans, because large epidemiological studies generally don't show artificial sweeteners to be risk factors for cancer. Yet this does not mean that these compounds are completely safe.

A 2010 study of 59,334 pregnant women from Denmark showed for the first time that consumption of artificially sweetened soft drinks significantly increased the risk for pre-term delivery, at less than thirty-seven weeks. This condition shouldn't be taken lightly, as it represents the leading cause of infant death. An interesting outcome of this study was that only artificially sweetened beverages increased the risk for pre-term delivery—and not sugar-sweetened soft drinks. I am not recommending that pregnant women consume sugary soft drinks, but this study indicates that they are much less harmful to your developing fetus than are artificially sweetened soft drinks. Any food additive that may cause migraine headaches, promote weight gain, and increase the risk for pre-term pregnancies should not be part of the Paleo Diet.

Cooking Advice for Contemporary Stone Agers

If you were to walk into your local physician's or general practitio- ner's office and ask him or her about the connection between nutrition and health, most doctors would toe the party line and tell you that a diet high in plant foods and low in animal proteins and fat is the way to go. If you were to ask your doctor about the glyce- mic index and how it influences your health, most would not have a good answer. It is not their fault—they simply were not taught this crucial dietary/health relationship in medical school. If you were to question your doctor about RAGEs, AGEs, and diet, almost none would know the answer. Although these terms are virtually unknown to most physicians, they have huge implications on our health and well-being that have only been recently recognized.

AGEs stands for *advanced glycation end-products*. These are compounds that naturally form in our bodies from the chemical reaction of sugars with proteins. If the concentration of AGEs becomes excessive in our bloodstream, they can cause damage to almost every tissue and organ in our bodies. In the past decade scientists have discovered that foods that contain AGEs may greatly contribute to the AGE burden in our bodies. The problem with AGEs is that they act like a key that permanently turns on low-level inflammation in our bodies by binding to cellular receptors known as RAGEs. AGEs also cross-link with proteins in our cells, altering their normal structure and function.

It is now becoming clear that high tissue levels of AGEs are associated with almost all chronic diseases that afflict us in the Western world. AGEs are directly involved with or accelerate the progression of numerous diseases, including the metabolic syndrome (type 2 diabetes, high blood pressure, cardiovascular disease), kidney failure, Alzheimer's disease, allergies and auto-immune diseases, cancers, cataracts, retinal degeneration, and gastrointestinal diseases. Additionally, excessive AGEs are known to speed up the aging process. In rodents, diets low in AGEs lengthen their life spans to the same degree that caloric restriction does. In human beings, restriction of dietary AGEs lowers markers of oxidative stress and inflammation. There is no reason to believe that our life spans cannot be increased in a manner similar to those of experimental animals by limiting our dietary AGEs.

The good news is that if you are already following the Paleo Diet, you won't have to tweak it much at all to make it a low-AGE diet. The following table lists the concentrations of AGEs found in many Paleo foods and in some non-Paleo foods. By closely examining this table, you can get a feel for foods that yield excessive AGEs and those that don't.

Advanced Glycation End-Product (AGE) Contents in Foods (kU per 100 grams)

Food Source	AGE Content	Food Source	AGE Content
Fruits		**Poultry**	
Apple	13	Chicken breast, raw	769
Avocado	1,577	Chicken breast, boiled (1 hr.)	1,123
Banana	9	Chicken breast, boiled with lemon	957
Cantaloupe	20	Chicken breast, poached (7 min.)	1,101
Dates	60		
Raisins	120	Chicken breast, microwaved (5 min.)	1,524
Vegetables		Chicken breast, pan fried	4,938
Carrots	10		
Celery	43	Chicken breast, broiled (15 min.)	5,828
Cucumber	31	Chicken breast, deep fried (20 min.)	9,722
Olives	1,670		
Onion	36		
Tomato	23	**Fish/Seafood**	
Grilled vegetables (broccoli, carrots, celery)	226	Salmon, microwaved (1 min.)	954
		Salmon, poached (7 min.)	1,801
Beef		Salmon, fried in olive oil	3,083
Beef, raw	707		
Beef, microwaved (6 min.)	2,687	Salmon, broiled	3,347
		Shrimp, raw	1,003
Beef, ground (pan browned)	4,928	Shrimp, grilled on BBQ	2,089
Beef, hamburger fast food	5,418		
Beef, roast	6,071	Trout, raw	783
Beef, steak (broiled)	7,479	Trout, baked (25 min.)	2,138
		Tuna, canned in water	452
Pork/Lamb			
Pork chop, raw	1,188	**Eggs**	
Pork chop w/vinegar BBQ	3,334	Poached	90
Pork chop, pan fried	4,752	Scrambled (med. low heat)	97
Lamb, raw	826		
Lamb, leg, boiled (30 min.)	1,218	Omelet (olive oil, low heat)	337

Food Source	AGE Content	Food Source	AGE Content
Dairy Products		Chicken crispy (McDonald's)	7,722
Butter	23,340	Chicken selects (McDonald's)	9,257
Parmesan cheese	16,900		
Philadelphia cream cheese	10,883	**Processed Foods**	
Cheese, American processed	8,677	Tub margarine	17,520
Cheese, feta	8,423	Mayonnaise	9,400
Cheese, Brie	5,597	Big Mac (McDonald's)	7,801
Cheese, cheddar	5,523	Pizza, thin crust	6,825
Cheese, mozzarella	1,677	Filet-O-Fish (McDonald's)	6,027
Nuts, Seeds		Toasted cheese sandwich	4,333
Almonds, roasted	6,650	Potato chips	2,883
Cashews, raw	6,730	Rice crispies	2,000
Chestnuts, raw	2,723	Oreo cookies	1,770
Pumpkin seeds, raw	1,853		
Sunflower seeds, raw	2,510	**Miscellaneous**	
Sunflower seeds, roasted	4,693	Olive oil, extra virgin	10,040
Processed Meats		Diet soda	3
Bacon, fried (5 min.)	91,577	Distilled spirits	0
Bacon, microwaved (3 min.)	9,023	Vinegar	40
Beef frankfurter, broiled (5 min.)	11,270	Beer	1
		Wine	11–33

Although we don't yet have clear guidelines regarding healthful dietary limits for AGEs, we do know that the typical American adult consumes about 14,700 kU of AGEs per day. Based on animal studies, if we can cut this number in half (7,350 kU per day), it may reduce inflammation and oxidative stress—and potentially increase our life spans. You can use the table to get an idea of your daily AGEs consumption.

An important element missing from this table is fructose. You remember that most Americans ingest this sugar in the form of processed foods, particularly soft drinks sweetened with high-fructose corn syrup. We also obtain fructose from the metabolism of table sugar (sucrose). When we digest sucrose, half of it is converted into fructose in our intestines. When all of these processed dietary sugars are added up, the average American consumes a staggering 59 pounds of fructose per year.

Because the concentration of AGEs in fructose is negligible (0–3 kU per 100 grams), you might think it is a minor contributor to our bodies' total AGE load. Nothing could be further from the truth. Studies from Dr. Takeuchi's laboratory at Hokuriku University in Japan show that fructose, once in our bodies, produces ten times more AGEs than the usual sugar found in our bloodstream, glucose, does. The message here is clear—although table sugar and high-fructose corn syrup contain virtually no AGEs, they dramatically elevate the concentrations of these noxious compounds in our bodies.

Notice that fruits and veggies and staples of the Paleo Diet are very low in AGEs, as are eggs. In contrast, most dairy products and fast and processed foods are loaded with these harmful substances. In their raw state, meat and seafood contain relatively few AGEs, but these chemicals become increasingly concentrated in our diets depending on the method of cooking.

I do not advocate that we always eat our meat and seafood raw— the risk for bacterial infection with E. coli and other bacterial contaminants is greatly magnified when we eat raw meat or seafood. Nevertheless, if you can find sources of untainted meats and seafood, eating these foods raw may represent a healthy alternative when it comes to AGEs. Sushi bars (raw fish and seafood) and restaurants serving steak tartare (raw beef) have been popular for decades.

Raw meats and fish contain much lower concentrations of AGEs, but so do animal foods that are prepared using slow cooking methods, and cooked meats are generally free from bacteria that may produce disease. As a Paleo Dieter, be aware that slow cooking methods, such as stewing, poaching, steaming, and slow roasting, reduce the AGE content of meats, while simultaneously preventing bacterial contamination.

When it comes to AGEs, the worst way to cook your meats and seafood is by high heat: searing, broiling, frying, and high-temperature roasting.

I would never be one to ruin a wonderful summer evening dinner at a close friend's home by saying that I couldn't eat the char-crusted barbecued London broil that my friend generously served onto my plate. By slicing off the burned surface and eating the pink inner layers, however, I can reduce my AGE intake nearly to the levels found in raw, uncooked beef. This is a table strategy that you may want to consider for all meats—being on the rare side is a good thing when it comes to AGEs.

Whenever possible, try to replace high-temperature searing techniques with long slow-cooking procedures. I love tender beef stew chunks slowly cooked all day long with carrots, celery, onions, and spices in a crock pot. Similarly, poached salmon with basil and tender, fresh asparagus don't get much better for me. A final tip: cooking with lemon juice can significantly reduce the AGEs in your meat or fish, while simultaneously enhancing its flavor. Bon appetit.

Paleo Bottom Line

Attempt to emulate our Stone Age ancestors in the food groups they ate by choosing everyday foods available in grocery stores, farmer's markets, and supermarkets. Avoid starches, processed foods, and overcooked meats.

PART TWO

Paleo Pitfalls

From Vegetarian to Paleo Dieter:
Tom's Story

As a health professional and a former long-time vegetarian, I have been following the Paleo Diet for about two years and am delighted with the results. My weight has returned to normal and remained normal; my HDL has increased to 50 from 35; my LDL, which was at the upper range of normal, has decreased to healthy levels; my VLDL [very low-density lipoprotein] has also returned to healthy levels (around 12); my triglycerides have plummeted from 250 to 60; and my fluctuating high blood pressure is now consistently within safe parameters. The tendonitis in my knee has cleared up completely. I now recommend this diet to many of my patients in my acupuncture practice, the majority of whom have symptoms of metabolic syndrome.

4

Vegetarianism Can Be Hazardous to Your Health

I started the Paleo Diet about two years ago because the low-fat vegetarian thing that I'd been doing for twenty years just wasn't working. Within weeks, I'd lost three dress sizes (not so many pounds, but who's counting?), and my muscle tone had visibly improved. But the most amazing change was in my personality and health. It was as if someone had lifted a dark veil from my head. I sleep less but better, wake up happy, and look forward to my daily challenges. My hair loss and skin problems have vanished. My teeth are stronger, and my gums don't bleed. My thyroid (which I claimed was enlarged, but doctors disagreed) has gone back to its normal size. I could go on and on.

—Suzanne

Undoing Decades of Damage: Trevor's Story

I had two heart attacks at forty-seven; it was downhill after that: Glaucoma, chronic lymphatic leukemia about fourteen years ago. Open heart surgery eight years ago. Type 2 diabetes four years ago. I had to take early retirement at age fifty-eight.

45

I converted to the Paleo Diet more than a year ago.

I am now better than I have been for many years. The steady downturn has been reversed. On my last six monthly visits to see my hematologist, I was told, "You will almost certainly never require any therapy [chemo, radiation]. You will die of something else. Go out and enjoy the next twenty years of your life!"

On my last visit to see the endocrinologist, for diabetes two months ago, he almost took me off insulin, so well controlled were my blood sugars. I am expecting this to happen at my next visit in December. I began to use emu oil because of crippling effects of statin drugs. Emu oil has kept my cholesterol at the same levels as statin drugs, allowing me to quit statin drugs for about four years now.

The Paleo Diet is adding to this improvement. Virtually the only cereals I eat are some healthful whole-grain breads. I quit eating what I thought were the loves of my life—pasta, rice, dairy products—and now don't miss them. I am doing light manual work around the grounds here, quite impossible for me in the past.

One final advantage: I could not lose weight under the diabetic diet. Only when I went on the Paleo Diet did I lose weight and not feel deprived or hungry. My weight dropped 9 pounds to 145 pounds. Quitting bread is on my agenda.

I eat mostly chicken, grilled fish, vegetables, salad, a little canned salmon, and lots of fruit. Certainly well within the 85 percent rule—I think about 90 percent-plus compliant.

Since the publication of my first book, I have been asked time and again if there is a vegetarian version of the Paleo Diet. I say emphatically, *No!* I'll explain why.

Vegetarian diets are a bit of a moving target because they come in at least three major versions. We all know in principle that vegetarians do not eat meat, poultry, or fish—this is the first and foremost characteristic of vegetarian diets. Less restrictive are lacto/ovo vegetarians, who limit their animal food choices to dairy products and/or eggs, whereas vegan vegetarians eat plant foods exclusively. A 2008 study published by *Vegetarian Times* magazine revealed that 3.2 percent of U.S. adults, or 7.3 million people, follow a vegetarian-based diet. Approximately 0.5 percent, or one million Americans, are vegans. The study also indicated that more than half (53 percent) of current vegetarians follow their plant-based diet to improve overall health. Additional reasons underlying their vegetarian lifestyles were:

1. Animal welfare—54 percent
2. Environmental concerns—47 percent
3. Natural approaches to wellness—39 percent
4. Food safety issues—31 percent
5. Weight loss and weight maintenance issues—25 percent

I respect everyone's choice and believe that people have the right to follow whatever diet they like and to eat foods that they feel are best suited for themselves and their families. I also respect people's decisions to abstain from meat eating for religious, moral, or ethical reasons. Nevertheless, as a scientist I hope that we all try to make dietary decisions based not only on philosophical and ethical issues, but also on knowledge about foods that are good for our bodies and our long-term health. I can't lend my support to any version of a vegetarian diet that people may adopt for the mistaken idea that these diets improve overall health, because they don't.

The Evolutionary Evidence

Although vegetarianism has deep historical roots dating back at least to 500 BC with such ancient Greeks as Pythagoras, Porphyry, and Plutarch, this manner of eating has only been with us for a blink of an eye on an evolutionary time scale. In our comprehensive analysis of 229 hunter-gatherer diets, my research group and I showed

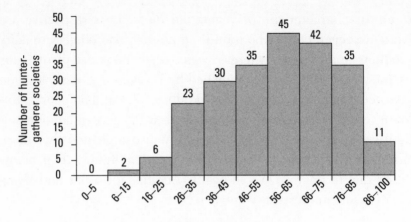

% subsistence on animal foods

Hunter-Gatherers and Animal Foods

beyond question that no historically studied foragers were vegetarians. In fact, whenever and wherever animal foods were available, they were always preferred over plant foods. The graph above shows the overwhelming preference for animal foods in all 229 hunter-gatherer societies that we studied. Notice that not a single foraging society fell into the 0–5 percent animal subsistence category. Most (73 percent) of the 229 hunter-gatherers consumed 46 percent or more of their daily calories as animal food.

The compelling reason for our Paleo ancestors' preference of animal foods over plant foods was that they got more bang (food calories) for the buck—their energy expended to obtain the food.

Human beings' preference for, and attraction, to meat, marrow, and animal food has a very long history in our ancestral line. Fossils of butchered animals with stone tool cut marks on their bones have been discovered in Africa dating back 2.5 million years. These smoking guns in the archaeological record leave little doubt that all human species ate animal foods from the beginning of our existence. Scientists are able to determine the relative percentage of plant and animal foods in extinct human species by analyzing elements called isotopes within their fossilized bones. Every single hominid skeleton examined since the emergence of *Homo sapiens*

2.5 million years ago shows an isotopic signature characteristic of meat-based diets. Furthermore, if we compare our biochemical and anatomical machinery to cats', which are carnivores, we both share evolutionary enzyme pathways characteristic of processing lots of meat. If you are interested in these details, I have written about them in my debate with the noted vegetarian Dr. T. Colin Campbell, the author of *The China Study*. The full debate can be downloaded from: www.cathletics.com/articles/article.php?, article ID=50.

If we accept the idea that vegetarianism represents an ideal human diet, then vegetarianism must be part of a much larger mechanism governing human biology. What I'm getting at is the why question: Why would a vegetarian diet represent an optimal nutritional road map for our species? Any unified theory of human nutrition is a detective story in which scientists attempt to reveal or uncover biological systems that have been designed and put into place by evolution through natural selection. Therefore, hypotheses regarding what we should and shouldn't eat must be consistent with the system and the ancient environments that engineered our genes. If we are to buy into vegetarianism, the system that shaped our present genome—evolution via natural selection—necessarily had to be conditioned over eons by a plant-based vegetarian diet. Otherwise, there is no rational hypothesis to explain why humans would "prosper and thrive" on vegetarian diets.

Bottom line: there is no credible fossil, archaeological, anthropological, or biochemical evidence to show that any hunter-gatherers or pre-agricultural human beings ever consumed exclusively plant-based diets. This information should be a major clue that there may be some problems with vegetarian dietary recommendations created by human beings for human beings.

We are all human; we all make mistakes, the saying goes. As I have suggested throughout this book, let's not depend on human frailties for dietary advice—rather, let's rely on the wisdom of the system that designed the diet to which we are all genetically adapted.

The Experimental Evidence

If you are currently a vegetarian or a vegan, one of the most powerful health expectations for adopting this lifestyle is that you will outlive your hamburger-eating neighbors by escaping cancer, heart disease, and other causes of death. If the truth be known, your lifelong dietary deprivations will not prolong your life span but rather will produce multiple nutrient deficiencies that are associated with numerous health problems and illnesses.

In their 2009 "Position Statement on Vegetarian Diets," the American Dietetic Association tells us,

> Appropriately planned vegetarian diets including total vegetarian or vegan diets are healthful, nutritionally adequate, and may provide health benefits in the prevention and treatment of certain disease. Well-planned vegetarian diets are appropriate for individuals during all stages of the life cycle, including pregnancy, lactation, infancy, childhood, and adolescence, and for athletes.

I don't know where the authors of this paper came from or what scientific journals they have been reading, but these statements simply are not supported by the data.

First, if vegetarian diets are so healthful, any reasonable person might expect that people eating plant-based diets would have lower death rates from all causes than their meat-eating counterparts. This question was never fully answered until 1999, when Dr. Key and colleagues at Oxford University conducted a large meta analysis comparing overall death rates between 27,808 vegetarians and 48,364 meat eaters. I quote Dr. Key's study: "There were no significant differences between vegetarians and non-vegetarians in mortality from cerebrovascular disease, stomach cancer, colorectal cancer, lung cancer, breast cancer, prostate cancer *or all other causes combined.*" I have italicized the last words of this sentence to emphasize the fact that vegetarians do not fare any better than their hamburger-eating counterparts when death rates for all causes are considered.

A more recent 2009 analysis, the EPIC-Oxford Study employing the largest sample of vegetarians (33,883) ever examined, came up with identical conclusions: "Within the study mortality from circulatory diseases and all causes is not significantly different between vegetarians and meat eaters." The results of this study and the earlier meta analysis fly directly in the face of the American Dietetic Association's suggestion that vegetarian and vegan diets may provide health benefits in the prevention and treatment of certain diseases.

Vegetarian Diets and Nutritional Deficiencies

The American Dietetic Association's view that appropriately planned vegetarian diets, including total vegetarian or vegan diets, are healthful and "nutritionally adequate" is shared by the USDA MyPyramid guidelines, which have recently (June 2011) been renamed MyPlate and which counsel us, "Vegetarian diets can meet all the recommendations for nutrients."

The American Dietetic Association's quote is a craftily written statement that is misleading and one-sided. Taken at face value, it would appear that all vegetarian diets, including vegan diets, are nutritionally sound all by themselves and don't require any additional nutritional supplements.

In order to get to the true meaning out of the ADA's position statement, we need to dig deeper and determine what they mean by an "appropriately planned vegetarian diet." The ADA tells us, "Key nutrients for vegetarians include protein, n-3 fatty acids, iron, zinc, iodine, calcium, and vitamins D and B12. A vegetarian diet can meet current recommendations for all of these nutrients. In some cases, supplements or fortified foods can provide useful amounts of important nutrients."

Let's dissect this statement. The last line informing us that supplements and fortified foods *sometimes* are useful is outlandish. In reality, it is not only in *some cases* that supplements and vitamin-fortified foods are required, but rather in *all cases* for vegan diets and in most cases for lacto/ovo diets. Without supplementation, vegetarian diets simply don't work and invariably cause multiple nutrient deficiencies that adversely affect not only our health and well-being but our children's as well.

Vegetarian Diets and Vitamin B12

Even informed vegetarians won't argue that plant foods contain no vitamin B12 and that meat and animal foods are the only significant dietary source of this crucial nutrient. Additionally, we can't synthesize B12 in our bodies. If you decide to become vegan, by default you will become vitamin B12 deficient unless you supplement your diet with this essential vitamin or eat B12-fortified foods.

Any lifelong dietary plan that requires nutrient supplementation on a regular basis makes no sense from an evolutionary perspective. You don't have to be an evolutionary biologist to realize that wild animals don't take nutritional supplements, nor do they normally develop vitamin deficiencies when living in their native environments. If our ancestral foragers didn't eat B12-containing animal foods, they developed vitamin B12 deficiencies, which in turn impaired their health and survival, worsening their chances of reproducing. Any behavior that favored all-plant diets would have been quickly weeded out by natural selection because of our genetic requirement for vitamin B12. Unlike modern-day vegetarians, hunter-gatherers couldn't simply pop a vitamin pill to make up for nutritional shortcomings in their diets.

I want to emphasize that this flaw in nutritional logic is not just a minor point to be shuffled under the rug, as the ADA and the USDA have done, but rather represents a huge error in judgment for recommending vegan diets. To fully appreciate this breakdown in reasoning, let's examine the history of vitamin B12. Because it was the last vitamin to be discovered, in 1948, vitamin B12 only became available as a commercial supplement in the 1950s. Consequently, every person on the planet who consumed a strict lifelong vegan diet before the discovery of B12 would have been deficient in this essential nutrient. Unfortunately, most of the world's vegetarians and vegans have not been able to figure out just exactly what an "appropriately planned" vegetarian diet consists of, as almost all of them maintain deficient or marginal vitamin B12 concentrations in their bloodstream. A 2003 study by Dr. Hermann and colleagues of ninety-five vegetarians revealed that 77 percent of lacto/ovo vegetarians were deficient in vitamin B12—and a staggering 92 percent of the vegans had deficiencies in this essential vitamin.

And the EPIC-Oxford study, which examined simple B12 concentrations in the blood of 231 ovo/lacto vegetarians and 232 vegans, verified that B12 deficiencies were widespread in these groups. If we use the normal cutoff point (150 pmol/liter) as the measure for vitamin B12 deficiency in the blood, then the data from this study shows that 73 percent of the vegans and 24 percent of the lacto/ovo vegetarians had vitamin B12 deficiencies.

These two scientific papers are representative of nearly all other studies reporting vitamin B12 levels in vegetarians. When this many people who follow vegetarian or vegan diets become vitamin B12 deficient, it is beyond comprehension to me why governmental agencies and national dietary organizations still stubbornly cling to the belief that plant-based diets are healthful.

Even more disturbing is a report by Dr. Corinna Koebnick and coworkers in Germany showing that long-term ovo/lacto vegetarian diets impair vitamin B12 status in pregnant women. Maternal B12 deficiencies can then be handed down to the unborn fetus and to nursing infants, who frequently have no other source of nutrition except for their mothers' vitamin B12–depleted milk. Clearly, B12 deficiency in pregnant women is not just a simple, benign nutritional problem—it has potentially disastrous health outcomes for both mother and child.

B12 deficiency in pregnant women is known to cause spontaneous abortions, weak labor, premature and low-birth-weight deliveries, birth defects, and preeclampsia (maternal high blood pressure and damage to the liver, the kidneys, and the blood vessels). Infants born from mothers with vitamin B12 deficiency frequently suffer from congenital malformations, irritability, failure to thrive, apathy, mental retardation, and developmental problems. This data hardly supports the ADA's position that "well-planned vegetarian diets are appropriate for individuals during all stages of the life cycle, including pregnancy, lactation, infancy, childhood."

Vegetarian Diets and Homocysteine

Vitamin B12 deficiencies caused by vegetarian or vegan diets are just as devastating to adults as they are to infants and pregnant women. Vitamins technically are defined as "organic catalysts"— meaning that without their presence in our diets, our metabolic machinery slows or is sufficiently damaged to eventually cause illness and disease. One of the most destructive changes in our bodies caused by vitamin B12 deficiency is the appearance of a toxic substance in our bloodstream known as homocysteine. Without sufficient dietary sources of vitamin B12, a chemical reaction within our bodies is impaired and causes blood concentrations of homocysteine to rise.

Homocysteine is a toxin for almost every cell in our bodies. It increases the risk for birth defects, infertility, dementia, psychological illness, stroke, heart attacks, blood vessel disease, blood clots, osteoporosis, and overall death rates. Worldwide studies of vegetarians and vegans show that the less animal food they eat, the higher their blood concentrations of homocysteine are. Let's take a look at how vegetarian diets raise blood concentrations of homocysteine and increase the risk for numerous diseases.

Homocysteine and Cardiovascular Disease

It is widely assumed that vegetarian diets reduce the risk for cardiovascular disease and heart attacks because they lower the total amount of fat and saturated fats in our diets. Unfortunately, this simplistic explanation is only part of the story. As discussed in chapter 2, total fat and saturated fat have been shown in large meta analyses to have little effect on the atherosclerotic process that clogs the arteries and causes heart and blood vessel disease. In contrast, meta analyses published in the last ten years have confirmed that homocysteine is an independent risk factor for cardiovascular disease and heart attacks. The higher your blood levels of homocysteine, the greater will be your risk of having a stroke or a heart attack.

Homocysteine is particularly dangerous when high concentrations build up in our bloodstream because it damages the cells that line the blood vessels. This initial injury to the blood vessels represents one of the first steps in the artery-clogging process. If blood concentrations of homocysteine remain high and the blood vessel damage goes on unabated for decades, it may result in fatal strokes and heart attacks.

A meta analysis in 2008 by Dr. Humphrey and colleagues indicated that for each (5 micromol/L) rise in blood homocysteine levels, the risk for cardiovascular disease events increased by approximately 20 percent. Because vegetarian diets cause vitamin B12 levels in the bloodstream to plummet, which in turn makes homocysteine levels rise dangerously, you might expect to find high rates of cardiovascular disease in strict lifelong vegetarians. One of the problems in examining cardiovascular disease in vegetarians from the United States and Europe is that many of them aren't strict vegetarians and typically haven't consumed vegetarian diets for their entire lives. All of these variables tend to confound the results of epidemiological studies. Given this scenario, what better place to examine vegetarian diets and cardiovascular disease than in India? With a population of 1.17 billion people, 31 percent (362,700,000) of whom are vegetarians, India represents the perfect country to study cardiovascular disease and plant-based diets. Unlike most vegetarians in the United States and Europe, Indian vegetarians are committed to lifelong vegetarian diets due to their religious convictions and family conventions.

If vegetarian diets provide protection from cardiovascular disease, as the ADA suggests, you would expect to find a low prevalence of heart disease and stroke in India because almost one-third of its population are vegetarians. Unfortunately, this is not the case. In reality, the incidence of cardiovascular disease is much higher in India than anywhere else in the world. Moreover, Indians develop cardiovascular disease at a much earlier age than do people from other countries. In the largest study ever of 368 lifelong Indian vegetarians with cardiovascular disease, Dr. Kumar and coworkers showed that heart disease was higher in vegetarians and that they had lower blood levels of vitamin B12. Dr. Kumar wrote, "We believe that the beneficial effect of a vegetarian diet in this population is circumvented by deficiency of vitamin B12."

Homocysteine and Neurological Diseases

Numerous studies have found that homocysteine adversely affects brain function, behavior, and mood. People with higher blood concentrations of homocysteine have a greater risk for Alzheimer's disease, dementia, depression, Parkinson's disease, and stroke. In a comprehensive 2010 review of 1,627 articles on high blood levels of homocysteine and low levels of vitamin B12, Dr. Werder concluded, "Hyperhomocysteinemia (high blood levels of homocysteine) with or without hypovitaminosis B12 (low blood levels of vitamin B12) is a risk factor for dementia." Another B vitamin, folate, when deficient can cause blood concentrations of homocysteine to rise, but in a study involving 2,403 older people, Dr. Clarke found that "the relative importance of vitamin B12 deficiency as a determinant of homocysteine concentrations and cognitive impairment is probably greater than that of folate deficiency in older adults."

A recent study by Dr. Selhub's research group showed that a high dietary intake of folate seems to make B12 deficiencies worse by further increasing blood concentrations of homocysteine. This is precisely the dietary pattern found in the blood of most vegetarians—low B12 and adequate or elevated folate. Is it any wonder why so many vegetarians and vegans have dangerously high blood levels of homocysteine?

Homocysteine and Bone Disease

The list of chronic diseases associated with high blood concentrations of homocysteine has recently been extended to bone disease.

By raising blood homocysteine levels, vegetarian diets increase bone fracture risk. The notion that vegetarians have weaker bones than their meat-eating counterparts was verified in the largest study ever undertaken in a vegetarian population (9,420 vegetarians and 1,126 vegans). The authors of the study concluded, "The higher fracture risk in the vegans appeared to be a consequence of their considerably lower mean calcium intake." Low calcium and vitamin D intake are well-known risk factors for bone fractures and osteoporosis, and these nutritional deficiencies are common in vegan and vegetarian populations. Since 2003, more than a dozen studies have identified low B12, low folate, or high homocysteine blood levels as risk factors for poor bone density, fractures, or osteoporosis.

Although we don't completely understand how high blood levels of homocysteine adversely affect bone, tissue studies have identified a number of mechanisms. Homocysteine seems to impair the normal bone mineralization process. It also causes an accelerated breakdown of bone and inhibits the formation of new bone cells. Some of the best evidence implicating homocysteine in bone disease comes from human dietary interventions. In a two-year study of 559 elderly women in Japan, Dr. Sato showed that supplementation of vitamin B12 and folate (*not* folic acid) reduced blood concentrations of homocysteine by 38 percent. Yet more important, women in the vitamin-supplemented group suffered thirty-three fewer hip fractures than women in the unsupplemented control group.

One of the best ways you can prevent hip fractures is to follow the Paleo Diet. Because you will be eating meat and fish at virtually every meal, you won't have to worry about vitamin B12 deficiencies, as these two foods are our best sources of this essential vitamin. The other mainstay of the Paleo Diet is fresh fruit and veggies, which are rich sources of the B vitamin folate. The combination of lots of meat and fish, along with plenty of fruits and vegetables at every meal, will ensure that you do not develop vitamin B12 or folate deficiencies and that your blood homocysteine levels will remain low throughout your life—as nature intended.

Homocysteine and Infertility

Elevated blood concentrations of homocysteine result primarily from too little vitamin B12 and folate in our diets. When adequate stores of these two B vitamins are present from nutritious foods in our diet (including meats, fresh fruits, and veggies), our cells can defuse the poisonous effects of homocysteine and convert it into less toxic compounds. When B12 is lacking or deficient, however, as it almost always is in vegetarian and vegan diets, homocysteine builds up in our bloodstream and literally infiltrates nearly every cell in our bodies. Healthy egg cells in women and healthy sperm cells in men are essential requirements for getting pregnant, staying pregnant, and producing normal embryos, vigorous infants, and healthy children. A diet deficient or marginal in vitamins B12 and folate can severely reduce your chances for successful fertilization and conception. Infertility is a huge problem in both the United States and Europe and affects at least six million people in the United States, about 7.4 percent of the reproductive-age population.

Many environmental and genetic factors may be involved, but one thing is certain. As a couple, if you or your partner's blood levels of vitamin B12 and/or folate are low and your homocysteine is elevated, your chances for normal conception will be significantly reduced.

The injurious effects of homocysteine in our bones and cardiovascular and nervous systems have been much better studied than in our reproductive systems, but it is becoming increasingly evident that the low vitamin B12 and folate status responsible for elevated homocysteine is toxic to both sperm and egg cells and may represent a major previously unrecognized risk factor for infertility. More than thirty years ago, at least one group of researchers pointed out that Indian vegetarian men maintained lower vitamin B12 concentrations in their sperm than nonvegetarians did and attributed these values to their vegetarian diet. A number of these earlier studies in Asian populations hinted that vitamin B12 supplementation could improve sperm function and vigor and boost male fertility.

Similar nutritional patterns have been discovered in Western populations. In a 2009 study of 172 men and 223 women who were unable to conceive, 36 percent of men and 23 percent of women had vitamin B12 deficiencies. Almost 40 percent of the infertile men had abnormal semen that was directly related to their vitamin B12 deficiencies. Other recent studies in men show that low dietary folate and vitamin B12 are associated with high blood concentrations of homocysteine that likely underlie abnormal sperm function.

Women with compromised dietary B12 and folate intake frequently have elevated blood levels of homocysteine, which prevents them from becoming pregnant. We are not completely sure how these blood chemistry changes impede successful pregnancies in women, but tissue studies suggest that egg cells that are infiltrated by homocysteine and are deficient in vitamin B12 and folate become fragile and unable to continue with a normal pregnancy once fertilized.

Menstrual Problems Caused by Vegetarian Diets

Vegetarian diets are frequently associated with menstrual problems known to affect fertility. A total of five studies have compared the incidence of menstrual irregularities between vegetarians and meat eaters. Four out of these five studies demonstrated significantly higher rates of menstrual complications in vegetarians.

Not all types of scientific experiments have equal clout in establishing cause and effect. Of the five studies, four were epidemiological (population) studies, and one was an experimental intervention. Because dietary interventions represent the most powerful experimental procedure for determining whether dietary changes improve health or cause illness, they carry more weight than epidemiological studies do. Let's take a look at the only dietary intervention investigating vegetarian diets on menstrual health. Dr. Pirke at the University of Trier in Germany randomly divided eighteen young women with normal menstrual periods into either vegetarian or nonvegetarian diet groups. After six weeks, seven of the nine women assigned to the vegetarian diet stopped ovulating, whereas only a single woman in the meat-eating group experienced this problem. In other words, within only six weeks of consuming a vegetarian diet, 78 percent of healthy, normally cycling women ceased ovulating. The take-home message is this: if you are trying to get pregnant, one of your best strategies is to avoid vegetarian diets. While you're at it, make sure your husband or partner does the same.

Zinc Deficiencies Impair Sperm Function

One of the most frequent nutritional shortcomings of vegetarian and vegan diets is that they fall short of recommended intake for zinc. In the largest epidemiological study of vegetarians, Dr. Davey noted that vegans had "the lowest intakes of retinol [vitamin A], vitamin B12, vitamin D, calcium and zinc" when compared to meat and fish eaters. More important, with zinc it's not just how much is present in your food, but how much is actually absorbed in your body. Although dietary zinc intake in vegetarian diets sometimes appears to be adequate on paper, in the body it actually results in deficiencies because most plant-based zinc is bound to phytate and therefore unavailable for absorption. Phytate is an antinutrient found in whole grains, beans, soy, and other legumes that prevents normal assimilation of many minerals. Laboratory experiments show that vegetarians absorb about half as much zinc as meat eaters do because zinc from animal food is much better assimilated than zinc from plant foods.

Based on this information, you might expect blood concentrations of zinc to be lower in vegetarians than in meat eaters. Sometimes scientists have found this to be the case, but not always. The problem here has to do with where zinc ends up in our bodies after we ingest it. Most zinc finds its way into the interior of cells and does not accumulate in the liquid portion (plasma) of blood. So unless scientists examine zinc concentrations within cells, readings obtained in blood plasma frequently do not accurately reflect body stores of this essential mineral. In virtually every study of vegetarians that measured zinc levels inside various cells (red blood cells, hair cells, and skin cells in saliva), plant-based diets caused zinc deficiencies. In one study, 12 meat-eating women were put on a lacto/ovo vegetarian diet, and after only twenty-two days Dr. Freeland-Graves reported that zinc concentrations in the women's salivary cells plunged by 27 percent. Similar results were described by Dr. Srikumar from a longer-term experiment in which twenty meat-eating men and women adopted a lactovegetarian diet for an entire year. In this study, both hair cells and blood levels of zinc sharply declined and remained low throughout the twelve-month experiment.

Because of their low zinc content and bioavailability, long-term vegetarian diets almost always cause zinc deficiencies. Numerous epidemiological studies have shown that infertile men had poor sperm counts that were associated with reduced zinc levels in their semen. Virtually every well-controlled experimental study ever conducted shows that men put on zinc-deficient diets ended up with reduced sperm counts, impaired sperm health, and often depressed blood testosterone levels. The good news is that these deleterious changes in male reproductive function can be reversed if zinc-rich diets such as the Paleo Diet are followed, or if zinc pills are supplemented. Dr. Steegers-Theunissen in the Netherlands showed dramatic improvements in the reproductive health of 103 subfertile men when zinc and folic acid supplements were added. Following the six-month supplementation program, sperm counts increased significantly in the subfertile men, while sperm abnormalities declined by 4 percent. A similar study of 14 infertile men from India also indicated that zinc supplementation increased sperm health and sperm counts and shortly thereafter resulted in three successful conceptions by the men's wives.

Whether you are a man or a woman, if you want to sidestep infertility problems, the best advice I can give you is to abandon vegetarian diets and adopt the nutritional patterns that have sustained our hunter-gatherer ancestors for the last 2.6 million years. There are no known risks to adopting the Paleo Diet, and, in fact, regular consumption of meat, seafood, and fresh fruit and vegetables, at the expense of cereals, dairy, and processed foods, will prevent vitamin B12 and folate deficiencies. In turn, these essential vitamins will ensure that your blood levels of homocysteine will return to normal—effectively reducing your risk for cardio-vascular, neurological, bone, and reproductive diseases.

You don't have to look any further than the ADA's "Position Statement" or the USDA's recommendations on vegetarian diets to discover additional nutrient shortcomings caused by plant-based diets. The ADA matter-of-factly states, "Key nutrients for vegetar-ians include protein, n-3 fatty acids, iron, zinc, iodine, calcium, and vitamins D and B12." The USDA notes, "Vegetarians may need to focus on . . . iron, calcium, zinc, and vitamin B12."

These subtle admissions of potential nutrient deficiency problems associated with vegetarian diets represent the tip of a nutritional nightmare. Just as was the case with vegetarian diets and vitamin B12 deficiency, there is little credible scientific evidence to show that people adhering to a lifelong plant-based diet without taking supplements or eating fortified foods can achieve an ade-quate dietary intake of omega 3 fatty acids (EPA and DHA), iron, zinc, iodine, calcium, and vitamin D. To this list, you can also add vitamin B6 and taurine, an amino acid.

Mineral Deficiencies in Vegetarian Diets

One major complication with the assessment of dietary nutrient adequacy in any diet has to do with whether the vitamins and the minerals measured in certain foods actually get absorbed into our bodies. The bioavailability of vitamins and minerals in foods is just as important in how they affect our health as is the simple content of the nutrients in food.

Phytate is not a good thing because it prevents the absorption of essential minerals. Whole grains and legumes are rich sources of phytate, and our bodies have great difficulty extracting certain minerals from these foods because they are tightly bound to phytate. As mentioned earlier, phytate in whole grains impairs calcium absorption and may adversely affect bone health; phytate also binds zinc, interfering with its assimilation and incorporation into our cells. To this list, you can add iron and magnesium.

Because vegetarian diets are virtually impossible to follow without including lots of whole grains, beans, soy, and legumes, they are inherently high in phytate. This is why it is difficult or impossible for vegetarians and vegans to maintain adequate body stores of calcium, zinc, and iron.

Zinc Deficiencies in Vegetarian Diets

Zinc is required for good health and disease resistance in virtually every cell in our bodies, whether you are a man or a woman. Marginal zinc status impairs our immune systems, slows wound healing, adversely affects glucose and insulin metabolism, and damages our bodies' built-in antioxidant systems. Without adequate dietary zinc, we experience more upper-respiratory illnesses that last longer. Zinc lozenges can slow or prevent common cold symptoms and zinc oxide creams applied topically can speed healing. If you have ever experienced painful cracked heels or nose bleeds that just wouldn't stop, try rubbing zinc oxide ointments into these wounds—you will be amazed at how rapidly zinc can heal these stubborn sores.

People who eat excessive amounts of whole grains and/or legumes and do not eat meat, fish, or animal products on a regular basis put themselves at risk for all of the illnesses and health problems associated with borderline or deficient zinc intake.

Iron Deficiencies in Vegetarian Diets

The same types of diets that produce zinc deficiencies also create iron deficiencies. High-phytate vegetarian diets based on whole grains, beans, soy, and other legumes invariably cause iron deficiencies, the most common nutrient deficit worldwide. In the United States 9 percent of all women between twelve and forty-nine years of age are iron deficient, while 4 percent of three- to five-year-old children have insufficient stores of this crucial mineral. If you are pregnant, low-iron status increases your child's risk of dying during childbirth and frequently causes low birth weights and preterm deliveries. Even more disturbing is the potential for iron deficiencies to prevent normal mental development in our children.

As a parent, I would never wish on my child or anyone else's a diet that causes nutritional deficiencies known to impair brain development and normal mental function. Yet this is just what you're doing if you follow a vegetarian diet and make your children eat that way as well. Plant-based diets not only increase the risk of impaired cognitive function in your children but will also hamper your own mental functioning. Numerous experimental studies show that inadequate iron stores in adults can slow or impair tasks that require concentration and mental clarity.

Diets that cause iron deficiencies make us fatigued and tired. If you are an athlete or have a demanding job that requires physical exertion, low iron stores will invariably worsen your performance. A 2009 experiment involving 219 female soldiers during military training showed that iron supplements increased blood iron stores, improved performance for a 2-mile run, and enhanced mood. Similarly, a study by Dr. Hinton demonstrated that iron supplements in iron-deficient male and female athletes improved their endurance, performance, and efficiency. Whether you are an athlete, a laborer, or an office worker, your best nutritional strategy to boost your iron stores, add vigor to your life, and improve your performance is to eliminate whole grains and legumes from your diet by adopting the Paleo Diet.

You might expect that the experimental evidence surrounding vegetarian diet recommendations would be convincing and overpowering. Nothing could be further from the truth, particularly when it comes to iron deficiencies and vegetarian diets.

Scientists who believe that vegetarian diets don't adversely affect our iron stores often cite scientific papers that show no difference between blood iron concentrations in vegetarians and meat eaters. What they don't tell us is how iron measurements were performed in the experiments they quote to support their viewpoint—information that is essential in knowing whether iron deficiencies exist. Any study examining blood levels of iron in vegetarians using measurements of either hemoglobin (an iron-carrying substance in red blood cells) or *hematocrit* (the concentration of red blood cells) is an unreliable indicator of long-term iron status. A much better marker is an iron-carrying molecule called *ferritin*. Virtually all epidemiological studies of vegans or ovo/lacto vegetarians show them to be either deficient or borderline iron deficient when blood ferritin levels are measured. Given this nearly unanimous finding, you might think that either the USDA or the ADA would become concerned and reexamine its endorsement of vegetarian diets. Unfortunately, these organizations have not done so. We still live with governmental and institutional dietary recommendations that may do considerable harm to our health.

The most convincing type of experiments to reveal whether vegetarian diets may cause our iron stores to nosedive are dietary interventions. Why not put a large group of nonvegetarians on a plant-based diet for an extended period and see what happens to their blood iron levels? A great idea, but unfortunately no such study has ever been conducted.

In order to once and for all know whether vegetarian diets cause iron deficiencies, we would need to perform a rigorous experiment for at least a year with more subjects and a control group and monitor changes in women's menstrual periods. You would think that this kind of very basic experimental evidence would have already been in place before any governmental or institutional organization told us that vegetarian diets were safe and didn't cause nutritional deficiencies. Unfortunately, these precautionary steps have never been taken, and millions who adhere to vegetarian diets with the mistaken belief that they will benefit health-wise will suffer.

Iodine Deficiencies in Vegetarian Diets

Numerous epidemiological studies have consistently reported that vegetarian and vegan diets greatly increase the risk for iodine deficiency. One study from Europe demonstrated that 80 percent of vegans and 25 percent of ovo/lacto vegetarians suffered from iodine deficiency. Additionally, a dietary intervention by Dr. Remer in 1999 confirmed the often-reported epidemiological evidence. After six healthy adults spent only five days on ovo/lacto vegetarian diets, their iodine status and function became impaired.

The primary reason why vegetarian diets cause iodine deficiencies is that plant foods—except for seaweed—are generally poor sources of iodine compared to meat, eggs, and fish. Gross deficiencies of iodine cause our thyroid glands to swell, producing a condition known as goiter, and in pregnant women result in severe birth defects called cretinism. Because salt is fortified with iodine, most people in the United States and Europe rarely develop gross iodine deficiencies. Yet moderate to mild iodine deficiencies are common in Westernized countries, particularly among vegetarians and vegans. Moderate iodine deficiency impairs normal growth in children and adversely affects mental development. A large meta analysis revealed that moderate childhood iodine deficiency lowered IQ by 13.5 points. Paleo diets are not only good medicine for adults, but they also ensure normal physical and mental development in our children because of their high iodine content.

One of the problems with plant-based diets is that they may put into play a vicious cycle that makes iodine deficiencies worse. When the thyroid gland's iodine stores become depleted, as often happens with vegetarian diets, certain antinutrients found in plant foods can gain a foothold and further aggravate iodine shortages.

Soy beans and soy products are frequently a mainstay in vegetarian diets. Unfortunately, soy contains certain antinutrients (isoflavones) that impair iodine metabolism in the thyroid gland, but only when our body stores of iodine are already depleted. Other plant foods, such as millet, cassava root, lima beans, sweet potatoes, and cruciferous vegetables (broccoli, cauliflower, turnips, kale, cabbage), also contain a variety of antinutrients that hinder normal iodine metabolism, although these foods are fine to eat as part of a Paleo diet. Plant-based diets put us at risk for developing iodine deficiencies in the first place, and when this happens, our bodies become vulnerable to plant antinutrients that worsen the preexisting deficiency.

The good news is that antinutritional compounds have virtually no effect on our thyroid glands when our bodies' stores of iodine are normal and full. Because meats, fish, eggs, and poultry are rich sources of iodine, you will never have to worry about this nutrient when you eat Paleo style.

Vitamin D and Vitamin B6 Deficiencies in Vegetarian Diets

Excessive consumption of whole grains negatively affects vitamin D status in our bodies. Vitamin D deficiencies run rampant in vegetarians because it is nearly impossible to become a full-fledged vegetarian without eating lots of grains. In the largest study of vegetarians ever undertaken (9,420 vegetarians and 1,126 vegans), Dr. Crowe reported that blood concentrations of vitamin D were highest in meat eaters and lowest in vegans and vegetarians. Nearly 8 percent of the vegans maintained clinical deficiencies of vitamin D. Vitamin D is not really a vitamin at all but a crucial hormone that affects virtually every cell of our bodies. Vegetarian diets are clearly a nightmare. The number of nutritional deficiencies and negative health effects related to vegetarianism far outweighs any supposed health effects of this very unnatural way of eating.

One of the biggest-kept secrets about vegan or vegetarian diets is that they frequently cause vitamin B6 deficiencies. If you recall, neither the ADA nor the USDA has given us any warning that meatless diets increase our risk for vitamin B6 deficiencies.

On paper, it would appear that vegetarian diets generally meet daily recommended intakes for vitamin B6. This assumption comes primarily from population surveys that examined the foods that vegans and vegetarians normally eat. When blood samples were analyzed from people relying on plant-based diets, though, they unexpectedly revealed that long-term vegetarians and vegans frequently are deficient in vitamin B6. A recent study of ninety-three German vegans by Dr. Waldman showed that 58 percent of these men and women suffered from vitamin B6 deficiencies despite a seemingly adequate intake of this essential nutrient. It turns out that the type of vitamin B6 (pyridoxine glucoside) found in plant foods is poorly absorbed and never makes it into our bloodstream in a usable form. The presence of pyridoxine glucoside in plant foods reduces the bioavailability of vitamin B6 so that only 20 to 25 percent is absorbed and completely utilized. In contrast, vitamin B6 found in animal foods is easily assimilated, and an estimated 75 to 100 percent fully makes its way into our bloodstream.

Compelling evidence that vegetarian diets that rely on the plant forms of vitamin B6 adversely affect our bodies' overall vitamin B6 stores comes from Dr. Leklem's laboratory at Oregon State University. Nine women were put on diets either high or low in the plant form of vitamin B6 (pyridoxine glucoside). After only eighteen days, the high–pyridoxine glucoside diets consistently lowered blood concentrations and other indices of vitamin B6 status. Deficiencies in this vitamin elevate blood homocysteine concentrations and increase our risk for cardiovascular disease, similar to shortages of folate and vitamin B12. Vitamin B6 is also an important factor in normal immune system functioning, and shortfalls of this crucial nutrient have been identified in depression and pancreatic cancer.

Omega 3 Fatty Acid Deficiencies in Vegetarian Diets

There are telltale indicators of omega 3 fatty acids in our bloodstream that reveal whether we have regularly consumed fish, seafood, or other good sources of these healthy fats. The three main types of omega 3 fatty acids we need to concern ourselves with are EPA, DHA, and ALA. EPA and DHA are called long-chain omega 3 fatty acids and are found in high amounts only in fish, seafood, certain meats, and other foods of animal origin. Plant foods contain no EPA or DHA. On the other hand, ALA is called a short-chain fatty acid and is found in both plant and animal foods. Both EPA and DHA in our red blood cells are markers of these important fatty acids in our diet. Without good dietary sources of EPA and DHA such as are found in fish, seafood, and certain meats, our blood levels of EPA and DHA will decline. Just as salt in the urine is an indicator for dietary salt intake, EPA and DHA concentrations in our red blood cells are markers for our dietary intake of these long-chain omega 3 fatty acids. It is virtually impossible to achieve high blood levels of EPA and DHA without regularly consuming fish, seafood, and certain meats, especially grass-fed meats.

One of the major nutritional shortcomings in vegans is that they obtain absolutely no EPA or DHA from their diets. They are totally dependent on plant-based ALA, supplements, or fortified foods to obtain these healthful long-chain omega 3 fatty acids. Without supplements or fortified foods, all vegans will become deficient in DHA because plant-based ALA is inefficiently converted into these long-chain fatty acids in our bodies. The liver converts less than 5 percent of ALA into EPA and less than 1 percent of ALA into DHA.

Virtually every epidemiological study that has ever been published shows that vegans who do not supplement or consume long-chain omega 3–fortified foods are deficient in both EPA and DHA. Lacto/ovo vegetarians don't fare much better because milk- and egg-based vegetarian diets do not supply sufficient DHA or EPA to maintain normal blood concentrations.

Vegan or vegetarian diets cause reductions in blood concentrations of DHA and EPA, which in turn represent a potent risk factor for many chronic diseases. Perhaps the single most important dietary recommendation to improve your health and prevent illness is to increase your dietary intake of EPA and DHA. Thousands of scientific papers covering an assortment of diseases clearly show the health benefits of these fatty acids. In randomized clinical trials in patients with preexisting heart disease, omega 3 fatty acid supplements significantly reduced cardiovascular events. Omega 3 fatty acids lessen the risk for heart disease through a number of means, including a reduction in heartbeat irregularities called arrhythmias, a decrease in blood clots, and reduced inflammation, which is now known to be an chief factor causing atherosclerosis or artery clogging.

In addition to lowering the risk for heart disease, regular consumption of fish or supplemental omega 3 fatty acids may be useful in averting, treating, or improving a wide range of diseases and disorders, including virtually all inflammatory diseases, such as the following:

- Rheumatoid arthritis (and any other disease ending with "itis")
- Inflammatory bowel disorders (Crohn's disease, ulcerative colitis)
- Periodontal disease (gingivitis)
- Mental disorders (autism, depression, postpartum depression, bipolar disorder, borderline personality disorder, impaired cognitive development in infants and children)
- Asthma

- Exercise-induced asthma
- Many types of cancers
- Macular degeneration
- Pre-term birth
- Psoriasis
- Insulin resistance
- Type 2 diabetes
- Cancer cachexia
- Intermittent claudication
- Skin damage from sunlight
- IgA nephropathy
- Lupus erythematosus
- Type 1 diabetes
- Multiple sclerosis
- Migraine headaches

Taurine Deficiencies in Vegetarian Diets

Taurine is an amino acid in our bloodstream that has multiple functions in every cell of our bodies. Unfortunately, this nutrient is not present in any plant food and is found in low concentrations in milk (6 mg per cup). In contrast, all flesh foods are excellent sources of taurine. For example, ¼ pound of dark meat from chicken provides 200 mg of taurine. Shellfish are richer still, with more than 800 mg per quarter pound. The daily taurine intake in nonvegetarians is about 150 mg, whereas lacto/ovo vegetarians take in about 17 mg per day and vegans get none. Although our livers can manufacture taurine from precursor molecules, our capacity to do so is limited— so much so that this amino acid is fortified in infant formulas.

As you might expect, studies of vegans show that their blood taurine levels are 22 percent lower than in meat eaters. How depleted blood concentrations of taurine affect our overall health is not entirely understood. Nevertheless, shortages of this amino acid and omega 3 fatty acids (EPA and DHA) may cause platelets in our blood to clot more rapidly, which in turn increases our risk for cardiovascular disease. Despite their meat-free diets, vegetarians almost always exhibit abnormal platelets that excessively adhere to one another. In one dietary intervention, Dr. Mezzano demonstrated that after eight weeks of EPA and DHA supplementation, normal platelet function was restored in a group of eighteen lacto/ovo vegetarians. Obviously, compromised taurine status will never become a problem in Paleo diets, because meat, fish, and animal products are consumed at nearly every meal.

If you have adopted or are considering adopting a plant-based diet for reasons of improving your health, make sure you reread this chapter and look up all of the references I have provided. The evidence that vegetarian and vegan diets almost always cause a multitude of nutritional deficiencies is overwhelmingly conclusive.

During the course of a lifetime, vegetarian diets will not reduce your risk of developing chronic diseases and will not allow you to live longer. Rather, this abnormal way of eating will predispose you to a host of health problems and illnesses. Vegetarianism is an unnatural way of eating that has no evolutionary precedent in our species. No hunter-gatherer society ever consumed a meatless diet—nor should you.

The ADA has labeled the Paleo Diet a fad diet because it eliminates "two entire food groups"—grains and dairy. Yet hypocritically, the ADA exempts vegan diets from this characterization, despite the fact that vegan diets eliminate two food groups (dairy and meats/fish).

If the Paleo Diet is a fad diet, it is the world's oldest fad diet—a fad for good health.

Paleo Bottom Line

Eat meat and fish daily. Avoid dairy products, grains, legumes, and processed foods.

5

Just Say No to the Milk Mustache

Healing Gastrointestinal Problems: Annie's Story

I have to share what an altering life change the Paleo Diet has been for me. As far back as I can remember, I have had GI [gastrointestinal] problems. I remember going to the hospital to receive barium treatments and always being mortified. I was constantly drinking castor oil, having Metamucil with my orange juice, and suppositories at four years old.

As I became an adult, I had terrible acid reflux, but I just assumed that the reflux was due to my pregnancies. At twenty years old, I started to have severe abdominal cramping—food would run through my body faster than it took to consume it. I was always exhausted and could gain ten pounds at a time.

Finally, when my weight was up to 163 pounds, I was not able to hang onto anything I ate, and I was always so tired I felt drugged, I made an appointment with one of my state's top gastroenterologists. He immediately gave me a prescription for an antispasmodic because he believed that I had IBS [irritable bowel syndrome], and then scheduled a day to do an EDG [esophagogastroduodenoscopy]. I came back for my EDG, and the doctor found that I have GERD [gastrointestinal reflux disease] and a hiatal hernia; he suspects IBS. I still seemed to have a difficult time with eating anything baked or dairy, and I was still gaining weight and still "dumping" my food.

A month later, I went in to see my GI doctor. He told me not to drink any mixed drinks, white wines, or beer. I thought, Well, that is okay. I do not drink that often.

Two months went by. A coworker suggested the Paleo Diet. I immediately started it and eventually began hiking four miles every morning—I am now up to running, and I am not a runner!

My results: since the middle of March, I have lost 44 pounds. I am now 119 pounds and a size 2! I have energy again and feel fabulous. Oh yes, I have a flat tummy again!

The food I was eating was slowly killing me. That sounds so dramatic, but it seriously was. My doctor said my body was in starvation mode and would hang onto anything it could. My belly was always distended, and I appeared to be six months pregnant.

I love the Paleo Diet and cannot say enough about it. I truly believe my tummy issues are genetic, and I have been dealing with celiac symptoms, lactose intolerance, GERD, and IBS all of my life. I have bought *The Paleo Diet* for everyone in my family.

My signature lecture, "Origins and Evolution of the Western Diet: Health Implications for the 21st Century," is based on a scientific paper I published in the *American Journal of Clinical Nutrition* in 2005. In this lecture, I trace the chronological introductions of all of the food groups and the foods that have become part of the contemporary U.S. and Western diet. When I lecture, I like to engage the audience so that it becomes not just a one-way presentation by me but rather an interactive give-and-take conversation. When I get to the part about milk and dairy products, I pose a question: "How do we know that our hunter-gatherer ancestors never ate this food group?" In the ensuing pause before a few people raise their hands and give the correct answer, I flip to the next slide. Immediately appears an unruly herd of about thirty African Cape buffalo, snorting and pawing the earth with powerful hooves supporting their one-ton bodies, crowned by enormous menacing horns.

Have you ever tried to approach a wild animal? How about milking one? This is an impossible task, to say the least. Until the dawn of agriculture ten thousand years ago and the subsequent domestication of dairy animals, milk, butter, cheese, and yogurt were never part of our ancestors' menu.

Although ten thousand years ago seems unimaginably distant compared to a single human life span, it is very recent on an evolutionary time scale. Only 333 human generations have come and gone since we first domesticated animals and began to consume their milk. As a species, we have had scant evolutionary experience to adapt to a food that now makes up about 10 percent of the calories in the American diet. Milk and dairy products have the enormous potential to disrupt our health and well-being through a variety of means that I barely touched on in *The Paleo Diet*. If you had any prior doubts about whether you should eat dairy foods, the information contained in this chapter should help you make an informed decision in the best interest of your health.

Milk and dairy products became part of the current Western diet during the period known as the Neolithic or New Stone Age, which began about 10,000 years ago and ended 5,500 years ago. The following graph shows just how recent dairy foods and other staples of the Western diet really are, when evaluated in an evolutionary time frame.

Unless you are lactose intolerant, have an allergy to milk and dairy products, or have been a devoted follower of the Paleo Diet,

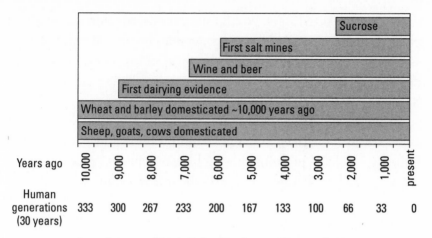

Introduction of Non-Paleo Foods into Human Diets

you probably don't give a second thought to whether you should consume a food group that seems to be found nearly everywhere in the Western diet. Your favorite dairy foods may include ice cream, chocolate milk, fruit-flavored yogurt, or fancy imported cheeses. You may think that you are doing your body a favor by eating these calcium-rich foods. But remember this: we are the only species on the planet to consume another animal's milk throughout our adult lives.

An increasing body of scientific evidence supports the evolutionary caution that this dietary practice is not necessarily harmless. The table below shows the sources and amounts of dairy foods in the U.S. diet.

These figures don't tell the entire story, as dairy products are put into almost all processed foods. Take some time to read labels. If you are a milk chocolate addict, you are eating dairy, and the

Dairy Products	% Total Calories in U.S. Diet
Whole milk	1.6
Low-fat milks	2.1
Cheese	3.2
Butter	1.1
Other	2.6
Total	**10.6**

same goes for latté lovers. Nonfat milk solids, a major ingredient in chocolate, are also put into candy, cereal, bread, salami, bologna, sausages, baked goods, salad dressings, chips, condiments, soft drinks, and many other foods that come in a can, a jar, a bottle, a bag, or a plastic wrapper.

Even though these tiny residues of milk in processed foods seem to be trivial, don't fool yourself. Milk proteins and peptides (the building blocks of proteins) have a high potential to promote heart disease, cancer, allergies, and other health problems.

The Dairy Advertising Hype

Let's take a step back and look at the vast advertising campaign that the milk-processing industry has shoved down our throats for nearly twenty years. This glitzy promotional crusade with the "Got Milk" slogan depicts movie stars, sports personalities, politicians, and other public figures with a wet, white film of what appears to be milk on their upper lips. Implied in magazine ads, TV and radio commercials, and social media is the notion that all public figures with "milk mustaches" endorse dairy products, presumably because these are healthy and nutritious foods. Let's stop for a minute and touch base with reality.

I haven't drunk a glass of milk in nearly forty years, but if I were to, I certainly wouldn't spill it all over my upper lip. This issue really doesn't matter and is simply part of the industry's advertising strategy—if the movie stars and the sports heroes do it, so should you. My question: why would a Wimbledon tennis champion, an Oscar-winning actress, and an Indy 500 race car driver blindly support a product they know virtually nothing about?

These public figures have spent their lifetimes honing talents, skills, and knowledge specific to their life callings. Yet when it comes to understanding milk's intricate influence on our metabolism, hormonal function, and long-term health, most of these people are novices operating completely outside their areas of expertise, without knowledge or understanding of the facts. Like the public, they have bought into the milk-processing industry's ad campaign, which portrays milk right along with motherhood, apple pie, and the American way.

This is exactly the message the milk-processing industry wants to convey to consumers because it sells more milk and dairy products, plain and simple. Is there a conspiracy by dairy industry middlemen, executives, and CEOs to sabotage our health and promote disease? Of course not. By and large, these people, just like the movie stars and the sports figures who endorse milk, are uninformed and blindly believe in their product. To them, the Got Milk and Milk Mustache advertising campaigns simply represent a logical corporate tactic to increase sales and maximize profits of a supposedly nutritious and healthful product.

As was the case with saturated fats, whether people should consume dairy products is divisive within the scientific community because the human experimental and epidemiological evidence is not necessarily conclusive and still can be interpreted in a variety of ways. Does milk prevent disease or does milk promote disease— or is the answer somewhere in between?

In an ideal world, this question could be decisively answered by well-controlled human experimental studies conducted during entire lifetimes. Unfortunately, these hypothetical lifelong experiments in real people will never be carried out because they would be impossible to control, incredibly expensive, and unethical. In lieu of these studies, conventional nutrition researchers are left with four scientific procedures to unravel the milk-drinking dilemma: (1) epidemiological studies, (2) animal studies, (3) tissue studies, and (4) short-term human experiments.

Unfortunately, traditional nutrition researchers are unaware of or don't appreciate the most powerful research tool in all of biology. This concept could point them in the right direction when it comes to deciphering all of the conflicting information about dairy products and human health: the evolutionary template. Anybody who doesn't use it might just as well do calculations with a pencil and paper, rather than with a computer. When the evolutionary template is combined with the four procedures scientists use to establish causality between diet and disease, we can make sense of all of the contradictory data and be sure of arriving at the correct answer.

Evolutionary Clues

George Santayana's famous quote has influenced my thinking about life, as well as diet, for decades: "Those who cannot remember the past are condemned to repeat it."

I am not the first scientist to recognize that milk and dairy consumption may have adverse effects on our health. One of the most vocal opponents to milk drinking was a physician, Frank Oski, M.D. (1932–1996), who was the department chairman of pediatrics at Johns Hopkins University from 1985 until 1996. He was a member of the National Academy of Sciences and the author or coauthor of three hundred academic papers and twenty books. A book he wrote in 1977, *Don't Drink Your Milk*, was decades ahead of its time. Here is an excerpt:

> The fact is: the drinking of cow milk has been linked to iron-deficiency anemia in infants and children; it has been named as the cause of cramps and diarrhea in much of the world's population, and the cause of multiple forms of allergy as well; and the possibility has been raised that it may play a central role in the origins of atherosclerosis and heart attacks. . . . In no mammalian species, except for the human (and the domestic cat), is milk consumption continued after the weaning period [the period of breast-feeding]. Calves thrive on cow milk. Cow milk is for calves.

When you apply the evolutionary template to milk drinking, it becomes absolutely clear that cow's milk was never intended to nourish another species—us—throughout our entire adult lives. It was specifically designed by natural selection to encourage rapid growth, support immune function, and prevent disease in young suckling animals. Newborn calves, like most mammals, are nearly helpless for the first few hours after birth. They are unable to stand up, much less sprint away from potential predators. For the first few days and weeks after birth, they can't forage for food and are almost entirely dependent on their mothers' milk for nourishment.

Milk is designed to make young animals grow rapidly and to prime their immune systems and prevent disease by allowing hormones and other substances in their mothers' milk to enter their bloodstream. This is a brilliant evolutionary strategy to encourage survival for young suckling animals at the beginning of their lives, but it is a formula for disaster when adult humans consume a food intended only for the young of another species.

One of the telltale signs that there may be something wrong with milk drinking is that about 65 percent of all people on the planet can't do it without experiencing gas, bloating, and digestive distress. Maybe we should be listening to our bodies.

Milk is a mixture of carbohydrate, protein, and fat. Most of the carbohydrates in milk occur in the form of a sugar called lactose, which in turn is made up of two simple sugars: glucose and galactose. When we consume milk, ice cream, and other dairy products rich in lactose, it must first be broken down into these two simple sugars by an enzyme in our guts called lactase. About 65 percent of the world's people haven't inherited the genes to make lactase and are therefore lactose intolerant. The notable exceptions to this rule are people from Northern Europe and their descendants—because they maintain high gut lactase activity as adults, they can metabolize lactose into its two simple sugars and don't experience gastrointestinal upset after drinking milk. In the following graph, you can see that the percentage of people with Northern European ancestry who can digest lactose without discomfort is much higher than almost all of the world's other people.

The evolutionary explanation for the information in this illustration is simple. Most people on the planet can't drink milk without gastrointestinal upset because their genes haven't had enough time to adapt to this newcomer food. Milk is foreign fare that

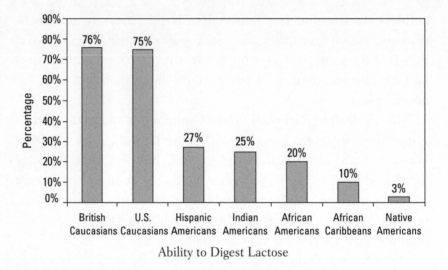

Ability to Digest Lactose

their bodies reject, as should we all, whether we can digest lactose or not. The lactose evidence is like a canary in a coal mine and hints at even greater health problems with milk and dairy consumption.

Dairy: A Nutritional Lightweight

Based on the dairy ad campaigns, cow's milk appears to be nothing less than an extraordinary food to perk up our health and avoid illness. This milky white liquid served cold is touted as "good for everybody" and high in nine nutrients, including calcium and vitamin D.

If the truth be known, milk is a lousy source of vitamin D, as well as of the top thirteen nutrients most lacking in the U.S. diet, as shown in the following table. Let's take a look at the facts.

In a paper published in the *American Journal of Clinical Nutrition*, my research group and I pointed out how dairy products were nutritional lightweights when compared to lean meats, seafood, fresh fruits, and vegetables. Based on the thirteen vitamins and minerals most lacking in the U.S. diet, our analysis showed that whole milk ended up near the bottom of the stack for all food groups.

Nutrient	% of the U.S. Population Not Meeting 100% of the Daily Recommended Requirement
Zinc	73.3%
Calcium	65.1%
Magnesium	61.6%
Vitamin A	56.2%
Vitamin B6	53.6%
Iron	39.1%
Vitamin C	37.5%
Folate	33.2%
Vitamin B1	30.2%
Vitamin B2	30.0%
Vitamin B3	25.9%
Protein	20.5%
Vitamin B12	17.2%

The highest sources of these thirteen nutrients are:

1. Fresh vegetables
2. Seafood
3. Lean meats
4. Fresh fruits
5. Whole milk
6. Whole grains
7. Nuts and seeds

To suggest that milk is a good source of vitamin D is a total stretch of the facts. In the last year, the official Institute of Medicine's recommended intake for vitamin D has increased from 400 IU to 600 IU per day for most people. Although this advice represents a substantial increase, it still falls far short of human experimental evidence showing that at least 2,000 IU per day is required to keep blood levels of vitamin D at the ideal concentration of 30 ng/ml.

An 8-ounce glass of raw milk (280 calories) straight from the cow, without fortification, gives you a paltry 3.6 IU of vitamin D. At this rate, you'd have to drink 167 8-ounce glasses of milk just to achieve the 600 IU daily recommendation. Because most of the milk we drink is fortified with vitamin D, an 8-ounce glass typically yields 100 IU of this nutrient. Even with fortification, you would have to drink six 8-ounce glasses (1,680 calories or around 75 percent of your daily caloric intake) of milk to meet the daily requirement for vitamin D. If you wanted to reach the 2,000 IU level as suggested by the world's best vitamin D researchers, you would have to drink twenty 8-ounce glasses of fortified milk, amounting to 5,600 calories. No one in his or her right mind would drink twenty glasses of milk a day, even if it was possible.

As you can see from these simple calculations, whether fortified or raw, milk is a very poor source of vitamin D. The best way to get your vitamin D is not by drinking milk, but rather by getting a little daily sun exposure as nature intended.

Milk, Ulcers, and Heart Disease

One of the more remarkable tales in recent medical history involves peptic ulcers. This is a chronic condition in which the linings of the stomach or the small intestine are eroded away, causing painful internal wounds. Complications include bleeding and perforation of the gastrointestinal tract, which are potentially life threatening.

For the better half of my adult life, peptic ulcers were routinely attributed to excessive stomach acid production caused mainly by stress, spicy foods, or too much gum chewing. Even as recently as the mid 1980s, ulcer patients were advised to take antacids, make lifestyle changes to reduce stress, cut back on spicy foods, and stop chewing gum. Yet this advice didn't do much to alleviate symptoms or cure the problem.

One of the more unusual ideas that surfaced to treat peptic ulcers came from an early twentieth-century doctor, Betram Sippy, M.D. Dr. Sippy authored an influential paper that appeared in the *Journal of the American Medical Association* in 1915 suggesting that peptic ulcers could be effectively treated by feeding patients milk and cream on a regular basis throughout the day. The doctor's advice became known as the Sippy Diet and was employed widely across the United States to care for patients with ulcers, even as recently as twenty-five to thirty years ago.

One of the downsides to the Sippy Diet, first recognized by Dr. Hartroft in 1960, was that it noticeably increased fatal heart attacks in ulcer patients. In Dr. Hartroft's study, three groups were examined at autopsy: (1) subjects with peptic ulcers who followed the Sippy Diet, (2) subjects with peptic ulcers who didn't follow the Sippy Diet, and (3) subjects without peptic ulcers. The fatal heart attack rate was similar between subjects without peptic ulcers and those with peptic ulcers who hadn't been on the Sippy Diet; however, the fatal heart attack rate in ulcer patients who had adhered to the Sippy Diet was a staggering 42 percent. *Close to half of all ulcer patients following the Sippy Diet had died of heart attacks!* Thank goodness for us all that the medical community no longer recommends the Sippy Diet.

The reason that physicians no longer recommend the Sippy Diet or any other dietary regime for the treatment of ulcers is one of the most unlikely tales in modern medicine. For almost a hundred years, peptic ulcers were looked on as a disease of excessive stomach acid production caused by stress, spicy food—whatever. No one considered that this condition might be caused by an infectious organism until the publication of two revolutionary papers in 1983 and 1984 by two Australian scientists, Barry Marshall and Robin Warren, showing that 70 to 90 percent of peptic ulcers resulted from infection by the bacterium *Helicobacter pylori*. At first, these innovative publications were generally dismissed and discredited by the medical community. Yet it didn't take long for practicing physicians to realize that ulcers could be effectively cured simply by giving their patients a good dose of antibiotics.

Unfortunately, it took about a decade for these brilliant scientists' ideas to be accepted worldwide. Now, because of their groundbreaking insights, antibiotics are routinely used to successfully treat and cure almost all peptic ulcer cases. In 2005, Drs. Marshall and Warren were awarded the Nobel Prize in medicine for their discoveries.

The information about Sippy Diets and the risk of heart attacks has been buried in the scientific literature for nearly fifty years and is virtually lost to contemporary scientists. I would no longer necessarily hang my hat on fifty-year-old studies than I would drink a cup of milk, but the knowledge, wisdom, and insight of our parents', grandparents', and great-grandparents' generations shouldn't be swept under the rug. Is it possible that they were on to something?

Dairy and Heart Disease: Contemporary Studies

The data from the early 1960s studies on milk and heart attacks bears further scrutiny. As we move forward from the past, numerous studies support the view that milk and dairy products may not be heart healthy and good for everybody. A 1993 epidemiological study involving forty countries worldwide demonstrated that milk and its components—calcium, protein, and fat—had the highest relationship with cardiovascular death rates for any food or nutrient examined. Similar results implicating milk consumption as a cause for high mortality from heart disease were reported by Drs. Renaud and De Lorgeril in 1989, by Dr. Appleby in 1999, by Dr. Segall in 2002, and by Drs. Moss and Freed in 2003.

Milk isn't simply a creamy white liquid that is good for everybody but rather is a complex mixture of many substances suspected of causing heart disease, including its high calcium content, saturated fats, lactose, and certain proteins. Because milk contains so many compounds that could potentially promote heart disease, it is difficult or impossible for epidemiological studies to sort out all of the facts. Let's take a closer look at some specific elements in milk that may promote heart disease.

Most people know that milk and dairy products are one of our best sources of calcium. The dairy-manufacturing industry has pounded this message into our brains for decades—so much so, that many women fear they will develop osteoporosis if they don't consume dairy foods. Until recently, the prevailing knowledge was that if a little calcium was good for us, then more certainly must be even better. Not necessarily so.

In 2002, I wrote a scientific paper covering this topic, and my analysis showed that modern-day Paleo diets provide us with only about 70 percent of the daily recommended calcium intake, no matter what we eat. Given this evolutionary clue, it is not surprising to find that the supra normal intake of calcium that can be achieved by milk and dairy consumption may cause unexpected health problems.

A 2010 meta analysis published in the *British Journal of Medicine* by Dr. Bolland from the University of Auckland confirmed the health hazards of too much calcium. His comprehensive analysis involving twenty-six separate studies and more than twenty-thousand participants revealed that calcium supplementation significantly increased the risk for heart attacks and sudden death. High blood levels of calcium from either supplementation or from excessive milk consumption are likely involved in atherosclerosis—the artery-clogging process—because too much calcium promotes the formation and fragility of the plaque that blocks our arteries.

High dietary calcium also tends to cause imbalances in magnesium, and this mineral is generally protective against heart disease for many reasons. In 1974, Dr. Varo pointed out in one study that high dietary calcium-to-magnesium ratios were a better predictor of heart disease than was high calcium intake alone. The bottom line is that if you get too much calcium and not enough magnesium in your diet, it put you at an increased risk for heart disease. Because milk's calcium-to-magnesium ratio is quite high (about 12:1), the inclusion of dairy products in our diets can easily raise the overall calcium-to-magnesium ratio to about 5:1, thereby reducing cellular magnesium stores and promoting heart disease. Our studies of hunter-gatherers confirm that the dietary calcium-to-magnesium ratio was much lower—close to 2:1.

Supplementation studies of magnesium show that it reduces heart disease risk via multiple mechanisms. It improves our blood lipid profiles, prevents heartbeat irregularities called arrhythmias, improves insulin metabolism, and lowers markers of inflammation. When you consume dairy products, you effectively negate each of these therapeutic effects of magnesium, either fully or in part.

Let's consider just a few other nutritional features in milk that further promote heart disease. In the 1950s and the early 1960s, when nutritional researchers were just beginning to understand how atherosclerosis and heart attacks developed, it was assumed to be a simple plumbing problem. Eat too much saturated fat and cholesterol, and your total blood cholesterol levels skyrocketed, clogging your arteries and thereby predisposing you to a heart attack or a stroke. Unfortunately, these simplistic views did not stand up well to the test of time, as hundreds of studies beginning in the 1990s showed that inflammation and immune reactions were just as important as or more important in the artery-clogging process than the consumption of either saturated fat or cholesterol.

What elements in the diet may be responsible for causing the chronic low-level inflammation that is now known to underlie not only heart disease, but also cancer and autoimmune diseases? The evolutionary template again brings us back to foods we never consumed in our ancestral past. Is there any possibility that these recent foods, such as milk and dairy, grains, and legumes, may cause chronic low-level inflammation and promote immune responses that lead to heart disease?

Milk is an amalgamation of nutrients, proteins, and hormones that have only recently been discovered and appreciated. It certainly is not the pure white liquid, high in calcium, vitamin D, and other vitamins and minerals, portrayed by milk manufacturers and their lobbyists. Milk is essentially nothing more than filtered cow's blood. It contains almost all of the hormones, immunological factors, and body-altering proteins that are found in bovine blood.

Let's not get too alarmed at this information; most of these compounds in milk have very short half-lives and are spontaneously degraded within minutes or hours after the manufacture of modern dairy foods, so they should not enter our bloodstream. Furthermore, a healthy human gut lining rarely allows intact large proteins such as those found in milk hormones to bypass its protective barrier.

So why should we worry? Are there proteins or hormones in cow's milk that bypass the gut barrier and eventually get into our bloodstream to wreak havoc with our immune systems and promote atherosclerosis?

Although no smoking gun has yet been found that implicates milk in the pro-inflammatory and immune processes that underlie atherosclerosis, a suspect substance is well known. One of the more important cow's milk proteins that may penetrate the gut barrier and get into our bloodstream is an enzyme in milk called *xanthine oxidase*. Numerous human studies show that our immune systems recognize this bovine enzyme as a foreign protein and produce antibodies to fight off this perceived foreign invader. Because we have a molecular duplicate of bovine xanthine oxidase located in the endothelial cells lining our arteries, it may also become a simultaneous target for the immune system's attack and may promote atherosclerosis. Even though we don't know for sure whether milk is involved in this process, there are no known health risks to not drinking milk, whereas the health benefits from abstaining might be enormous.

Milk, Insulin Resistance, and the Metabolic Syndrome

The glycemic index gauges how much a food raises our blood glucose concentrations. Processed foods such as white bread, candies, breakfast cereals, cookies, and potatoes have high glycemic indices because they cause rapid and marked increases in our blood glucose levels. These foods tend to promote the metabolic syndrome, a condition that includes diseases of insulin resistance such as type 2 diabetes, hypertension, cardiovascular disease, obesity, gout, and detrimental blood chemistry profiles. Natural foods such as lean meats, fish, eggs, fresh fruits, and nonstarchy veggies typically have moderate to low glycemic indices and are not associated with the metabolic syndrome.

Normally, when our blood-sugar levels soar after we consume high-glycemic-index carbohydrates, our blood insulin concentrations also rise. Shortly after the glycemic index was developed in the early 1980s, it was discovered that milk, yogurt, and most dairy foods had low glycemic responses. Presumably, these foods should be healthy and should help prevent the metabolic syndrome. About *five to ten* years ago, however, experiments from our laboratory and others unexpectedly revealed that low-glycemic dairy foods paradoxically caused huge rises in blood insulin levels. The table below shows that despite their low glycemic indices, dairy foods maintain high insulin responses similar to white bread.

This information posed a challenge to nutritional scientists. It was unclear whether milk's insulin-stimulating effect but low glycemic response was healthful or harmful. To date, only one human study conducted by Dr. Hoppe in 2005 has addressed this question; it put twenty-four eight-year-old boys on either a high-milk or a high-meat diet for seven days. The high-milk diet worsened the boys' insulin response almost 100 percent, and the entire group became insulin resistant in only a week's time. In contrast, the high–meat eating group's insulin levels did not change, and the boys' overall insulin metabolism remained healthy.

The results of this experiment are alarming, particularly if future studies also demonstrate this effect in teenagers and adults. As insulin resistance is the fundamental metabolic defect underlying the metabolic syndrome, it would not be surprising to discover that drinking milk may cause other diseases of insulin resistance.

Food	Glycemic Index	Insulin Index
White bread	70	100
Skim milk	32	90
Whole milk	27	90
Reduced-fat yogurt	27	115
Nonfat yogurt	24	115
Fermented milk (3% fat)	11	90

Milk and Acne

Until 2002, the official party line of the mainstream dermatology community was that diet had nothing to do with acne. This viewpoint was expressed time and again in all of the major dermatology textbooks and became the doctrine taught to new dermatologists. If you didn't know any better, you might think that this perspective was based on hundreds or even thousands of carefully controlled scientific studies.

When I first started to examine the link between diet and acne more than ten years ago, this is exactly what I had expected. How wrong I was! As it turned out, the dogma that diet didn't cause acne was based solely on two poorly conceived experiments conducted in 1969 and 1971. In a series of papers from 2002 to 2006, I pointed out this flawed assumption to the dermatology community.

My research rekindled the entire diet/acne debate, but more important, we showed that acne was completely absent in two non-Westernized populations who didn't drink milk or eat processed foods. We suspected that both milk and foods with high glycemic indices caused blood insulin levels to rise steeply and remain high all day long. In turn, elevated insulin levels set off a hormonal cascade that triggered the known cellular events that caused acne. My hypothesis that milk in part caused acne was verified by a series of recent epidemiological studies from scientists at the Harvard School of Public Health. Even more convincing was an experimental study carried out by Dr. Neil Mann in Australia showing that low-glycemic-index, high-protein diets improved acne symptoms.

I'm including in this book some of the many unsolicited e-mails I have received from patients whose acne symptoms were completely cured by the Paleo Diet.

Healing Adult Acne: Ray's Story

I took antibiotics for twenty-five years to fight my acne. I also tried many changes to my diet but never saw results until

I read and tried *The Paleo Diet.* For the last six weeks, I ate an almost entirely Paleo diet. In addition to my newfound energy, I am off my medication for the first time. I have found that if I eat any dairy (milk, cream, ice cream, or milk chocolate), it is only a matter of hours until I get pimples. It only took three or four days for me to realize that I didn't need my medicine. It took another two weeks for me to start believing that it really worked.

I have not determined what it is exactly that causes the acne—milk, hormones, or the high glycemic load—but I know that if I eat Paleo, I don't get acne. I will probably experiment to see if things like muffins and other grain-based foods have the same effect. But then again, I might not, because I don't see any reason to eat those foods. Ice cream is another matter. I can stay off it most of the time, but I don't think I am willing to say I won't ever eat it again!

As it has been fewer than ten years since my study in the *Archives of Dermatology* revived the diet/acne debate, scientists worldwide have not completely worked out how milk drinking promotes acne. Some researchers share our view that milk's exaggerated insulin response sets off a hormonal cascade that causes acne. Others suggest that hormones found in cow's milk may be responsible, whereas some scientists believe that both mechanisms are involved.

Milk Is Filtered Cow's Blood

Milk may be advertised as a squeaky-clean white liquid, high in vitamin D and calcium, but if the truth be known, it is filtered cow's blood and as such contains almost all of the hormones and the bioactive peptides (protein building blocks) found in blood itself. Take a look at the following lists. You can see the incredible profusion of biologically active substances found in milk, even in these incomplete lists.

Growth Hormones Found in Milk

- Insulin
- Insulin-like growth factor 1 (IGF-1)
- Insulin-like growth factor 2 (IGF-2)
- Insulin-like growth factor binding proteins, 1 to 6 (IGFBP-1, 2, 3, 4, 5, 6)
- Betacellulin (BTC)
- Growth hormone (GH)
- Growth hormone releasing factor (GHRF)
- Transforming growth factor alpha (TGF α)
- Transforming growth factor beta 1 (TGF-β1)
- Transforming growth factor beta 2 (TGF-β2)
- Platelet-derived growth factor (PDGF)

Steroid Hormones Found in Milk

- Estrogens (estrone, estradiol-17β, estriol, and estrone sulfate)
- Progesterone
- 20 α-dihydropregnenolone
- 5α androstanedione
- 5 α pregnanedione
- 20α- and 20β-dihydroprogesterone
- 5α-pregnan-3β-ol-20-one
- 5α-androstene-3β17β-diol
- 5α-androstan-3β-ol-17-one
- Androstenedione
- Testosterone
- DHEA acyl ester

Bioactive Proteins and Peptides Found in Milk

- Relaxin
- Thyrotropin-releasing hormone (TRH)
- Luteinizing hormone-releasing hormone (LHRH)
- Somatostatin (SIH)
- Gastrin-releasing peptide (GRP)
- Calcitonin
- Adrenocorticotropic hormone (ACTH)

- Prolactin
- Thyroid-stimulating hormone (TSH)
- Lysozyme
- Lactoperoxidase
- Lactoferrin
- Transferrin
- Immunoglobulins (IgA, IgM, IgG)
- Proteose-peptone
- Glycomacropeptide
- Plasmin
- α Casein
- β Casein
- κ Casein
- α Lactoglobulin
- β Lactoglobulin
- Bovine serum albumen (BSA)
- Gastric inhibitory polypeptide (GIP)
- Glucagon-like peptide-1 (GLP-1)
- Antitrypsin, plasminogen activator inhibitor-1
- α(2) antiplasmin
- Butyrophilin
- Xanthine oxidase
- Mucin-1
- Mucin-15
- Adipohilin
- Fatty acid binding protein
- CD36
- Periodic acid Schiff 6/7

Bioactive Peptides Formed in the Human Gut from Milk Proteins

- Casomorphins
- α Lactorphin
- β Lactorphin
- Lactoferroxins
- Casoxins

- Casokinins
- Casoplatelins
- Immunopeptides
- Phosphopeptides

The trick for any of these elements to harm our health and well-being is for them to end up fully intact and present in our bloodstream. To accomplish this feat, these hormones, proteins, and peptides must first survive pasteurization (the quick heating of milk to destroy micro-organisms), homogenization, and other processing procedures applied to dairy foods. Next, they must survive the digestion process and resist breakdown by our gut enzymes. Finally, they must cross the intestinal barrier, which normally blocks the entry of whole proteins, hormones, and large peptides into our bloodstream. It now seems quite probable that cow hormones in milk do indeed enter our bloodstream, particularly if we have a leaky gut—more about that later.

For a young suckling calf, it is a good thing for its mother's hormones, peptides, and immune factors to cross the intestinal barrier. This process ensures that the calf will get a healthy start in life, grow rapidly, and develop resistance to disease. To ensure that mother's hormones and peptides are not degraded in the calf's gut by various enzymes, milk contains substances called protease inhibitors that prevent this breakdown. The downside of milk's protease inhibitors is that they also prevent our own gut enzymes from destroying cow hormones and peptides.

Many hormones and bioactive peptides in milk do survive pasteurization and food processing. They also resist enzymatic breakdown in our guts because compounds in milk protect them. Ultimately, in order to adversely affect our health, these substances must bypass the gut barrier and enter our bloodstream.

It is apparent that this final hurdle is routinely overcome because so many people have allergies and immune reactions to milk. When intact hormones, proteins, or peptides cross the intestinal barrier, the immune system takes immediate steps to destroy any particle that is perceived as a foreign invader. Part of this process is to form antibodies against milk proteins, which later are involved in allergic and autoimmune reactions. Many of the proteins and the substances I have listed show up as specific milk allergens—meaning that they had to cross the gut barrier and interact with the immune system.

Unsafe Milk Hormones

Of all of the milk hormones and the bioactive peptides listed previously, very few have been examined directly in human experiments. Nonetheless, evidence from animal, tissue, and epidemiological studies suggest that the consumption of milk and cow hormones at best may be unwise and at worst may be responsible for a number of life-threatening diseases. Let's take a look at the most problematic of these hormones.

Bovine Insulin

The regular, everyday milk you buy at the supermarket is loaded with bovine insulin. This cow hormone not only survives your gut's digestive enzymes, it seems to frequently cross the gut barrier and make its way into the bloodstream, as revealed by telltale signs from our immune systems. Because the structure of bovine insulin varies from the human form, if it enters circulation, it is immediately recognized as a foreign particle and flagged by the immune system. The large number of children who display immune system flags (antibodies) to bovine insulin means that it has indeed crossed the gut barrier intact and has caused an immune reaction. Although the mechanism is not entirely clear, the presence of bovine insulin antibodies in our bloodstream is associated with a greatly increased risk for type 1 diabetes.

Type 1 diabetes is an autoimmune disease in which the immune system destroys beta cells in the pancreas so that it can no longer make insulin. Type 1 diabetic patients must take insulin injections for the remainder of their lives. This devastating disease most frequently strikes children before their teen years. Epidemiological studies have time and again identified cow's milk as a major risk factor for the disease, particularly if children are exposed to milk or milk-containing formula before the age of three. The bottom line: milk is a potentially lethal toxin for infants and young children.

Insulin-like Growth Factor 1

Another hormone found in milk that may have disastrous effects on our health and well-being is insulin-like growth factor 1 (IGF-1). As implied from its name, this hormone encourages growth. Unfortunately, it promotes growth not only in healthy tissues and organs but also in cancerous growths. Like all milk hormones, IGF-1 is a large protein molecule that normally should not breach the gut barrier and get into our bloodstream. Nevertheless, recent meta analyses of fifteen epidemiological studies and eight human dietary interventions by Dr. Qin have shown without a doubt that milk drinking robustly elevates IGF-1 in our bloodstream. This effect may result directly from the additional ingested bovine IGF-1 that crosses our gut barriers or via indirect mechanisms. Milk drinking causes our blood insulin levels to rise sharply, and whenever blood insulin concentrations increase, a series of connected hormonal events simultaneously cause IGF-1 to increase. During a twenty-four-hour period, blood insulin concentrations are a good marker for IGF-1 concentrations. When one increases, so does the other.

Whether IGF-1 in our blood is increased either directly from ingested bovine IGF-1 or indirectly from milk's insulin-raising effects doesn't really matter. The end result is the same—milk raises our total blood levels of IGF-1. This particular consequence of milk drinking is especially ominous because it encourages the growth of many types of cancer. Numerous worldwide meta analyses during the last forty years show that high blood levels of IGF-1 strongly increase the risk for prostate and breast cancer. If this outcome doesn't alarm you, additional meta analyses will: these comprehensive studies show that milk drinking also increases the risk for ovarian cancer in women.

If you or any close relatives have a history of cancer, one of the best lifestyle changes you can make to reduce your risk of developing these life-threatening diseases is to wipe your upper lip clean of the milk mustache and get milk and dairy completely out of your life.

Estrogen

By now, you can see that milk isn't simply an innocuous high-calcium food that builds strong bones, but rather is a concoction of body-altering hormones, enzymes, and proactive peptides whose wide-ranging effects promote cardiovascular disease, insulin resistance, cancers, allergies, and autoimmune diseases. Another dangerous cancer-promoting hormone in milk is the female hormone estrogen. Cow's milk is chock full of it. It is present in bovine milk in a variety of forms, including estrone, estradiol-17β, estriol, estrone sulfate, and progesterone.

Modern dairy farmers maximize milk production from their cows. Dairy farmers are in the business to make money, and the more milk they can get from a single cow in a year, the more money they make. Female cows, like all mammals, produce milk only in the latter half of pregnancy and during the suckling period. The trick for modern dairy farmers is to get cows to make large amounts of milk during the early months of pregnancy when milk is normally not produced. Dairy farmers achieve this goal by artificially inseminating cows within three months after they have just given birth. In effect, these unfortunate cows become pregnant once again while they are still nursing the young of their previous birth. This totally contrived interference by humans causes the mother cow to produce milk 305 days out of the year. From an economic perspective, this strategy makes perfect sense—more milk means more money. From a dietary and health perspective, this practice is disastrous for us because it strikingly increases the estrogen content in the milk we drink.

The main form of estrogen in cow's milk is estrone sulfate, which also happens to be the most frequently prescribed hormone replacement therapy for menopausal women. This pharmaceutical form of estrogen has high oral bioactivity—meaning that when you ingest it in pill form, it readily gets into your bloodstream. There is no reason to believe that estrone sulfate from cow's milk acts any differently. So, whether you are a man, a woman, or a child, if you drink milk and eat other dairy products, your blood concentration of female hormones will be higher than if you don't drink milk. This situation is not good.

For women, elevated blood estrogen and its metabolites increase your lifetime risk for developing breast and ovarian cancers. For men, milk's added estrogen may increase your risk for getting prostate and testicular cancers.

Food Allergies and Colic

Here are the eight most common food allergies in the U.S. population. These foods account for 90 percent of all food allergies. Notice that milk tops this list.

1. Milk
2. Eggs
3. Peanuts
4. Tree nuts
5. Fish
6. Shellfish
7. Soy
8. Wheat

Milk is also the most common childhood food allergy, where it afflicts from 2 to 3 percent of children between the ages of one and three. Symptoms include stomach pain, diarrhea, skin rashes, hives, wheezing, infantile colic, and anaphylactic shock, which can be life threatening. By age three, 85 to 90 percent of children grow out of their milk allergy. This change may appear to be a good thing, but the problem is that a childhood milk allergy predisposes children to other food allergies for the rest of their lives.

One study by Dr. Høst alarmingly revealed that 50 percent of all infants and young children who were allergic to milk later developed allergies to a wide variety of other foods before puberty. As was the case with type 1 diabetes, early exposure to milk proteins is the key to whether your child will develop allergies. The crucial period for restricting cow's milk is from birth until at least age two or three.

One of the more interesting disorders related to milk allergy is infantile colic. When a healthy baby cries, screams, or fusses intensely for more than three hours a day, three days a week, it probably has colic. Continual infant crying is considerably more than just a parental annoyance. Crying and its associated exhaustion to parents and infants may lead to serious problems, including stress to your marriage, breast-feeding failure, and shaken baby syndrome, which frequently results in death.

Twenty-five to thirty years ago, it was still possible to purchase infant formula that was manufactured with cow's milk proteins. Not so today, as it is almost universally recognized by pediatricians that infants should never consume milk or dairy products until at least age one or beyond. A series of human infant experiments carried out in the 1980s revealed that whey proteins in milk were largely responsible for colic. A powerful experiment by Drs. Lothe and Lindberg demonstrated that colic symptoms disappeared in 89 percent of all infants when they were given a cow's milk–free diet.

You may ask why this information is relevant in 2011 when cow's milk–based formula is no longer commercially available, and no pediatrician in his/her right mind would recommend giving cow's milk to your infant. An often forgotten but important offshoot of these 1980s double-blind crossover experiments was that they were also repeated in milk-drinking mothers who breast-fed their infants. Not surprisingly, infants whose moms drank milk became colicky, which indicated that certain elements in cow's milk may have caused an immunological response in the nursing mothers that was transferred to their milk, which in turn was transmitted to their babies, making them cry. Any food that causes such distress in infants should be a warning to us all. It may be possible that our babies are more in tune with their bodies than we are.

Asthma and Excessive Mucus Production

Too much milk consumption has long been associated with increased mucus production in the respiratory tract and the incidence of asthma. A few years back, I went to a high school cross-country meet and watched the young athletes cross the finish line. I noticed a few runners who were literally foaming at their mouths because they had so much mucus being produced from their respiratory system. I wondered whether milk drinking had anything to do with it, but at the time, the science hadn't yet caught up with my observation and those of others. An intriguing 2010 hypothesis by Drs. Bartley and McGlashan from New Zealand may have found the answer.

In my list of all of the hormones and bioactive substances found in milk, you will notice under the category "Bioactive Peptides Formed in the Human Gut from Milk Proteins" (see page 92) a substance called casomorphins. These compounds are produced in our guts from the breakdown of the milk protein casein. One of these casomorphins, beta-casomorphin-7, directly stimulates mucus production from specific glands located in the gut. If the gut becomes leaky, which it invariably does on a typical Western diet, beta-casomorhin-7 can enter our bloodstream and travel to our chests, where it stimulates mucus production from MUC5AC glands located in our lungs and respiratory tracts. A final piece of this puzzle is that beta-casomorphin-7 is much more likely to trigger mucous production if the lungs and the respiratory tract are inflamed by asthma. Many people's exercise-induced asthma symptoms disappear on the Paleo Diet.

Treating Asthma: Shannon's Story

I'm a trainer, and I work with a very overweight woman, Jenny, who recently started my boot camp. She weighs 260 pounds at present. Until recently, she also suffered from exercise-induced asthma. For the first week of boot camp, she could not get through a class without her inhaler. Although I admired her dedication, it was painful and a bit scary to watch.

Then I put her on the Paleo Diet. This week, after doing this for a little less than two weeks, she no longer needs her inhaler. Miraculous!

Jenny's also doing great on the diet—she's not hungry at all, so I know the weight will be coming off soon as well.

Parkinson's Disease

Parkinson's disease is a nervous system disorder that primarily affects areas of the brain that control movement. Disease symptoms include tremors, stiffness, and difficulty moving, and its two most famous victims are Muhammad Ali and Michael J. Fox. Although the cause of Parkinson's disease isn't known, both genetic and environmental elements seem to be involved. Like autoimmune diseases, it appears that environmental factors may be the most important triggers of this debilitating illness.

When we talk about environmental origins of any chronic disease with an unknown cause, diet is at the top of our list. The first items that we should examine are the foods that were not part of our ancestral human diet. This leads us once again to milk and dairy products.

A comprehensive 2007 meta analysis by researchers at the Harvard School of Public Health has identified a high intake of dairy foods as a prominent risk factor for Parkinson's disease. Men who consumed the highest quantities of dairy products had an 80 percent greater risk of developing the disease than did men who ate the lowest amounts. These results are consistent with a study of Japanese men showing that people who consumed more than 16 ounces of milk daily had a 130 percent greater risk of Parkinson's disease than non–milk drinkers. No one really knows how and why milk drinking increases the risk for this illness, but autoimmune mechanisms seem likely, particularly those directed at insulin. When you adopt the Paleo Diet, you will reduce your risk for developing Parkinson's disease and other conditions with autoimmune components because this lifetime nutritional plan eliminates milk and all other foods that are suspected of causing autoimmune diseases.

Milk and Cataracts

Senile cataracts are cloudy opacities that form in the lenses of the eyes as people age and can ultimately cause blindness. The bad news is that if you live long enough, you will probably develop cataracts. The good news is that you can probably forestall their appearance until very late in life by following the Paleo Diet. For people between fifty-two and sixty-two years of age, 42 percent develop cataracts. This percentage increases to 60 percent between ages sixty-five and seventy-five and rises further to 91 percent for people between seventy-five and eighty-five years of age. In the United States and other Westernized countries, cataracts are treated by surgical removal, whereas left untreated they are the leading cause of blindness in older adults worldwide.

Milk drinking has a lot to do with cataract formation. Scientists routinely produce cataracts in rats, pigs, and guinea pigs even before they reach old age simply by feeding them high-milk and -lactose diets. As you recall, the main sugar in milk is lactose, which is broken down into its two constituent sugars, glucose and galactose, by the gut enzyme lactase. Numerous epidemiological studies show that lactose and galactose are involved in premature cataract formation. Due to the way cataracts form, we can probably never prevent them completely, but chances are good that if you adopt a dairy-free diet, you can live most of your life, even into old age, without developing cataracts.

Milk Impairs Iron and Zinc Absorption

As you saw earlier in the chapter in the list of the top thirteen missing nutrients in our diets, zinc is number one: more than 73 percent of all people in the United States don't get enough of this essential mineral. Iron is number six, and about 40 percent of the population are deficient in this nutrient. Milk and dairy products are lousy sources of both iron and zinc, and the high concentration of calcium in cow's milk strongly interferes with the absorption of both iron and zinc. If you were to add a slice of melted cheese to your burger, it would severely reduce the amount of iron and zinc you could absorb from the burger.

Both zinc and iron are crucial minerals for our health and well-being. Low iron stores are the most frequent cause of anemia, and in children and teens, low iron can impair mental functioning. Pregnant women with iron deficiency are at greater risk for delivering pre-term babies, and low iron may adversely affect athletic performance and work ability. The list of health problems associated with zinc deficiency includes low sperm counts, reduced libido, reduced immune function, increased susceptibility to upper respiratory infections, acne, white spots on fingernails, rough skin, lack of sexual development, stretch marks, macular degeneration, reduced collagen, and increased wrinkling. When you follow the Paleo Diet, you will be eating meat at almost every meal, and meat is a primary source of the most highly absorbable forms of both zinc and iron.

Milk, Dairy, and Bone Health

One of the biggest selling points the milk manufacturers would like us to believe is that by drinking lots of milk, we can reduce our risk of osteoporosis and future hip fractures. The foremost danger associated with osteoporosis is hip fracture in the elderly. Between 18 and 33 percent of all elderly people who suffer hip fractures die within a year after breaking their hips—not a pretty statistic. Although most people, including dairy lobbyists, believe that a low intake of calcium is a risk factor for hip and other bone fractures, the data says that's not the case.

A 2007 meta analysis from the Harvard School of Public Health reported that high calcium intake had no therapeutic effect on hip fractures in 170,000 women and 68,000 men. In the same study, a pooled analysis of five human experimental trials showed no benefit of calcium supplementation on nonvertebrae fractures but, rather, showed that increased calcium intake actually increased the risk for hip fracture. A follow-up 2010 meta analysis specifically examining milk consumption and hip fracture risk in 195,000 women and 75,000 men also showed that low milk intakes didn't increase fracture risk, nor did a high intake prevent it.

These studies show that we have been misled by the dairy manufacturers' overhyped advertising and marketing campaigns. It's clear that dairy doesn't prevent bone fractures, and it might contribute to heart disease and cancer. I cannot come up with one single reason to drink milk or eat dairy products.

Paleo Bottom Line

Avoid dairy products.

6

Grains Are Antinutritious

I Don't Miss Grains One Bit!: Bob's Story

Here is my experience with removing virtually all grains and legumes from my diet for the last ninety days. I eat seafood at least twice a week and eat until I'm satisfied a good quantity of lean meats, whole fruits (great in smoothies), and nonstarchy vegetables. In between snacks are a trail mix of walnuts and other assorted nuts (all raw) and chopped dried fruits.

I am a fifty-four-year-old man in good overall health, except for having been on lisinopril for three years for blood pressure of 130/90 (unmedicated). My height is 5'7". Here are my before and after statistics:

Start

    Weight: 178

    BMI: 27.9

Total Cholesterol 182, HDL 48, Ratio Total
Cholesterol/HDL 3.79, LDL 109, Triglycerides 128,
Glucose 92 (fasting)

After 90 days

Weight: 158

BMI: 24.9

Total Cholesterol 180, HDL 60, Ratio Total
Cholesterol/HDL 3.00, LDL 105, Triglycerides 77,
Glucose 93 (not fasting)

My doctor and I were very pleased with the 20 pound
weight loss, reduction in blood pressure (about 10 points),
and significant improvement in HDL and triglycerides after
ninety days. He is reducing the lisinopril dosage, and I should
be off it in a month. I'm also looking forward to continuing
to drop more weight.

This is the first time in my adult life that I have felt in
control of my weight and blood chemistry.

Bob's follow-up

My wife and I are now at the seven-month point in eating
mostly Paleo. (We include some milk and cheese in our
diet but no starches or processed sugars.) I'm down 28
pounds to 150 pounds, with a BMI of 23.5, and am off
blood pressure medication now. She decreased two dress
sizes. Here is my blood chemistry profile:

After 7 months

Weight: 150

BMI: 23.5

Total Cholesterol 157, HDL 47, Ratio Total
Cholesterol/HDL 3.3, LDL 103, Triglycerides "not
detected by test," Glucose 87.

We're very pleased with this eating plan and have
absolutely no problem staying with it.

In the United States, a number of governmental, institutional, and private organizations determine official national nutritional policy. The United States Department of Agriculture's (USDA) MyPyramid, recently renamed MyPlate, is probably the most visible governmental program that attempts to sway our perspective on what is and is not a healthy diet. The MyPyramid/MyPlate guidelines tell us that we must consume foods from *all five* of their self-proclaimed food groups—grains, vegetables, fruits, dairy, and meat/beans. The Pyramid/MyPlate cautions us, *"For good health, eat a variety of foods from each food group every day."*

The USDA suggests that women between the ages of nineteen and thirty should eat at least 6 ounces of grains daily, and half should come from whole grains. For men, this figure is increased to 8 ounces of daily grains. Implicit in these recommendations is the notion that cereal grains represent an essential component of human nutrition. In other words, healthy human diets are difficult or impossible to achieve without cereal grains because they are nutrient-rich foods that we all require.

As a scientist, I can tell you that we should never blindly trust recommendations from the USDA or anyone else without first examining the data. The data speaks without the overtones of either charismatic individuals or rigid governmental organizations.

Grains are not part of the Paleo Diet. In this chapter I'm going to meticulously show you the science underlying why cereal grains are inferior foods, and why they should be avoided. In the decade since the publication of my first book, startling new information has surfaced about wheat consumption and human health. So much so, that the National Institutes of Health, the Food and Drug Administration, and the Centers for Disease Control have now taken an active interest in this newly recognized public health threat.

The USDA's MyPyramid/MyPlate encourages us to replace refined grains—white bread, white flour, white rice, and degermed corn meal—with whole grains because refined grains have been stripped of fiber, vitamins, and minerals. In the following chart, you can see how the refining process reduces the nutrient content of whole wheat.

Percentage of Vitamins and Minerals in Whole-Wheat versus White Flour

	Whole-Wheat Flour	White Flour
Calcium (Ca)	100%	50%
Chromium (Cr)	100%	33%
Copper (Cu)	100%	20%
Iron (Fe) (enriched)	100%	20%
Magnesium (Mg)	100%	18%
Manganese (Mn)	100%	10%
Selenium (Se)	100%	75%
Zinc (Zn)	100%	20%
Potassium (K)	100%	22%
Biotin	100%	20%
Vitamin B6	100%	17%
Vitamin E	100%	2%
Folic acid (enriched since 1998)	100%	25%
Vitamin B3 (enriched)	100%	20%
Vitamin B2 (enriched)	100%	33%
Vitamin B1 (enriched)	100%	18%
Pantothenic acid	100%	50%
Vitamin K	100%	24%

At least on paper, compared to refined grains, it may appear that whole grains are indeed nutrient-rich foods packed with vitamins and minerals. Unfortunately, it just isn't so. What we need to do is to compare whole grains on a calorie-by-calorie basis to other foods such as fresh fruit, veggies, lean meats, and seafood, which are the staples of the Paleo Diet.

In a paper I published in 2005 in the *American Journal of Clinical Nutrition*, I examined the thirteen nutrients most lacking in the U.S. diet and then ranked seven food groups—whole grains, milk, fruits, veggies, seafood, lean meat, and nuts/seeds—for each of these thirteen vitamins and minerals in 100-calorie samples. Food groups were ranked from 7 to 1—where 7 represented the highest-nutrient-density food group for a particular vitamin or mineral and 1 the lowest. We then summed up all of the rank scores to determine the most nutrient-dense food groups. The next table shows the results of our analysis. Fresh veggies were far and away the most nutrient-rich foods, followed by seafood, lean meats, and fruits. If you consider the sum rank scores, whole grains and milk are in fifth and sixth place, respectively. So much for the USDA's suggestion that whole grains are a nutrient-rich food essential for good human nutrition! From a practical perspective, you can see that the inclusion of either refined or whole grains in our diets lowers its overall vitamin and mineral content whenever these foods displace fresh fruit, veggies, lean meat, and seafood.

18 Vegetables Tested: Iceberg lettuce, tomato, onion, carrot, celery, broccoli, green cabbage, cucumber, bell pepper, cauliflower, leaf lettuce, sweet potato, zucchini, mushroom, green onion, radish, summer squash, asparagus

20 Types of Seafood Tested: Shrimp, cod, pollack, catfish, scallop, salmon, flounder, sole, oyster, orange roughy, mackerel, ocean perch, rockfish, whiting, clam, haddock, blue crab, rainbow trout, halibut, lobster

4 Lean Meats Tested: Beef (sirloin tip roast trimmed of visible fat), chicken (breasts without skin and trimmed of visible fat), pork (loin roast trimmed of visible fat), turkey (breasts without skin)

20 Fruits Tested: Banana, apple, watermelon, orange, cantaloupe, grapes, grapefruit, strawberry, peach, pear, nectarine, honeydew melon, plum, avocado, lemon, pineapple, tangerine, sweet cherry, kiwi fruit, lime

8 Whole Grains Tested: Whole wheat, whole corn meal, brown rice, barley, rye, oats, sorghum, millet

10 Nuts and Seeds Tested: Almonds, walnuts, pecans, filberts, Brazil nuts, pistachio nuts, macadamia nuts, coconut, sunflower seeds, pumpkin seeds

Vitamin B12

Food Group	Ranking	Nutrient Amount (µg)
Seafoods	7	7.42
Lean meats	6	0.63
Whole milk	5	0.58

Vitamin B12

Food Group	Ranking	Nutrient Amount (µg)
Vegetables	4	0.00
Fruits	4	0.00
Whole grains	4	0.00
Nuts/seeds	4	0.00

Vitamin B3

Food Group	Ranking	Nutrient Amount (mg)
Lean meats	7	4.73
Seafoods	6	3.19
Vegetables	5	2.73
Whole grains	4	1.12
Fruits	3	0.89
Nuts/seeds	2	0.35
Whole milk	1	0.14

Phosphorus

Food Group	Ranking	Nutrient Amount (mg)
Seafoods	7	219
Vegetables	6	157
Whole milk	5	152
Lean meats	4	151
Whole grains	3	90
Nuts/seeds	2	80
Fruits	1	33

Vitamin B2

Food Group	Ranking	Nutrient Amount (mg)
Vegetables	7	0.33
Whole milk	6	0.26

(continued)

Vitamin B2 (*continued*)

Food Group	Ranking	Nutrient Amount (mg)
Lean meats	5	0.14
Seafoods	4	0.09
Fruits	3	0.09
Whole grains	2	0.05
Nuts/seeds	1	0.04

Vitamin B1

Food Group	Ranking	Nutrient Amount (mg)
Vegetables	7	0.26
Lean meats	6	0.18
Whole grains	5	0.12
Nuts/seeds	4	0.12
Fruits	3	0.11
Seafoods	2	0.08
Whole milk	1	0.06

Folate

Food Group	Ranking	Nutrient Amount (µg)
Vegetables	7	208.3
Fruits	6	25.0
Nuts/seeds	5	11.0
Seafoods	4	10.8
Whole grains	3	10.3
Whole milk	2	8.1
Lean meats	1	3.8

Vitamin C

Food Group	Ranking	Nutrient Amount (mg)
Fruits	7	221.3
Vegetables	6	93.6
Whole milk	5	74.2

Vitamin C

Food Group	Ranking	Nutrient Amount (mg)
Seafoods	4	1.9
Whole grains	3	1.53
Nuts/seeds	2	0.4
Lean meats	1	0.1

Iron

Food Group	Ranking	Nutrient Amount (mg)
Vegetables	7	2.59
Seafoods	6	2.07
Lean meats	5	1.10
Whole grains	4	0.90
Nuts/seeds	3	0.86
Fruits	2	0.69
Whole milk	1	0.08

Vitamin B6

Food Group	Ranking	Nutrient Amount (mg)
Vegetables	7	0.42
Lean meats	6	0.32
Fruits	5	0.20
Seafoods	4	0.19
Whole grains	3	0.09
Nuts/seeds	2	0.08
Whole milk	1	0.07

Vitamin A

Food Group	Ranking	Nutrient Amount (RE)
Vegetables	7	687
Fruits	6	94
Whole milk	5	50

(continued)

Vitamin A (*continued*)

Food Group	Ranking	Nutrient Amount (RE)
Seafoods	4	32
Nuts/seeds	3	2
Whole grains	2	2
Lean meats	1	1

Magnesium

Food Group	Ranking	Nutrient Amount (mg)
Vegetables	7	54.5
Seafoods	6	36.1
Nuts/seeds	5	35.8
Whole grains	4	32.6
Fruits	3	24.6
Whole milk	2	21.9
Lean meats	1	18.0

Calcium

Food Group	Ranking	Nutrient Amount (mg)
Whole milk	7	194.3
Vegetables	6	116.8
Seafoods	5	43.1
Fruits	4	43.0
Nuts/seeds	3	17.5
Whole grains	2	7.6
Lean meats	1	6.1

Zinc

Food Group	Ranking	Nutrient Amount (mg)
Seafoods	7	7.6
Lean meats	6	1.9
Vegetables	5	1.04
Whole grains	4	0.67

Zinc

Food Group	Ranking	Nutrient Amount (mg)
Whole milk	3	0.62
Nuts/seeds	2	0.6
Fruits	1	0.25

Sum Rank Scores	
Vegetables	81
Seafoods	65
Lean meats	50
Fruits	48
Whole grains	44
Whole milk	44
Nuts/seeds	38

How about fiber? Almost everyone, including the USDA, assumes that whole grains are a good source of fiber. Traditional, dyed-in-the-wool nutritionists may ask, "If you eliminate whole grains from your diet, how in the world will you ever get enough fiber?" In the following graph, I depict the average fiber content in a 1,000-calorie serving of three refined cereals, eight whole-grain cereals, twenty fresh fruits, and twenty nonstarchy vegetables. Although

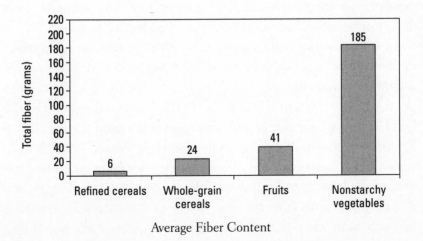

Average Fiber Content

whole grains have four times more fiber than refined grains do, they are lightweights when compared to either fresh fruits or veggies. Furthermore, the insoluble fiber found in every whole grain except oats does not have a blood cholesterol–lowering effect as does the soluble fiber present in fresh fruits and vegetables.

Phytate: One Antinutrient in Grains

Another piece of the whole-grain story that the USDA's MyPyramid/MyPlate doesn't mention is nutrient availability. It may seem as if whole grains are great sources of calcium, magnesium, iron, and zinc. Not true. All whole grains contain an antinutrient called *phytate* or phytic acid, which binds these minerals and makes them unavailable for absorption in our gastrointestinal tracts. Phytate binds these nutrients in a dose-dependent manner, meaning that the more whole grains you eat, the more likely you will become deficient in these minerals.

Just such an effect was verified in rural Iranians who frequently consume about 50 percent of their daily calories from a whole-wheat flat bread called tanok. A series of studies in the early 1970s by Dr. Reinhold demonstrated that excessive consumption of tanok caused zinc deficiency in young boys and teenagers, which resulted in a condition called hypogonadal dwarfism. This nutritional disease prevents normal growth and development, reduces stature, severely delays puberty, and adversely affects reproductive function.

By following the USDA guidelines, whole grains can easily make up a third or more of your caloric intake. A twenty-five-year-old sedentary woman has an energy requirement of about 1,600 calories per day. If she consumes 6 ounces of grain, as recommended by the USDA, this amount of cereal translates into about 29 percent of her daily calories. If this woman considers herself "health conscious" and purchases only whole-grain breads and cereals and has made a decision to reduce or completely eliminate meat, eggs, and other animal foods from her diet, whole grains can easily compose 50 percent or more of her diet. Like many Americans, she thinks she is following a healthy plant-based diet that will reduce her risk of developing many chronic diseases and nutritional deficiencies. In reality, most likely she will develop both iron deficiency anemia and zinc deficiency. Her whole-grain-based diet, because of its high phytate and antinutrient content, will also promote calcium loss and osteoporosis.

Whole Grains and Bone Health

One of the best-kept secrets about excessive whole-grain consumption is that it adversely affects skeletal health by impairing vitamin D and calcium metabolism. If you take a look at the table showing the vitamin and mineral contents of various food groups (see page 108), notice that the average amount of calcium in a 100-calorie serving of whole grains is a paltry 7.6 mg, whereas the same serving of fresh vegetables gives you fifteen times more calcium (116.8 mg). More important, vegetable calcium is well assimilated, whereas calcium in whole grains is virtually unabsorbable because it is bound to phytate. The more whole grains you include in your diet, the less calcium will be available to build and maintain a healthy skeleton.

If an extremely low calcium content that is poorly absorbed were not bad enough, whole grains have other adverse nutrient characteristics that harm calcium metabolism and bone health. Whole grains have a calcium/phosphorous ratio that is quite low (0.08). Consumption of excess phosphorus when calcium intake is adequate or low leads to a condition called secondary hyperparathyroidism, which causes progressive bone loss. The recommended, ideal calcium/phosphorous ratio is 1.00, whereas it averages 0.64 for women and 0.62 for men in the United States. High-grain diets such as those recommended by the USDA's MyPyramid/MyPlate (around 30 percent of your total calories) will further reduce the calcium/phosphorous ratio in your diet and increase your risk for developing osteoporosis.

Whole grains are bad news not only for adults' calcium metabolism but also for children's. In an experiment involving infants, Dr. Zoppi and coworkers showed that wheat bran given to infants for just one month caused their blood calcium to plummet. Most consumers believe that whole grains are vastly superior to refined grains in every respect. This assumption is simply untrue, particularly when it comes to calcium metabolism and bone mineral health. Animal experiments show that whole-grain oats and wheat are worse for your health than their refined counterparts for a variety of reasons, including their adverse effect on vitamin D metabolism.

Whole Grains Impair Vitamin D Metabolism

One of the most disturbing effects of whole grains is their capacity to impair vitamin D metabolism. Besides calcium, vitamin D is one of the most important nutrients when it comes to our bone health. Within the last ten years, scientists have determined that vitamin D deficiency spans the globe and has turned into a worldwide epidemic. Scores of studies indicate that anywhere from 40 to 100 percent of elderly men and women in the United States and Europe are vitamin D deficient. This epidemic is not limited only to the elderly. A study in Maine revealed that 48 percent of preteen girls had deficiencies in this important nutrient, while a study in Boston indicated that 52 percent of Hispanic and black teenagers were vitamin D depleted. Other studies have demonstrated that vitamin D deficiency is common in middle-aged adults, with as many as 60 to 90 percent of them maintaining inadequate blood concentrations of this crucial vitamin. Moreover, if you follow government guidelines and consume a third of your calories as grains and whole grains, you will make the potentially severe health problem of vitamin D deficiency even worse.

In 1919, Dr. Edward Mellanby of London University experimentally demonstrated that excessive whole-grain consumption caused rickets in puppies. Rickets is a debilitating bone disease that afflicts puppies and human children by causing a softening of bones that leads to fractures and deformities that may persist throughout life. Since Dr. Mellanby's pioneering work, numerous experiments in other laboratory animals and even humans have shown without question that whole grains impair vitamin D metabolism.

There appear to be at least two elements in whole grains and whole wheat in particular that undermine vitamin D metabolism in our bodies. Most of us are either borderline or vitamin D deficient to start with, so any losses caused by whole-grain consumption exacerbate the problem. A study of vitamin D in human beings who consumed 60 grams of wheat bran daily for thirty days demonstrated an increased elimination of vitamin D from the intestines. It is not entirely clear how whole grains promote losses of vitamin D from our bodies, but they may interrupt the normal recycling process of vitamin D between the intestines and the liver.

Recent work from our research group suggests that one substance found in whole wheat may play an even more important role in disrupting normal vitamin D metabolism than previously suspected substances do. Wheat contains a lectin known as *wheat germ agglutinin*, or WGA, that has been shown to easily penetrate the gut barrier of rats and enter their bloodstream. Experiments from our laboratory, as well as those from Dr. Roberto Chignola and coworkers at the University of Verona, support the view that WGA from whole and refined wheat bypasses the gut barrier and enters human circulation as well. This is definitely not a good thing because WGA is a lectin that can bind to almost any cell in our bodies and disrupt normal cellular function.

Lectins are protein molecules found in plant and animal cells that firmly bind to carbohydrate and sugar molecules. They were originally discovered when researchers noticed lectins' ability to cause red blood cells to clump together in test tubes. In plants, their main function is to act as an antinutrient to discourage potential predators such as insects, birds, and small animals from eating their various leaves, seeds, and roots. Most plant lectins in our food supply are harmless because they can't bind to cells in our gastrointestinal tract and therefore can't get into our bloodstream. Two notable exceptions are cereal grain and legume lectins, which bind to cells in our intestines and enter circulation.

Once WGA finds its way into the bloodstream, it attaches itself to red blood cells and is carried to almost every cell in our bodies. At this point, WGA crosses cell membranes and binds to a structure on the cell nucleus called the nuclear pore. This action effectively blocks the entry of many hormones into the nucleus and prevents their intended cellular actions.

Vitamin D is actually not a vitamin at all. It is classified as a hormone because it affects so many of our body's cells and organs. In order for vitamin D to produce its beneficial effects in our bodies, it normally must enter the cell nucleus through the nuclear pore. Unfortunately, this process can't occur when WGA binds and blocks the nuclear pore. This series of events has been experimentally demonstrated in tissue studies in vitro but has yet to be confirmed in living human experiments in vivo. Yet the bottom line remains the same—excessive whole wheat and grain consumption disrupts vitamin D metabolism and disturbs normal bone health.

Whole Grains and Celiac Disease

One of the most shortsighted aspects of the USDA's population-wide recommendation for all of us to consume grains is its failure to recognize that wheat, rye, and barley are troublesome to a large percentage of the U.S. population. In a landmark paper published in 2003, Dr. Alessio Fasano at the University of Maryland determined that 1 in 133 people in the United States has celiac disease, an autoimmune disease triggered by the consumption of gluten proteins found in all wheat, rye, and barley food products. Celiac disease arises when the immune system does not recognize the body's own intestinal tissues as itself and mounts an attack on them. In celiac patients, the range of symptoms runs the spectrum from intense inflammation, tissue destruction, diarrhea, and malabsorption of nutrients to virtually no symptoms at all. In infants and children, celiac disease can stunt normal growth and in adults increases the risk of developing other autoimmune diseases and associated illnesses, with outcomes that range from inconsequential to lethal.

At least 2,316,000 Americans have celiac disease. Unfortunately, most are unaware that they have the disease, because about 80 percent of all celiac patients remain undiagnosed. If we do the math, you can see that at least 1,852,800 people in the United States don't have a clue that they have celiac disease and that they shouldn't be eating wheat, barley, and rye. Despite these compelling figures, the USDA has completely failed us with its MyPyramid/MyPlate recommendation for every man, woman, and child in the United States to eat grains on a daily basis.

At first, these numbers may seem trivial because they imply that most people have no trouble whatsoever when eating gluten-containing grains. Not true. Until very recently, the classical medical view of gluten was that it caused only one autoimmune illness (celiac disease) or possibly one other (dermatitis herpetiformis—an itchy skin rash). In the last five years, a few of the most well-recognized celiac researchers in the world, including Drs. Alessio Fasano and Marios Hadjivassiliou, have completely demolished this traditional perspective on gluten. These scientists have coined the term "gluten sensitivity" and have shown that celiac disease is just one of many illnesses and autoimmune diseases caused by gluten-containing grains. Intriguing evidence uncovered by these researchers and others show that gluten sensitivity may underlie an extraordinary number of health problems and disorders, including those shown below.

Diseases and Disorders Linked to Gluten Sensitivity

Acid reflux
Addison's disease (adrenal disease)
Alopecia (hair loss)
Anemia
Aphthous ulceration (canker sores)

Asthma

Ataxias (a nervous system dysfunction causing grossly uncoordinated movements)

Attention deficit disorder (ADD)

Atopic diseases (flaky, itchy skin)

Autism

Autoimmune thyroid diseases

Dementia

Dental enamel defects

Depression and anxiety

Dermatitis herpetiformis (itchy skin disease)

Eating disorders

Epilepsy with cerebral calcifications

Graves' disease

Hashimoto's thyroiditis

Hyperactivity

Infertility

IgA nephropathy (kidney inflammation)

Irritable bowel syndrome

Liver disease

    Chronic active hepatitis

    Primary biliary cirrhosis

    Primary sclerosing cholangitis

Migraine headaches

Peripheral neuropathies (nerve damage causing pain, muscle weakness, tingling, spasms, cramps)

Psoriasis

Rheumatoid arthritis

Schizophrenia

Selective IgA deficiency (immune system dysfunction)

Sjögren's syndrome (dry eyes, mouth)

Systemic lupus erythematosus (whole body autoimmune disease)

Type I diabetes

Uveitis (autoimmune eye disease)

Vitiligo (skin depigmentation)

If even a small percentage of these diseases and disorders are directly caused by the consumption of gluten-containing grains, we really need to rethink governmental recommendations for all of us to eat cereals. In a recent interview, Dr. Fasano estimated that twenty million people nationwide are sensitive to gluten. These numbers are truly staggering and represent an epidemic—so much so, that the Centers for Disease Control now considers celiac disease and gluten sensitivity a major public health threat.

One of the greatest improvements you can make in your physical and mental health will be to eliminate not only wheat from your diet, but the other seven major cereal grains as well: rye, barley, oats, corn, rice, millet, and sorghum.

Pseudo Grains

All eight of the commonly consumed cereal grains are true cereals because they are the seeds of grasses that botanically belong to the Poaceae family of plants. By now, there should be little doubt in your mind why true cereal grains are inferior foods and should be avoided. Yet what about starchy seeds that are frequently used by celiac patients and others to replace gluten-containing grains? Technically, these seeds are not true grasses because they are not members of the Poaceae family. They include chia seeds, buckwheat, quinoa, and amaranth. Let's take a look at the nutritional pros and cons of these seeds.

Antinutrients in Seeds

As with all aspects of human nutrition, we first need to look at the evolutionary clues before we come to sweeping conclusions about which foods and food groups we should regularly include in, or omit from, our diets. From what we know about historically studied foragers, they hunted, gathered, and fished for foods in a manner that maximized their caloric intake versus the energy they expended to obtain these foods. This food-gathering strategy is referred to as the *optimal foraging theory* by anthropologists. Based on the optimal foraging theory, hunter-gatherers typically maintained the following order of food preferences:

1. Large animals
2. Medium-size animals
3. Small animals, birds, and fish
4. Roots and tubers
5. Fruit
6. Honey
7. Nuts and seeds
8. Grass seeds (cereals)

You can see from this list that hunter-gatherers always preferred large animals if they were available—simply because they got more food calories for their caloric expenditure. Notice that seeds and cereals were at the bottom of the list. There is no doubt that for-agers were opportunists, and if something was edible, it was probably consumed, but only if preferred foods couldn't be acquired first. So yes, the evolutionary evidence supports the notion that if pseudo grains or even cereal grains were available, they would have been occasionally consumed.

Nevertheless, seeds and grains would never have been eaten on a daily basis as staple foods that make up 25 to 50 percent of one's daily energy. In support of this conclusion is my 2000 analysis of 229 hunter-gatherer diets revealing that animal foods—not plant foods—were the preferred staples. Moreover, most wild plant foods, particularly seeds, are not available on a year-round basis but can be harvested and consumed seasonally for only a few weeks or months out of the year. Let's see how this evolutionary insight is an important nutritional concept that has relevance today.

Seeds of any mature plant represent their reproductive future. If they are entirely consumed by animals such as insects, birds, rodents, or mammals or are destroyed by fungi and microorganisms, the seeds can't make their way into the soil, germinate, and produce the next generation of plants. In other words, plants don't produce seeds simply to feed other animals or microorganisms—if they did, they would rapidly become extinct.

Natural selection has come up with a number of strategies to ensure that a plant's seeds are not completely eaten or destroyed by predators and microorganisms. First, the seed can be protected by a hard shell that makes it difficult or impossible for the predator to eat the inner seed. An example that comes to mind is a Brazil nut. Second, plants frequently evolve thorns, spikes, and other hazardous structures to keep animals away, such as what we find with cactus thorns. Another seed-saving strategy is the evolution of a very hard seed surrounded by sweet fruit. With this evolutionary solution, the predator is encouraged to eat the entire fruit, seed and all. The hard seed survives the predator's digestive system and exits fully intact in a nice pile of fertilizing dung. Strawberries and crab apples are a good example of this evolutionary approach.

One important strategy a plant can take to protect its seeds is the evolution of lethally toxic or moderately toxic compounds to discourage predation and damage by animals and microorganisms. These compounds are called *antinutrients*. Unfortunately, antinutrients not only adversely affect microorganisms, insects, birds, rodents, and animals, but they also cause varying degrees of harmful effects in our own bodies. The good news about antinutrients found in our food supply is that their toxicity is generally dose dependent, meaning that they become more and more poisonous as we eat more and more foods that contain antinutrients.

Not all food antinutrients affect us in exactly the same manner. Some have minimal or subtle effects, a few are lethally toxic, and others have long-term adverse health effects that we are only beginning to understand.

Pseudo grains such as chia seeds, amaranth, quinoa, and buckwheat are loaded with a variety of moderately toxic antinutrients that probably have minimal adverse health effects if we eat them occasionally, in limited quantities, or for only short periods. This dietary pattern mimics how hunter-gatherers would have consumed plant seeds. In the wild, plants produce seeds seasonally for only a few weeks or months out of the year. With the advent of agriculture and long-term storage technologies, we can now eat any plant seed that we like every single day of the year.

That's the problem. Repeated high exposure to seed antinutrients can undermine the nutrient quality of our diets but, more important, may impair intestinal function, promote chronic low-level inflammation, and increase our susceptibility to allergies and autoimmune and other inflammatory diseases.

Chia Seeds

Chia seeds are small and oval shaped, either black or white colored; they resemble sesame seeds. They are native to southern Mexico and northern Guatemala and were cultivated as a food crop for thousands of years in this region by the Aztecs and other native cultures. Chia seeds can be consumed in a variety of ways, which include roasting and grinding the seeds into a flour known as chianpinolli that can then be made into tortillas, tamales, and beverages. The roasted ground seeds are traditionally consumed as gruel called pinole.

In the last twenty years, chia seeds have become an increasingly popular item in co-ops and health food stores, primarily because of their high content of the healthful omega 3 fatty acid alpha linolenic acid (ALA). Chia seeds have also been fed to domestic livestock and chickens to enrich their meat and eggs with omega 3 fats. I can endorse feeding chia seeds to animals but have serious reservations when it comes to humans eating these seeds as staple foods. The next table shows the entire nutrient profile for a 100-gram serving of chia seeds.

At least on paper, it would appear that chia seeds are a nutritious food that is not only high in ALA but is also a good source of protein, fiber, certain B vitamins, calcium, iron, manganese, and zinc.

Unfortunately, as is the case with many other plant seeds, chia seeds contain numerous antinutrients that reduce their nutritional value. Notice the high phosphorus concentrations found in chia seeds. This revealing marker tells us that chia seeds are concentrated

Nutrients in Chia Seeds (100-gram serving)

Nutrient	Amount	% Dietary Reference Intake (DRI)
Kilocalories	490	25
Protein	15.6 g	31
Carbohydrate	43.9 g	15
Fat	30.8 g	47
Saturated Fat	3.2 g	6
Monounsaturated Fat	2.9 g	na
Polyunsaturated Fat	23.3 g	na
18:1 oleic acid	2.0 g	na
18:2n6 linoleic acid	5.8 g	na
18:3n3 alpha linolenic acid	17.6 g	na
Fiber	37.7 g	151
Vitamin A	36 IU	1
Vitamin B1	0.87 mg	58
Vitamin B2	0.17 mg	10
Vitamin B3	5.82 mg	29
Vitamin B6	0.69 mg	35
Vitamin B12	0	0
Folate	114 mcg	29
Pantothenic acid	0.94 mg	9
Vitamin C	15.7 mg	26
Sodium	19 mg	1
Potassium	100 mg	5
Phosphorus	948	95
Calcium	631 mg	26
Copper	0.19 mg	9
Iron	10.0	56
Magnesium	77 mg	19
Manganese	2.17 mg	108
Zinc	3.5 mg	23

sources of phytate, an antinutrient that binds to many minerals, such as calcium, iron, zinc, magnesium, and copper, making them unavailable for absorption. In our bodies, chia seeds actually become inferior sources of all of these minerals.

Similarly, the table suggests that chia seeds are good sources of vitamin B6. Unfortunately, in our bodies the utilization of this vitamin from plant foods such as chia seeds is quite low, whereas the bioavailability of B6 from animal products is quite high, approaching 100 percent.

One unusual characteristic of chia seed pinole or food products comes from a clear mucilaginous gel that surrounds the seeds. This sticky gel forms a barrier that impairs digestion and fat absorption and causes a low protein digestibility. Animal and human studies indicate that it is likely that other antinutrients, together with this gel, may promote a leaky gut, chronic systemic inflammation, and food allergies.

Amaranth, Quinoa, and Buckwheat

Many celiac patients or people who want to avoid gluten-containing grains frequently eliminate wheat, rye, and barley foods and substitute products that contain one or more pseudo grains—amaranth, quinoa, and buckwheat—or their flours. The market for gluten-free food items has become enormous in the last decade, with estimated consumer demand totaling sixty million people in the United States alone. If you have purchased gluten-free foods or are considering doing so, make sure that you read labels carefully, as sometimes the seed flours that replace gluten flours have nearly as many nutritional shortcomings as the foods they replace. The health problems associated with the habitual consumption of amaranth, quinoa, and buckwheat have not been as well studied as those for gluten-containing cereal grains. Nevertheless, there are important red flags that should grab your attention.

As I mentioned, all pseudo grains are chock full of antinutrients. These substances represent the plant's evolutionary defense mechanisms against predation by insects, birds, rodents, and other animals, as well as a means to discourage infection by microorganisms. When we examine the chemical composition of almost all seed antinutrients, whether they come from cereals, legumes, or pseudo grains, a familiar pattern of compounds emerges.

When you think about any poisonous or toxic substance, it has to follow a number of key steps in your body to do its poisoning and cause illness. First, it has to get into your body—this means that it has survive digestive processes and resist gut enzymes that normally break down toxic food proteins into their harmless amino acid components. We know from human and animal studies that almost all plant seeds contain protease inhibitors. These compounds neutralize predator gut enzymes that normally would degrade seed proteins/toxins into nonhazardous substances. If a plant seed is to deliver a lethal or partially lethal protein to a potential predator, the toxic compound has to survive the predator's digestive enzymes. Protease inhibitors found in plant seeds do precisely this. They allow plant seeds to deliver additional poisons to the host's next line of defense—its gut barrier.

In addition to protease inhibitors that protect seed toxins from the host's digestive enzymes, plant seeds have evolved a number of compounds that allow their toxins to penetrate the gut barrier. The most common gut-breeching chemicals are called *saponins*. Other gut-penetrating seed proteins are lectins; gliadin proteins from wheat, rye, and barley; and another category of substances known as *thaumatin-like proteins*. Each of these compounds works in a slightly different manner to compromise intestinal permeability, resulting in a condition known as leaky gut.

Once the gut barrier has been damaged, plant seed antinutrients can find their way into the bloodstream to disturb normal bodily functions, causing illnesses and disease. Antinutrient damage to the intestinal barrier allows toxins from bacteria and viruses found in the gut contents to enter the bloodstream as well.

Amaranth

As with all pseudo grains, unless you consume them as staples to replace cereals in your diet, they probably will have little adverse effects on your long-term health and well-being. Nevertheless, amaranth seeds and flour contain at least three potentially harmful antinutrients. First, the saponin content (790 mg/kg) of amaranth seeds is higher than in a variety of common human foods that have been shown to impair intestinal function and cause leaky gut, which can lead to an increased risk for allergies, autoimmune diseases, and chronic low-level inflammation.

Amaranth seeds are also concentrated sources of oxalic acid and contain four to five times more of this antinutrient than either cereals or legumes. Dietary oxalic acid is problematic because the more of it you consume, the greater your risk is for developing kidney stones.

The most disturbing antinutrient found in amaranth is a lectin abbreviated ACA. Experiments by Dr. Jonathan Rhodes have revealed that ACA is a potent promoter of cancer cell growth in the intestines.

Quinoa

Quinoa is a pseudo grain with origins in South America. Like amaranth and chia seeds, it contains numerous antinutrients, including saponins, protease inhibitors, phytate, and tannins. A potential health-threatening component in quinoa is its high saponin content—up to 5,000 mg/kg. In both rat and tissue experiments, saponins from quinoa seeds increased intestinal permeability.

As I mentioned, a leaky gut may lead to many health problems and is thought to be one of the essential triggers for autoimmune diseases. If you currently have an autoimmune disease or if you have a family history of these illnesses, I would definitely recommend that you avoid quinoa and all other pseudo grains.

Buckwheat

This plant produces a starchy seed that is ground into flour that is frequently made into noodles widely consumed in Japan, China, and Korea. It can be made into porridges or even mixed with yeast to produce pancakes. Because buckwheat contains no gluten, the flour and its products are often used by celiac patients as substitutes for wheat, rye, and barley.

From a health and nutrition perspective, buckwheat has not been examined in nearly the same detail as true cereal grains or even other pseudo grains, so the jury is still out on how it may affect our long-term health and well-being. Nevertheless, allergists worldwide have taken a great interest in buckwheat because it is such a potent and fatal allergen. Buckwheat allergy seems to be common in Asian countries and frequently causes life-threatening allergic reactions called anaphylactic shock that do not lessen after childhood.

Like other pseudo grains, buckwheat is a concentrated source of protease inhibitors, which are suspected in causing buckwheat's powerful allergic responses. One unusual detrimental health effect of buckwheat consumption is a damaging skin reaction frequently shown in many animal experiments. This response is caused when sunlight reacts with dietary buckwheat compounds that make their way into the skin. How this adverse effect occurs is currently unknown.

As with other pseudo grains, I cannot recommend that you eat buckwheat, except on an infrequent basis. You will be much better off by completely avoiding buckwheat and eating more fresh meats, seafood, fish, and fruits and veggies.

Paleo Bottom Line

Don't eat grains, which include wheat, rye, barley, oats, corn, rice, sorghum, and millet. Avoid pseudo grains such as buckwheat, chia seeds, amaranth, and quinoa.

7

The Trouble with Beans

Healing Inflammation:
Craig's Story

I had not been feeling well for several years. After I saw
several rheumatologists and many doctors, they were not
sure what was happening except I was exhibiting symptoms
of inflammation throughout my body (muscular and gut)—
minimal joint pain but back and hip stiffness. My energy
level was very low. I visited chiropractors and took Celebrex
on an as-needed basis.

I searched and found an article dated April 18, 2000, in
the WebMD archives that was written by Elizabeth Tracey
on possible (lectin) grain, pea, and bean/gut changes/
inflammation linkages to arthritis. Loren Cordain's name
was mentioned. Beans and peas cause me great digestive
and bowel issues.

I immediately stopped eating wheat, barley, peas, and
beans and then began to feel great! People even notice a

difference. It seems within a few days all of my symptoms have disappeared. My energy level and general feeling of well-being have increased dramatically! I am most relieved and hope I have finally found the answer.

One question that comes up time and again is, "Why can't I eat beans?" In this chapter I'll show you why legumes are inferior foods that should not be part of the Paleo Diet.

The Toxicity of Uncooked Beans

It may come as a surprise to you, but as recently as fifteen years ago, imports of red kidney beans into South Africa were legally prohibited because of "their potential toxicity to humans." Many people think about kidney beans as nutritious, plant-based, high-protein foods, but indeed they are toxic. Unless adequately soaked and boiled, kidney beans and almost all legumes produce detrimental effects in our bodies. Starting in the early 1970s, a number of scientific papers reported that consumption of raw or undercooked red kidney beans caused nausea, vomiting, abdominal pain, severe diarrhea, muscle weakness, and inflammation of the heart. Similar symptoms were documented in horses and cattle. Furthermore, raw kidney beans were lethally toxic to rats when fed at more than 37 percent of their daily calories.

These clues should make us proceed cautiously as we consider the nutritional benefits and liabilities of beans and legumes.

The Nutrient Content of Beans and Legumes

As a child growing up in Southern California in the 1950s, I was always playing around swimming pools and open water. My mother enrolled me in a swim class by the time I was a toddler. Later in my childhood, one of my great disappointments on hot summer afternoons was that Mom made me wait an entire hour after lunch before I could get back into the water. As did almost everyone else of that era, Mom assumed that if she didn't take this precaution, I could potentially end up with paralyzing stomach cramps, which in turn would cause me to drown. A decade later, as I trained to become a beach lifeguard, this same belief was repeated in the life-saving manual that was used to educate every lifeguard in the country. At the time, I never questioned this fundamental rule. I didn't even think about it. It simply was the way it was—yesterday, today, and presumably forever.

In nutrition we can frequently find these same dyed-in-the-wool beliefs, which, on careful scrutiny, make little sense. After the full story is presented to us in a logical and straightforward manner, we wonder why we ever believed in such silly ideas in the first place. If we examine the USDA's MyPyramid/MyPlate, governmental nutritionists have arbitrarily created five food groups: (1) grains, (2) vegetables, (3) fruit, (4) dairy, and (5) protein foods. I would agree that most common foods could logically be placed into one of these five categories, except for one glaring exception—protein foods.

The USDA has decided that protein foods should include: (1) meat, (2) poultry, (3) fish, (4) eggs, (5) nuts and seeds, and (6) dried beans and peas. I have little disagreement that meat, poultry, fish, and eggs are good sources of protein. The USDA, however, tells us that these six protein foods items are equivalent and can be used interchangeably with one another—that animal protein sources including meats, poultry, fish, and eggs are nutritionally comparable to plant protein sources: nuts, seeds, and dried beans and peas. I quote the USDA MyPyramid/MyPlate recommendations: "Dry beans and peas are the mature forms of legumes such as kidney beans, pinto beans, black-eyed peas, and lentils. These foods are excellent sources of plant protein, and also provide other nutrients such as iron and zinc. They are similar to meats, poultry, and fish in their contribution of these nutrients. Many people consider dry beans and peas as vegetarian alternatives for meat."

Let's see how "dry beans and peas" stack up to meats, poultry, fish, and eggs in terms of protein, iron, and zinc, as alluded to by the

USDA. In the graph below you can see that on a calorie-by-calorie basis, legumes are utter lightweights when compared to the protein content of lean poultry, beef, pork, and seafood. Nuts and seeds fare even worse. Beans, peas, and other legumes contain 66 percent less protein than either lean chicken or turkey and 61 percent less protein than lean beef, pork, and seafood. What the USDA doesn't tell us is that our bodies don't process bean and legume proteins nearly as efficiently as we do animal proteins—meaning that the proteins found in beans, peas, and other legumes have poor digestibility.

The Food and Agricultural Organization/World Health Organization of the United Nations have devised a protein quality index known as the Protein Digestibility-Corrected Amino Acid Score (PDCAAS). This index reveals that beans and other legumes maintain second-rate PDCAAS ratings that average about 20 to 25 percent lower than animal protein ratings. So legumes and beans not only contain about three times less protein than animal foods, but what little protein they do have is poorly digested. Their poor PDCAAS scores stem from a variety of antinutrients that impair protein absorption and from low levels of two essential amino acids, cysteine and methionine.

I have no idea how the USDA concluded that legumes are "excellent sources of plant protein . . . similar to meats, poultry, and fish in their contribution of these nutrients."

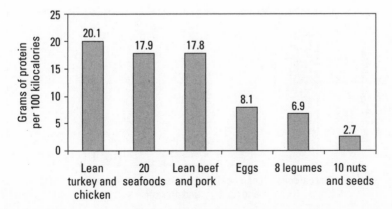

Protein in Various Foods

Let's take a look at the average zinc and iron content of eight commonly eaten legumes: green peas, lentils, kidney beans, lima beans, garbanzo beans (chick peas), black-eyed peas, mung beans, and soybeans. In the following graphs, I have contrasted the average zinc and iron content of these eight legumes to lean chicken, turkey, beef, pork, and seafood (the twenty types of seafood are shrimp, cod, pollack, catfish, scallop, salmon, flounder, sole, oyster, orange roughy, mackerel, ocean perch, rockfish, whiting, clam, haddock, blue crab, rainbow trout, halibut, and lobster).

Notice that the iron content of legumes appears to be similar to that of seafood and about twice as high as in lean meats and eggs. This data is misleading, though, because it doesn't tell us how legume iron is handled in our bodies. Experimental human studies from Dr. Cook in Switzerland and from Dr. Hallberg in Sweden have shown that only about 20 to 25 percent of the iron in legumes is available for absorption because it is bound to phytate.

In reality, the high iron content of legumes (2.2 mg/100 kcal) plummets by 75 to 80 percent when our bodies attempt to digest beans and peas, thereby making legumes a poor source of iron compared to animal foods. A similar situation occurs with zinc, as phytate and other antinutrients in legumes severely reduce its absorption in our bodies. Given that this information has been

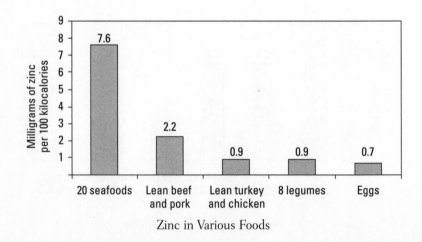

Zinc in Various Foods

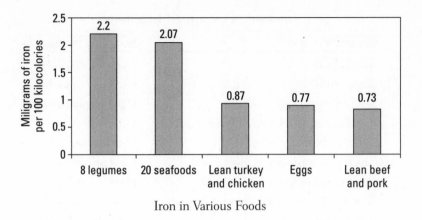

Iron in Various Foods

known for more than thirty years, it defies logic how the USDA could misinform the American public.

The Purpose of Antinutrients

You can see how misleading it is to evaluate the nutritional and health effects of beans and other legumes simply by analyzing their nutrient content on paper, as the USDA has done. Before we can pass nutritional judgment on any food, it is essential to determine how it actually acts within our bodies. Beans are not good sources of either zinc or iron, and they have low protein digestibility because legumes are chock full of antinutrients that impair our bodies' ability to absorb and assimilate potential nutrients found in these foods.

As was the case with the antinutrients found in whole grains, the primary purpose of most antinutrients in legumes is to discourage predation and prevent destruction of the plant's seeds, its reproductive materials, by microorganisms, insects, birds, rodents, and large mammals. We most frequently refer to legume seeds as beans. I've included peanuts here, which are not nuts at all; they are actually legumes. In the following table I have listed some of the more commonly known legume seeds, along with their scientific names.

Note that many different versions of the beans we frequently eat are actually the exact same species—and contain comparable

Commonly Consumed Legumes

Common Name	Scientific Name
Adzuki beans	*Phaseolus angularis*
Black beans	*Phaseolus vulgaris*
Black-eyed peas	*Vigna unguiculata*
Broad beans, fava beans, horse beans	*Vicia faba*
Canellini beans	*Phaseolus vulgaris*
Chick peas, garbanzo beans	*Cicer arietinum*
Great northern beans	*Phaseolus vulgaris*
Green beans, string beans, snap beans	*Phaseolus vulgaris*
Kidney beans	*Phaseolus vulgaris*
Lentils (brown, red, green)	*Lens esculenta*
Lima beans, butter beans	*Phaseolus lunatus*
Mung beans	*Vigna radiate*
Navy beans	*Phaseolus vulgaris*
Peanuts	*Arachis hypogaea*
Peas	*Pisum sativum*
Pinto beans	*Phaseolus vulgaris*
Soybeans	*Glycine max*
White kidney beans	*Phaseolus vulgaris*

concentrations of toxic antinutrients. Notice how many times you see the scientific name *Phaseolus vulgaris* repeated in the table. If you enjoy Mexican food, then you have probably tasted *Phaseolus vulgaris* as either refried beans or black beans, because these two beans are the same species, differing only by color. Great northern beans, green beans, kidney beans, navy beans, pinto beans, and white kidney beans are also members of the same species, *Phaseolus vulgaris*. All beans that are members of *Phaseolus vulgaris* contain some of the highest concentrations of antinutrients known.

The list of antinutrients found in legumes, beans, and soy includes lectins, saponins, phytate, polyphenols such as tannins and isoflavones, protease inhibitors, raffinose oligosaccharides, cyano-genetic glycosides, and favism glycosides. This list looks formidable at first because of all of the scientific terms, but don't worry—the concepts underlying how these toxins may impair our health are easily understood. Let's go through this list so that you can clearly understand why you should avoid legumes.

Lectins

Earlier in the book when I discussed cereals, I mentioned that almost all whole grains are concentrated sources of lectins. The same can be said for virtually all legumes. Lectins are potent antinutrients that plants have evolved as toxins to ward off predators. Raw or undercooked kidney beans have caused severe cases of food poisoning in humans and were shown to be lethally toxic in rats. Although several kidney bean antinutrients probably contributed to these poisonous effects, animal experiments indicate that a specific lectin found in kidney beans was the main culprit. Kidney beans and all other varieties of beans within the *Phaseolus vulgaris* species— black beans, kidney beans, pinto beans, string beans, navy beans and so on—contain a lectin called phytohemagglutinin (PHA). The more PHA we ingest, the sicker we become. This is why raw beans are so toxic—they contain much higher concentrations of PHA than cooked beans do. Cooking doesn't completely eliminate PHA, however, and even small amounts of this lectin are known to produce adverse health effects, providing they can penetrate our gut barrier.

The trick with lectins is that they must bypass our intestinal walls and enter into our bloodstream if they are to wreak havoc within our bodies. So far, no human studies of PHA have been conducted. Yet in laboratory animals, PHA easily breeches the gut barrier and enters into the bloodstream, where it may travel to many organs and tissues and disrupt normal cell function, causing disease.

Human tissue experiments reveal that PHA and other food lectins can cause a leaky gut. A leaky gut represents one of the first steps implicated in many autoimmune diseases. Impaired intestinal integrity produced by dietary lectins may also cause low-level inflammation in our bloodstream—a necessary precursor in developing atherosclerosis and cancer.

Besides kidney beans and other bean varieties within *Phaseolus vulgaris* species, all other legumes contain lectins with varying degrees of toxicity, ranging from mild to lethal. Soybean lectin (SBA) is also known to impair intestinal permeability and cause a leaky gut. Peanut lectin (PNA) is the only legume lectin to have been tested in living humans by Dr. Rhodes's research group in London. Within less than an hour after ingestion by healthy normal subjects, PNA entered their bloodstreams—not a good thing because it then had the capacity to interact with virtually every cell in the body.

The lectins found in peas (PSA) and lentils (LCA) seem to be much less toxic than PHA, SBA, or PNA, but they are not completely without adverse effects in tissue and animal experiments. Although no long-term lectin experiments have yet been conducted in humans, from animal and tissue studies we know that these antinutrients damage the intestinal barrier, impair growth, alter normal immune function, and cause inflammation.

Saponins

The word "saponin" is derived from the Latin word for "soap." Saponins are antinutrients found in almost all legumes. They have soaplike properties that punch holes in the membranes lining the exterior of every cell. As was the case with lectins, this effect is dose dependent—the more saponins we ingest, the greater will be the damage to our bodies' cells. Our first line of defense against any antinutrient is our gut barrier. Human tissue and animal studies confirm that legume saponins can easily disrupt the cells that line our intestines and rapidly make their way into our bloodstream. Once in the bloodstream in sufficient quantities, saponins can cause ruptures in our red blood cells in a process known as hemolysis, which can temporarily impair our blood's oxygen-carrying capacity. The main threat to our health from legume saponins stems not from red blood cell damage but rather from saponins' ability to increase intestinal permeability. A leaky gut likely promotes low-level inflammation because it allows toxins and bacteria in our guts to interact with our immune systems. This process is known to be a necessary first step in developing autoimmune diseases and may promote the inflammation necessary for heart disease and cancer to develop and progress.

The other major problem with legume saponins is that cooking does not destroy them. In fact, even after extended boiling for two hours, 85 to 100 percent of the original saponins in most beans and legumes remain intact. On the other hand, by eating fermented soy products such as tofu, tempeh, or sprouted beans, you can lower your saponin intake. The next table shows you the saponin content of some common beans, legumes, and soy products.

Saponin Content of Selected Beans, Legumes, and Soy Products

Legume or Product	Saponin Concentration (mg/kg)
Soy protein isolate	10,600
Textured vegetable protein	4,510
Navy beans	3,800
Soybeans	4,040
Soybean flour	3,310
Kidney beans	3,500
Broad beans (fava beans)	3,100
Chick peas (garbanzo beans)	2,300
Green peas	1,800
Soy tempeh	1,530
Bean shoot (sprouted)	1,100
Lentils	1,100
Canned baked beans	1,100
Lima beans	1,000
Green beans (snap beans)	1,000
Tofu	590
Mung beans	500
Soy milk	470
Peanuts	less than 100

Notice that the concentration of saponins in soy protein isolates is dangerously high. If you are an athlete or anyone else trying to increase your protein intake by supplementing with soy protein isolates, I suggest that you reconsider. A much healthier strategy would be to eat more lean meats and seafood. These protein-packed foods taste a lot better than artificial soy isolates and are much better for your body. If we eat legumes only occasionally, saponin damage to our intestines will quickly repair itself; however, when legumes or soy products are consumed in high amounts as staples or daily supplements, the risk for developing a leaky gut and the diseases associated with it is greatly increased.

Phytate

I discussed this antinutrient in great detail in chapter 4. Because phytate prevents the full absorption of iron, zinc, calcium, and magnesium in legumes and whole grains, reliance on these plant foods frequently causes multiple nutritional deficiencies in adults, children, and even nursing infants. Boiling and cooking don't seem to have much effect on the phytate content of legumes, whereas sprouting and fermentation can moderately reduce phytate concentrations. Also, vitamin C counteracts phytate's inhibitory effects on mineral absorption. That said, the best tactic to reduce phytate in your diet is to adopt the Paleo Diet—humanity's original legume- and grain-free diet.

Polyphenols: Tannins and Isoflavones

Polyphenols are antioxidant compounds that protect plants from UV sunlight damage and from insects, pests, and other microorganisms. Just as sunscreens protect our skin from ultraviolet damage, polyphenols are one of the compounds that plants have evolved to prevent the harmful effects of ultraviolet (UV) radiation from the sun, along with damage caused by animal and microorganism predators.

Polyphenols come in many different varieties and forms and are common throughout the plant kingdom.

When we eat these compounds, they seem to have both healthful and detrimental effects in our bodies. For instance, resveratrol is a polyphenol found in red grapes that may increase the life span in mice and slow or prevent many diseases. On the other hand, at least two types of polyphenols—tannins and isoflavones—in beans, soy, and other legumes may have adverse effects in our bodies.

Tannins are bitter-tasting polyphenols and give wine its astringent qualities. As with all antinutrients, the more tannin you ingest, the greater is the potential to disrupt your health. Tannins are similar to phytate, in that they reduce protein digestibility and bind iron and other minerals, preventing their normal absorption. Tannins damage our intestines, causing a leaky gut and allowing gut bacteria entry into our circulatory systems, thus encouraging low-level inflammation—a process intimately tied to heart disease, cancer, and autoimmune illnesses. By now you can see that legumes, beans, and soy represent a triple threat to our intestinal integrity because three separate antinutrients—lectins, saponins, and tannins—all work together to cause a leaky gut.

Isoflavones are some of nature's weirder plant compounds, in that they act like female hormones in our bodies. Certain isoflavones concentrated in soybeans and soy products are called phytoestrogens or "plant estrogens." Isoflavones from soy products can cause goiters, an enlargement of the thyroid gland, particularly if your blood levels of iodine are low. Two phytoestrogens in soy, genistein and daidzen, produced goiters in experimental animals.

You don't have to develop full-blown goiters by consuming these soy isoflavones to impair your health. In a study of elderly subjects, Dr. Ishizuki and colleagues demonstrated that when subjects with an average age of sixty-one were given 30 grams of soy daily for three months, they developed symptoms of low thyroid function—malaise, lethargy, and constipation. Half of these people ended up with goiters.

For women, the regular intake of soy or soy isoflavones may disrupt certain hormones that regulate the normal menstrual cycle.

In a meta analysis of forty-seven studies, Dr. Hooper demonstrated that soy or soy isoflavone consumption caused two female hormones, follicle-stimulating hormone (FSH) and luteinizing hormone (LH), to fall by 20 percent.

In chapter 4, I mentioned that seven of nine women who adhered to vegetarian diets for only six weeks stopped ovulating. One of the hormonal changes reported in this study, concurrent with the cessation of normal periods, was a significant decline in LH. Because Western vegetarian diets almost always contain lots of soy and soy isoflavones, it is entirely possible that soy isoflavones were directly responsible for the decline in LH and the disruption of normal menstrual periods documented in this study.

I have received e-mails from women all over the world whose menstrual and infertility problems subsided after they adopted the Paleo Diet. Their stories paint a credible picture that modern-day Paleo diets contain multiple nutritional elements that may improve or eliminate female reproductive and menstrual problems. Unfortunately, scientific validation of these women's experiences still lies in the future. But you don't have to wait—the potential benefits of the Paleo Diet are enormous, and the risks are minimal.

Perhaps the most worrisome effects of soy isoflavones may occur in developing fetuses with iodine-deficient mothers and in infants who receive soy formula. A 2007 paper by Dr. Gustavo Roman implicated soy isoflavones as risk factors for autism via their ability to impair normal iodine metabolism and thyroid function. Specifically, the soy isoflavone known as genistein may inhibit a key iodine-based enzyme required for normal brain development. Pregnant women with borderline iodine status can become iodine deficient if they have a diet that is high in soy. Their deficiency may then be conveyed to their developing fetuses, impairing growth in fetal brain cells known to be involved in autism. Infants born with iodine deficiencies are made worse if they are fed a soy formula.

Once again, the evolutionary lesson repeats itself. If a food or a nutrient generally was not a part of our ancestral diet, it has a high probability of disrupting our health and that of our children.

Protease Inhibitors

Very few people on the planet know about protease inhibitors. Yet I can tell you that when you eat beans, soy, or other legumes, you should be as aware of protease inhibitors as you are of a radar trap on the freeway.

When we eat any type of protein, enzymes in our intestines break the protein down into its component amino acids. These enzymes are called proteases and must be operating normally for our bodies to properly assimilate dietary proteins. Almost all legumes are concentrated sources of antinutrients called protease inhibitors, which prevent our gut enzymes from degrading protein into amino acids. Protease inhibitors found in beans, soy, peanuts, and other legumes are part of the reason why legume proteins have lower bioavailability than meat proteins. In experimental animals, ingestion of protease inhibitors in high amounts depresses normal growth and causes pancreatic enlargement.

Heating and cooking effectively destroy about 80 percent of the protease inhibitors found in most legumes, so the dietary concentrations of these antinutrients found in beans and soy are thought to have little harmful effects in our bodies. Yet at least one important adverse effect of protease inhibitors may have been overlooked.

When the gut's normal protein-degrading enzymes are inhibited by legume protease inhibitors, the pancreas works harder and compensates by secreting more protein-degrading enzymes. Consequently, the consumption of protease inhibitors causes levels of protein-degrading enzymes to rise within our intestines. One enzyme in particular, called trypsin, increases significantly. The rise in trypsin concentrations inside our gut is not without consequence, because elevated trypsin levels increase intestinal permeability, contributing to a leaky gut.

Raffinose Oligosaccharides

Here's another big scientific term for a little problem almost every one of us has had to deal with at one time or another after we ate beans: "Beans, beans, the musical fruit; the more you eat the more you . . . " Almost every schoolchild in the United States could complete this limerick. Plain and simple, beans cause gas or flatulence. Almost all legumes contain complex sugars called oligosaccharides. In particular, two complex sugars, raffinose and stachyose, are the culprits and are the elements in beans that give us gas. We lack the gut enzymes to break down these complex sugars into simpler sugars. Consequently, bacteria in our intestines metabolize these oligosaccharides into a variety of gases—hydrogen, carbon dioxide, and methane.

Beans don't affect everyone equally. Some people experience extreme digestive discomfort, with diarrhea, nausea, intestinal rumbling, and flatulence, whereas others are almost symptomless. These differences among people seem to be caused by varying types of gut flora.

Cyanogenetic Glycosides

Some of us have food dislikes that have been with us since childhood. Perhaps the world's most well-known food dislike comes from the forty-first president of the United States, George H. W. Bush: "I do not like broccoli and I haven't liked it since I was a little kid, and my mother made me eat it. And I'm president of the United States, and I'm not going to eat any more broccoli." My personal aversion is to coconuts. My father-in-law absolutely can't tolerate the thought of lima beans. His dislike is a good one that may involve heightened sensitivity to antinutrients in lima beans called cyanogenetic glycosides. When digested, these compounds are turned into the lethal poison hydrogen cyanide in our intestines. Fortunately, cooking eliminates most of the hydrogen cyanide in lima beans. Nevertheless, a number of fatal poisonings have been reported in the medical literature from people eating raw or undercooked lima beans.

Although most of us would never consider eating raw lima beans, the problem doesn't end here. When cooked, most of the hydrogen cyanide in lima beans is converted into a compound called thiocyanate, which, along with soy isoflavones, is a dietary antinutrient that impairs iodine metabolism and causes goiter. Remember that in iodine-deficient children, these so-called goitrogens are suspect dietary agents underlying autism.

Favism Glycosides

Most of us in the United States have never tasted broad beans, also known as fava or faba beans. In Mediterranean, Middle Eastern, and North African countries, broad beans are more popular. Unfortunately, for many people in these countries, particularly young children, the consumption of fava beans can be lethal. It has been intuitively known for centuries that fava bean consumption was fatal in certain people. Yet the biochemistry of the disease favism has been worked out only in the last fifty years or so.

Favism can only occur in people with a genetic defect called G6PD deficiency. This mutation is the most common human enzyme defect, which is present in more than four hundred million people worldwide. It is thought to confer protection against malaria. People whose genetic background can be traced to Italy, Greece, the Middle East, or North Africa are at a much higher risk for carrying this mutation.

If you or your children don't know whether you have the genes that cause favism, a simple blood test available at most hospitals and medical clinics can diagnose this problem. Consumption of fava beans in genetically susceptible people causes a massive rupturing of red blood cells that is called hemolytic anemia. It may frequently be fatal in small children unless blood transfusions are given immediately. Not all people with G6PD deficiency experience favism symptoms after they eat broad beans, but if your family background is from the Mediterranean region, you may be particularly susceptible.

Although it is not completely known how broad bean consumption causes favism, three antinutrient glycosides (divicine, isouramil, and convicine) found in these legumes likely do the damage. These compounds enter our bloodstream, and in people with the G6PD mutations they interact with red blood cells in a manner that causes them to rupture.

Peanuts and Heart Disease

What's wrong with peanut oil and peanuts? Most nutritional experts would tell us that they are heart-healthy foods because they contain little saturated fat and most of their fat is made up of cholesterol-lowering monounsaturated and polyunsaturated fats. On the surface, you might think that peanut oil would probably be helpful in preventing the artery-clogging process that underlies heart disease. Your thoughts were not much different from those of nutritional scientists—until they actually tested peanuts and peanut oil in laboratory animals.

Beginning in the 1960s and continuing into the 1980s, scientists unexpectedly found peanut oil to be highly atherogenic, causing arterial plaques to form in rabbits, rats, and primates. Only a single study showed otherwise. Peanut oil was found to be so atherogenic that it continues to be routinely fed to rabbits to produce atherosclerosis to study the disease.

Initially, it was unclear how a seemingly healthful oil could be so toxic in such a wide variety of animals. Dr. David Kritchevsky was able to show with a series of experiments that peanut oil lectin (PNA) was most likely responsible for its artery-clogging properties. Lectins are large protein molecules; most scientists had presumed that digestive enzymes in our guts would degrade lectins into their component amino acids. It was assumed that the intact lectin molecule would not be able to get into the bloodstream to do its dirty work. But they were wrong—it turned out that lectins were highly resistant to the gut's protein-degrading enzymes.

An experiment conducted by Dr. Wang and colleagues and published in the prestigious medical journal *Lancet* revealed that PNA got into the bloodstream intact in as few as one to four hours after subjects ate a handful of roasted, salted peanuts. Even though the concentrations of PNA in the subjects' blood were quite low, they were still at concentrations known to cause atherosclerosis in experimental animals. Lectins are a lot like super glue—it doesn't take much. These proteins can bind to a wide variety of cells in the body, including the cells lining the arteries. And indeed, it was found that PNA did its damage to the arteries by binding to a specific sugar receptor.

The takeaway is to stay away from both peanuts and peanut oil. There are much better options!

As you adopt the Paleo Diet or any diet, listen to your body. If a food or a food type doesn't agree with you or makes you feel ill or unwell, don't eat it. I should have listened to my own advice twenty-five years ago when I was experimenting with vegetarian diets. Whenever I ate beans or legumes, I experienced digestive upset and gas and frequently had diarrhea. Since I've embraced the Paleo Diet almost twenty years ago, these symptoms have become a thing of the past.

Paleo Bottom Line

Stay away from all beans, soy products, peanuts, and other legumes.

8

Potatoes Should Stay below Ground

S hould we be eating potatoes, sweet potatoes, yams, and other tubers, or not? Much new information has come out since I wrote *The Paleo Diet*. There was a time in my life back in the late 1970s and early 1980s when I thought that if I eliminated red meat, eggs, and other animal products and ate a mainly plant-based diet, I would become healthier, decrease my risk for developing heart disease and cancer, and live a longer, fuller life. Part of this conceptual package meant that I should replace meat proteins with whole grains, legumes, potatoes, and other tubers. I faithfully followed the recommendations of such vegetarian gurus of that time as Frances Moore Lappe, Dick Gregory, and others.

Once I started to eat in this manner, I immediately noticed gastrointestinal tract problems—bloating, gas, intermittent diarrhea, joint aches, back problems, increased upper respiratory illnesses, and an inability to train and run at higher intensities. The vegetarian diet books of that era simply told us that it would take time for our bodies to adjust to beans, legumes, whole grains, and tubers. Well, after months and months, my body never did adapt—my symptoms got worse, not better. I should have listened to my body, but no—I simply assumed that the nutritional experts of this era knew better than I, and that my symptoms must be some sort of anomaly.

Being a trusting soul, I continued with these nutritional experiments into my early and mid-thirties. Each and every time I went back to vegan/vegetarian dieting, everything about my health, well-being, and athletic performance declined. It took me a while to get it— diets based on whole grains, legumes, and tubers simply did not work in my body.

Even after all of these on-and-off-again experiments in my life, I tried plant-based diets one last time. Just before I got married and was approaching my fourth decade, I revisited vegetarian dieting. For breakfast, I would eat either brown rice, skimmed milk, and sliced bananas or a big bowl of boiled potatoes with salt and pepper. In those days, I typically got up and did a three- to five-mile run before 7:00 am and then ate breakfast. By 9:00 or 10:00 o'clock, I was famished and agitated, and it was all I could do to make it through until noon to put more high-starch, plant-based foods into my body. By 3:00 o'clock, I was in the same boat and couldn't wait to get home and eat more plant starch—brown rice, potatoes, chili beans—anything.

I'll never forget how bad early morning breakfasts of potatoes made me feel. They left me drained of energy and feeling nervous, agitated, and depressed—only a few hours after my morning meal. I lived with it.

In the early 1980s, a brand new concept called the glycemic index, developed by Dr. David Jenkins at the University of Toronto, had just emerged. It showed us that certain foods such as potatoes caused our blood sugar levels to precipitously rise and then dramatically fall. It was this effect that made me feel so bad. Potatoes for breakfast caused my blood sugar levels to spike—only to fall drastically below their original levels shortly thereafter.

Once I figured out how potatoes affected my body, I began to finally question whether vegetarian diets were nourishing or actually caused harmful effects. I now fully understand how potatoes are one of the worst foods we can eat. As with all plant foods, sporadic consumption of potatoes will have little impact on your overall health, but if you eat them regularly as the majority of your daily calories, your health will suffer. Let me explain why.

In the United States we eat a lot of potatoes. The per capita consumption of potato foods for every person in the United States in 2007 was 126 pounds. Out of that total, we ate

Frozen potatoes: 53 percent
Fresh potatoes: 44 percent
Potato chips: 16 percent
Dehydrated potatoes: 13 percent

From this breakdown, you can see that most of the potatoes consumed in the United States are highly processed in the form of french fries, mashed potatoes, dehydrated potato products, and potato chips. Processed potato foods typically are made with multiple additives—salt, vegetable oils, trans fats, refined sugars, dairy products, cereal grains, and preservatives—that may adversely affect our health in a variety of ways.

If we contrast this total consumption of potatoes with that of all refined sugars (137 pounds per capita) in the following list, you can see that as a country, we eat nearly as many potatoes as we do refined sugars:

Sucrose (table sugar): 62 percent
High fructose corn syrup: 56 percent
Glucose syrup and dextrose: 17 percent
Honey and other sweeteners: 2 percent

Let's take a look in the following table at the glycemic indices of various potato foods and contrast them with those of refined sugars, and you can clearly see that almost all potato products have glycemic indices that are substantially higher than sucrose—table sugar—or high-fructose corn syrup. Eating potatoes is a lot like eating pure sugars, but it's even worse for you because of the harm these starchy tubers do to your blood sugar levels.

Comparison of Glycemic Indices among Refined Sugars and Potato Foods

Item	Glycemic Index
Potato Foods	
Russet Burbank potatoes, baked without fat	111
Potato, white without skin, baked	98
Pontiac potato, peeled and baked	93
Red potatoes, boiled with skin	89
Sebago potato, peeled, boiled 35 min	87
Mashed potatoes	83
French fries, frozen, reheated in microwave	75
Potato chips	60
Refined Sugars	
Glucose (dextrose)	100
Sucrose	60–65
High-fructose corn syrup	60–65
Honey	48

It is obvious why those potato breakfasts I ate twenty-five years ago made me feel so awful. I may just as well have been consuming pure sugar or several candy bars for breakfast.

Because potatoes maintain one of the highest glycemic index values of any food, they cause our blood sugar levels to rise rapidly, which in turn immediately makes our blood insulin concentrations increase. When these two metabolic responses occur repeatedly for a week or two, we start to become insulin resistant—a condition that frequently precedes the development of a series of diseases known as the metabolic syndrome.

During the course of months and years, insulin resistance leads to a multitude of devastating health effects. The list of metabolic syndrome diseases is long: obesity, type 2 diabetes, cardiovascular disease, high blood pressure, high blood cholesterol and other abnormal blood chemistries, systemic inflammation, gout, acne, skin tags, and breast, colon, and prostate cancers. The Paleo Diet is your best medicine for the metabolic syndrome because it eliminates not only high-glycemic potatoes from your diet, but also virtually every other food that spikes your blood sugar levels. When you trade in potatoes, grains, dairy, and processed foods for fresh fruits, veggies, meat, and seafood, diseases of insulin resistance and the metabolic syndrome will no longer trouble you. A wonderful success story was sent to me by Dr. Lane Sebring M.D., a general practitioner whose first prescription for his metabolic syndrome patients is *The Paleo Diet*.

Curing Metabolic Syndrome: Dr. Lane Sebring's Story

About half of the new patients to my clinic know I am a strong proponent of the Paleo Diet before they get here, and about one-third have either read or just purchased *The Paleo Diet*. It truly is the best tool I have to help my patients. One day a forty-three-year-old, 5'8", 224 pound man—a pack-and-a-half-a-day smoker who had been on blood pressure meds for three years—was brought in by his wife, complaining of blurry vision. I noticed that he had lost 9 pounds since I last saw him, and his blood pressure was 170/100. I also noticed that his neck was smaller since I last saw him—more than you would expect with a 9-pound weight loss, something I've seen with new-onset diabetes. I asked him whether he had been getting up a lot in the middle of the night to go to the bathroom. He said, "Yes, how did you know?"

I checked his blood sugar, and it was 611. I increased his blood pressure medication and told him about diabetes. I started him on Avandia for diabetes and told him to read *The Paleo Diet*. Well, he didn't read it, but his wife did. She took away his lunch money and brought him lunch. At the two-week follow-up visit, he had lost about 3 more pounds and was complaining about no salt and no potatoes, but his blood pressure was fine, and his blood glucose was

254. I gave him some more samples and a script and told him to come back in eight weeks.

At follow-up, he had lost about 4 pounds, his blood glucose was 79, and blood pressure was 112/72, so I praised him and his wife for their good work. The wife then said almost apologetically, "Dr. Sebring, I'm sorry, but we just couldn't afford the prescription you gave us. He hasn't taken any pills at all in three weeks."

He weighs 178 pounds now and is no longer diabetic or hypertensive, and you couldn't get him off the diet.

Dr. Sebring's success in curing metabolic syndrome diseases in his patients are not isolated examples, as I have had people from all over the world and from all walks of life contact me.

Root and Tuber Vegetables

Approximately ninety-six vegetable crops are grown worldwide that fit under the catch-all phrase "roots and tubers." Root and tuber vegetables are actually the underground food-storage organs of various plants. These edible below-ground organs are classified into one of five categories:

1. Roots
2. Tubers
3. Rhizomes
4. Corms
5. Bulbs

Some commonly consumed roots are carrots, parsnips, radishes, beets, rutabagas, sweet potatoes, cassava, and celeriac. Frequently eaten tubers include potatoes and yams. Examples of edible rhizomes are arrowroot, ginger, and turmeric. Corms include taro and Chinese water chestnuts; common edible bulbs include onions and garlic. Crops with an enlarged stem, such as leeks and kohlrabi, even when located underground, are generally not classified as roots and tubers.

The table below lists fourteen roots and tubers that can be found in most well-stocked supermarkets or outlets specializing in produce.

Let's compare how other roots and tubers stack up to potatoes in regard to their glycemic indices and glycemic loads. The glycemic load is determined by multiplying the glycemic index by the carbohydrate content in a standard serving (100g). This calculation is a better overall measure than the glycemic index for how a food affects our blood glucose and insulin levels. Before the glycemic load was developed in 1997, foods with glycemic indices of greater than 70 were classified as high-glycemic foods. From the table, however, you can see that by applying the glycemic load concept,

Caloric Content, Carbohydrate Content, Glycemic Index, and Glycemic Load of Common Root Vegetables (100 g [around ¼ lb.] samples)

	Kcal(g)	CHO	Glycemic Index	Glycemic Load
Cassava (manioc, tapioca)	160	38.1	70	26.6
Potato, baked	109	25.2	85	21.4
Taro	142	34.6	55	19.0
Parsnips	81	19.5	97	18.9
Sweet potato, baked	103	24.3	61	14.8
Yam	116	27.6	37	10.2
Beet	44	10.0	64	6.4
Rutabagas	39	8.7	72	6.3
Carrots	45	10.5	47	4.9
Jerusalem artichoke	76	17.4	na	na
Chicory	73	17.5	na	na
Burdock root	72	17.4	na	na
Celeriac	42	9.2	na	na
Turnip	27	6.2	na	na

some roots and tubers with high-glycemic indices don't necessarily maintain high-glycemic loads.

My recommendation for overweight subjects or for people with diseases of insulin resistance—type 2 diabetes, hypertension, dyslipidemia (elevated triglycerides, low HDL, elevated small dense LDL), coronary heart disease, gout, and acne—is not to exceed a glycemic load of 10 for any given meal and to keep the day's glycemic load under 40. If you look at the table carefully, you can see that a 100g (around ¼ lb.) serving of baked potato would provide you with half of your daily glycemic-load allotment. Not a good choice, for many reasons. A similar serving of sweet potato would be a better choice, with a glycemic load of 14.8; better choices still would be beets, rutabagas, or carrots, which under normal circumstances you can basically eat until you are full, as it would be quite difficult to consume enough of these foods to exceed a daily glycemic load of 40. Although glycemic index and load values for celeriac have not yet been determined, the amount of carbohydrate per 100g (9.2g) is similar to that for beets, rutabagas, and carrots. It is likely that celeriac has a similar low glycemic load and presents no problems. The same goes for turnips. Enjoy these healthful root and tuber vegetables.

Remember the 85/15 rule—meaning that if one is 85 percent compliant with the diet most of the time, significant improvements in health could occur. I still adhere to this principle, and I believe that minor dietary indiscretions involving potatoes, sweet potatoes, or any other root or tuber on an occasional basis will have few unfavorable effects on your long-term health. In fact, for highly fit athletes or for healthy, normal-weight individuals who do a significant amount of exercise on a daily basis, sweet potatoes and yams represent a good source of carbohydrates, which are necessary to replenish your muscles' spent glycogen stores. All tubers are net base (alkaline) yielding vegetables; accordingly, they represent superior carbohydrate sources, compared to cereal grains, because they do not leach calcium from our bones or amino acids from our muscles, as do acid-yielding grains. Additionally, when fully cooked and peeled, these vegetables maintain low concentrations of antinutrients known to be harmful to our health. The two exceptions to this general rule are potatoes and cassava, both of which contain a number of antinutrients that, when present in high concentrations, can be either toxic or even lethal.

We rarely consume cassava in the United States except as tapioca, and you can see from the previous table that it has an exceptionally high glycemic load. This characteristic alone should make us shy away from eating this starchy root. Cassava, like lima beans, contains an antinutrient called cyanogenic glycoside, which, unless cooked sufficiently, can be converted into hydrogen cyanide, a deadly poison. Even when fully cooked, cassava root's cyanogenic glycosides are converted into thiocyanates, which may aggravate iodine deficiencies.

Potato Antinutrients

Cereal grains and legumes contain many antinutrients, which I discuss in the chapters devoted to those foods; these compounds may have far-reaching effects on the quality of our diet and health. Unfortunately, most nutritionists have zero knowledge of antinutrients—much less how they may impair body function and promote disease. Even governmental and private agencies that determine and influence national nutritional policy have largely ignored these toxic dietary elements. As was the case with whole grains and legumes, potatoes are laden with antinutrients including saponins, lectins, and protease inhibitors.

Saponins

I can almost guarantee that if you ask your family physician about dietary saponins and your health, he or she will draw a complete blank. The same can be said for ADA-trained nutritionists at your local hospital or clinic. Even astute complementary health-care practitioners are usually in the dark when it comes to saponins in our daily food supply. Despite a mountain of scientific evidence showing that these compounds can be potent and even lethal toxins, they are rarely considered dietary threats to our health.

Saponins derive their name from their ability to form soaplike foams when mixed with water. Chemically, certain potato saponins are commonly referred to as glycoalkaloids. Their function is to protect the potato plant's root (tuber) from microbial and insect attack. When consumed by potential predators, glycoalkaloids protect the potato because they act as a toxin. These compounds exert their toxic effects by dissolving cell membranes. When rodents and larger animals, including humans, eat glycoalkaloid-containing tubers such as potatoes, these substances frequently create holes in the gut lining, thereby increasing intestinal permeability. If glycoalkaloids enter our bloodstream in sufficient concentrations, they destroy the cell membranes of our red blood cells.

The following illustration shows how glycoalkaloids and saponins in general disrupt cell membranes, which leads to a leaky gut or red blood cell ruptures. These compounds first bind to cholesterol molecules in cell membranes, and in steps 1 through 4 you can see how saponins cause portions of the cell membrane to buckle and eventually break free, thus forming a pore or a hole in the membrane.

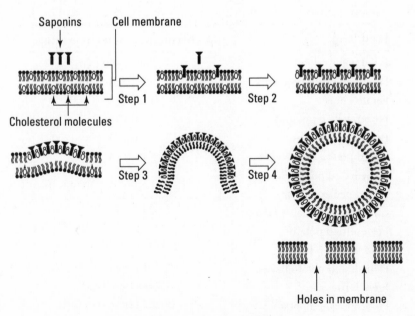

How Saponins Lead to Leaky Gut

Potatoes contain two glycoalkaloid saponins—α-chaconine and α-solanine—that may adversely affect intestinal permeability and aggravate inflammatory bowel diseases, including ulcerative colitis, Crohn's disease, and irritable bowel syndrome. Even in healthy normal adults, a meal of mashed potatoes results in the rapid appearance of both α-chaconine and α-solanine in the bloodstream. The toxicity of these two glycoalkaloids is dose dependent—meaning that the greater the concentration in the bloodstream, the greater is their toxic effect. At least twelve separate cases of human poisoning from potato consumption, involving nearly two thousand people and thirty fatalities, have been recorded in the medical literature. Potato saponins can be lethally toxic once in the bloodstream in sufficient concentrations because these glycoalkaloids inhibit a key enzyme, acetyl cholinesterase, which is required for nerve impulse conduction. The levels of both α-chaconine and α-solanine in a variety of potato foods are listed in the following table. Consumers beware!

Concentrations (mg/kg) of Total Glycoalkaloids (α-chaconine + α-solanine) in a Variety of Potato Foods

Food Item	α-chaconine + α-solanine (mg/kg)
Fried potato skins	567–1450
Potato chips with skins	95–720
Potato chips	23–180
Frozen baked potatoes	80–123
Frozen potato skins	65–121
Baked potato with jacket	99–113
Dehydrated potato flour	65–75
Boiled peeled potato	27–42
Canned whole new potatoes	24–34
Frozen fried potato	4–31
Frozen french fries	2–29
Dehydrated potato flakes	15–23
French fries	0.4–8
Frozen mashed potatoes	2–5
Canned peeled potato	1–2

Note that the highest concentrations of these toxic glycoalkaloids occur in potato skins. Fried potato skins filled with chili and topped off by sour cream and jalapeno peppers are a real gut bomb with devastating effects on your intestinal permeability. If you ate enough of these hors d'oeuvres, they could literally kill you.

The next logical question arises: should we be eating a food that contains two known toxins that rapidly enter the bloodstream, increase intestinal permeability, and potentially impair the nervous and circulatory systems?

In the opinion of Dr. Patel, "If the potato were to be introduced today as a novel food it is likely that its use would not be approved because of the presence of these toxic compounds."

In a comprehensive review of potato glycoalkaloids, Dr. Smith voiced similar sentiments:

> Available information suggest that the susceptibility of humans to glycoalkaloid poisoning is both high and very variable: oral doses in the range 1–5 mg/kg body weight are marginally to severely toxic to humans whereas 3–6 mg/kg body weight can be lethal. The narrow margin between toxicity and lethality is obviously of concern. Although serious glycoalkaloid poisoning of humans is rare, there is a widely held suspicion that mild poisoning is more prevalent than supposed.

The commonly accepted safe limit for total glycoalkaloids in potato foods is 200 mg/kg, a level proposed more than seventy years ago, whereas more recent evidence suggests this level should be lowered to 60–70 mg/kg. In the previous table, you can see that many potato food products exceed this recommendation.

I believe that far more troubling than the toxicity of potato glycoalkaloids is their potential to increase intestinal permeability during the course of a lifetime, most particularly in people with diseases of chronic inflammation—cancer, autoimmune diseases, cardiovascular disease, and diseases of insulin resistance. Many scientists now believe that a leaky gut may represent a nearly universal trigger for autoimmune diseases.

When the gut becomes leaky, it is not a good thing, as the intestinal contents may have access to the immune system, which in turn becomes activated, thereby causing a chronic low-level systemic inflammation known as endotoxemia. In particular, a cell wall component of gut gram negative bacteria called lipopolysaccharide (LPS) is highly inflammatory. Any LPS that gets past the gut barrier is immediately engulfed by two types of immune system cells. Once engulfed by these immune cells, LPS binds to a receptor on these cells, causing a cascade of effects that leads to increases in blood concentrations of pro-inflammatory hormones. Two recent human studies have shown that high-potato diets increase the blood inflammatory marker IL-6. Without chronic low-level systemic inflammation, it is unlikely that few of the classic diseases of civilization—cancer, cardiovascular disease, autoimmune diseases, and diseases of insulin resistance—would have an opportunity to take hold and inflict their fatal effects.

A final note on potatoes: This commonly consumed food is also a major source of dietary lectins. On average, potatoes contain 65 mg of potato lectins per kilogram. As is the case with most lectins, they have been poorly studied in humans, so we really don't have conclusive information on how potato lectins may affect human health. Yet preliminary tissue studies indicate that potato lectins resist degradation by gut enzymes, bypasses the intestinal barrier, and can then bind to various tissues in our bodies. Potato lectins have been found to irritate the immune system and produce symptoms of food hypersensitivity in allergenic and nonallergenic patients.

Root and tuber vegetables such as sweet potatoes, yams, beets, carrots, turnips, and others are nutritious, tasty additions to the Paleo Diet. These foods complement the staples of modern-day Stone Age diets, and I encourage you to regularly include them in your diet.

Paleo Bottom Line

Don't eat potatoes or cassava; all other root vegetables are generally okay.

9

The Food–Autoimmune
Disease Connection

M ost of us complete our education by our late teens or early
twenties and move on to our adult lives and careers. I took a
different track—I have never left school. I have returned to school
nearly every fall of my life since my mother first enrolled me in
kindergarten at Arthur Amos Noyes Elementary School in Altadena,
California in 1955.

As I look back on my fifty-six years of school, I have many fond
memories of the places I have visited and the people I have known.
Yet perhaps the most important aspect of my long academic career
are the people whose lives have been forever changed by the Paleo
Diet. I believe that one of the most important previously unrecognized effects of the Paleo Diet is its potential to ameliorate or cure
symptoms of autoimmune disease.

When I wrote *The Paleo Diet*, I was relatively certain that the
nutritional principles I laid out could powerfully improve people's
quality of life and cause the remission of many chronic diseases.
I knew that this lifetime way of eating might positively affect or
even cure certain autoimmune diseases. Together with my graduate

students, we wrote an innovative scientific paper published more than ten years ago in the *British Journal of Nutrition* describing how modern-day Paleo diets might be effective in combating rheumatoid arthritis and other autoimmune diseases.

At the time, we simply couldn't prove our case because we didn't have either anecdotal patient reports or scientific confirmation of our theories. In the ensuing decade since I wrote this scientific paper, I now know that diets devoid of cereals, dairy, and legumes can have positive and often dramatic outcomes in people suffering from these crippling, life-threatening diseases. Here are some stories sent to me by people afflicted with various autoimmune diseases.

Multiple Sclerosis in Remission: Linda's Story

In 1980, my husband, Dr. Rich Land, was handed an amazing gift of information that helped him recover from multiple sclerosis. At the time, we didn't know why the diet-restriction and supplement-based suggestions worked; we were simply grateful that they facilitated the full remission. Years later, when I learned that our children might be genetically predisposed to the cluster effect of autoimmune diseases, I began to look for research that could explain my husband's recovery and possibly lead to preventative measures. The quest initially located, as with most puzzle work, a few perimeter pieces. The bulk of the puzzle pieces fell into place, however, when I was introduced to Dr. Cordain.

I had heard of Dr. Cordain's research in the area of autoimmune disease and was invited to attend a consultation with him for someone newly diagnosed with MS. He had the cutting-edge research that validated the recovery strategy from all of those years ago, and I had two thirty-year-long recovery examples affirming his work. On completion of the puzzle, by locating the other factors that contributed to my husband's health crash, I felt an enormous responsibility to share the discoveries.

Because of Dr. Cordain's validating research, we've been able to suggest to our children that they proactively modify their diets as a preventative measure. And, with the recent publication of my book *The Gift of Remission*, I can pass along the gift of hope and healing to those who need it immediately and raise awareness of those who might be setting themselves up for a devastating illness. I will always be incredibly grateful to Dr. Cordain for his research and will look forward to funding autoimmune disease research from the book's proceeds.

Ulcerative Colitis: Beth's Story

I started the Paleo Diet eight months ago. I have lost 52 pounds, and I went from a size 22 to a size 12. While I'm thrilled with the weight loss, the thing that I am most happy about is my health. I had been suffering with irritable bowel syndrome (IBS) for five years and ulcerative colitis for two years. Both of these conditions have virtually disappeared since I have started eating Paleo.

I used to deal with IBS on a daily basis, and it was beginning to interfere with my work and social environments. Now I never experience the embarrassing and painful attacks that I suffered after every meal. (I have to be careful with any Open Meals because they can sometimes bring about an episode of IBS that serves as my incentive to stick to the diet.)

I am still taking my ulcerative colitis medication; however, I intend to discuss stopping it at my next visit with my doctor. My doctors have told me that the only cure for ulcerative colitis is surgery, but I truly believe that this diet is the cure for me. My family, friends, and coworkers are amazed at what this diet has done for me. Many of them are trying out the Paleo Diet themselves!

Rheumatoid Arthritis: Bill's Story

I have just recently read your article "Modulation of Immune Function by Dietary Lectins in Rheumatoid Arthritis" (*British Journal of Nutrition* 83 [2000]: 207–217) and find this is the best explanation of the joint problems I've been having for the last two and a half years. The attacks I've had are of arthritic characteristics, red hot, swollen, and very painful. The attacks are random and becoming more frequent to the point where I have been bedridden. Since reading your article, I have stopped eating grains and now find my joints are beginning to feel much better, so much so, that I have stopped taking prescription anti-inflammatory drugs.

Ankylosing Spondylitis: Peter's Story

I am a medical scientist (specializing in infectious diseases) based in Johannesburg, South Africa. My wife is an M.D. who has suffered from ankylosing spondylitis [a systemic autoimmune disease mainly involving the joints] for many years. As a family we made a decision to adopt a Paleo diet, and we are astounded by the results. My wife has essentially gone into remission and has gone off all medication for the last three years. She can now carry a 20-pound toddler up a mountain without any physical problems or inflammation. For myself, my antithyroid antibodies and inflammatory markers have dropped to zero. We are so astounded by the improvement in quality of life that this diet has caused for us and other friends and family members, we have become a bit like religious zealots in singing its praises for all manner of autoimmune disorders and ADD. I must thank you for some excellent and thorough research in the form of your books and peer-reviewed articles.

These stories are amazing. I have heard them time and again over the years. Not only have Paleo Dieters written to me—so have their physicians. These medical professionals have repeatedly informed me that when they put their patients on Paleo diets, many of their clients experienced improvements or even complete remission of various autoimmune disease symptoms. In science, nonexperimental information doesn't get you very far in the refereed scientific literature, and rightly so—without rigorous experimental control, it is difficult or impossible to show cause and effect. Still, it is hard for me to ignore the personal victories achieved by auto-immune patients all over the world when they adopt modern-day Paleo diets.

I would prefer to offer my scientific colleagues meta analyses (comprehensive summaries of all studies) of randomized controlled human trials showing that contemporary Paleo diets improve autoimmune disease symptoms. Unfortunately, these analyses have yet to be conducted and lie years in the future—long after I will retire from academic life. So the best evidence I can give you about autoimmune diseases and diet comes from animal, tissue, and epidemiological studies.

I want to share with you experiences I have directly witnessed that support the viewpoint that modern-day Paleo diets may improve or cure some autoimmune diseases.

In September 2009, I was privileged to speak before a large audience of CrossFit enthusiasts in San Diego, California. One of the organizers of the event, Joe, had been eating Paleo for more than two years and was loving it. His blood pressure and cholesterol levels had normalized for the first time in years, and he told me that he now slept "like a rock" and was fully energized throughout the day. He was so impressed with the benefits of this way of eating that he had recommended it to his mother, almost a year earlier. Joe's mom is a wonderful lady who came up to the podium and congratulated me after my talk. She proudly informed me of her brand-new head of thick, full hair. Her stylishly coiffed locks looked great to me. Little did I know that a year earlier, she had been suffering from an autoimmune disease, alopecia areata, that causes splotchy hair loss. For me, Joe's mom's triumph over alopecia epitomizes the life-altering elements that the Paleo Diet may bring to many people.

As I left the stage and began to mingle with the overflowing crowd, a fit young woman approached me with her little daughter. I glanced to my right and immediately saw that the mother's eyes were welling up with tears as she reached out to shake my hand. She came closer, hugged me, and said, "Thank you, your diet has saved my little girl's life." This woman was JoAnne, and her daughter's success story and remission are included in chapter 14. I was overwhelmed.

I finally made my way through the audience, took my tie off, and began to joke around with Joe, Robb Wolf, and John Welbourne, the other speakers at this event. Just when I thought things couldn't get any better, a young man who knew Robb approached us and introduced himself.

James was a CrossFitter who had adopted the Paleo Diet solely to improve his physical fitness. Originally, he had no idea that diets free of grains, dairy, and legumes could improve a condition called vitiligo that had plagued him for years. Vitiligo is an autoimmune disease that causes the skin to turn a blotchy white color as skin pigmentation is progressively destroyed by the immune system.

James proudly showed me before and after photographs of his body. Ten months earlier, about 75 percent of his skin had been mottled with blotchy white spots, but photos taken a week before my lecture revealed an extraordinary improvement after nearly a year on the Paleo Diet. Less than 20 percent of his skin remained afflicted by this disease.

An afternoon that started with my PowerPoint presentation about the therapeutic health advantages of modern-day Paleo diets had ended with three remarkable success stories of people whose lives were forever changed by returning to our ancestral way of eating. For me, these heartwarming, life-changing accounts are more gratifying than all of the academic and professional awards that I have received in my career.

Autoimmune Diseases: Medical Science's Black Box

One of the last great frontiers for medicine is to unravel the underlying causes of autoimmune disease. Although scientists have made enormous gains in understanding how dietary and environmental factors may promote heart disease and cancer, we are still in the dark ages with our knowledge of how environment may influence the development of autoimmune diseases.

More than a hundred specific diseases are known to be autoimmune in nature. The table below shows some common ones.

After cardiovascular disease and cancer, autoimmune diseases are the most common group of illnesses in the United States, affecting between 14.7 and 23.5 million people, or 5 to 8 percent of the population. The burden of these diseases disproportionately falls on women, who sustain 78.8 percent of all cases of autoimmune

Disease	Tissue/Organ Affected	Prevalence in Population
Alopecia areata	Hair follicle	170 per 100,000
Ankylosing spondylitis	Spine and sacroiliac joints	129 per 100,000
Autoimmune uticaria	Skin	330 per 100,000
Celiac disease	Small intestine	400 per 100,000
Crohn's disease	Gastrointestinal tract	184 per 100,000
Diabetes, type 1	Pancreas	120 per 100,000
Graves' disease	Thyroid gland	1,120 per 100,000
Hashimoto's thyroiditis	Thyroid gland	9,460 per 100,000
Lupus erythematosus	Any tissue in the body	510 per 100,000
Multiple sclerosis	Brain, nerves	140 per 100,000
Psoriasis	Skin	2,020 per 100,000
Rheumatoid arthritis	Joints	920 per 100,000
Scleroderma	Skin, other organs	110 per 100,000
Ulcerative colitis	Colon	35–100 per 100,000
Uveitis	Anterior eye	850 per 100,000
Vitiligo	Skin	740 per 100,000

diseases. These diseases collectively are among the top ten leading causes of death for women in every age group up to age sixty-four.

Autoimmune diseases occur when the body's immune system loses its capacity to discriminate between "self" and "non-self," attacking healthy tissues and organs as if they were foreign invaders. One unexpected fact about autoimmune diseases is that environmental factors represent 70 percent of the risk for developing these illnesses. Genetics play a smaller role, with 30 percent of the risk being attributed to inherited elements.

Up until the last five to ten years, autoimmune diseases were the black boxes of the medical world. We really had no idea how or why environmental factors triggered these illnesses in genetically susceptible people. Some remarkable developments have occurred in the last five years, chiefly from Dr. Alessio Fasano at the University of Maryland Center for Celiac Research, which have helped unravel the mysteries underlying autoimmune diseases. Work by Dr. Fasano's group, as well as by other scientists worldwide, shows that a leaky gut or increased intestinal permeability plays a vital initial step in initiating some, if not all, autoimmune diseases.

I quote from Dr. Fasano's paper on celiac disease in the August 2009 issue of *Scientific American*: "Surprisingly, essentially the same trio—an environmental trigger, a genetic susceptibility and a leaky gut—seem to underlie other autoimmune disorders as well." Dr. Fasano's revealing conclusion dovetails with the results of my scientific publication on rheumatoid arthritis more than ten years earlier, in which I also suggested that a leaky gut precedes and initiates many autoimmune diseases in genetically predisposed people.

Grains and Leaky Gut

When I was a little boy, I remember my mother reading fairy tales to me. One that has struck me to this day was Hans Christian Andersen's "The Emperor's New Clothes."

As a researcher, the lifelong message I have learned from this fairy tale is that stating the obvious—"The emperor is wearing nothing at all"—is frequently the most difficult admission for all of us, including scientists. When we engage in a specific behavior that doesn't immediately harm us or cause apparent disease, it is difficult to determine whether our communal practice is unsafe.

Case in point—cigarette smoking. In the United States, cigarettes were first commercially manufactured in 1864 and became wildly popular after World War II. Unfortunately, at that time, most people had no idea smoking was dangerous. Finally, after nearly a hundred years, with the publication of the "Surgeon General's 1964 Report on Smoking and Health," the obvious was plainly stated—cigarette smoking was disastrous to our health.

Let me be the first to state the obvious—eating wheat is disastrous to the health of all autoimmune patients. Incredibly, wheat—consumed by nearly every person on earth, has been found to be one of the chief perpetrators of a leaky gut, not only in autoimmune patients, but also in some healthy normal people. Wheat contains a protein called *gliadin* that interacts with gut receptors to set off a cascade of hormonal events, which ultimately allows the intestinal contents—food and bacteria—to interact with the immune system. Gliadin is not the only problem. Wheat contains two other compounds, wheat germ agglutinin (WGA) and thaumatin-like proteins, which also increase intestinal permeability. Withdrawal of wheat and all gluten-containing cereals (rye and barley) from celiac patients completely cures their disease symptoms.

Increasingly, scientific evidence shows that this strategy may work for many other autoimmune diseases. The elimination of gluten-containing grains from your diet may even have numerous favorable health effects that aren't necessarily limited to autoimmune illnesses.

Other Leaky Gut Dietary Triggers

With the discovery that a leaky gut probably represents an essential first step in the development of autoimmunity, it became apparent to me and my fellow researchers that any dietary element capable of increasing intestinal permeability should also be suspect in autoimmune illnesses. As we combed through the scientific literature, we discovered the following list of foods and substances, in addition to gliadin in wheat, rye, and barley, that also promote a leaky gut.

- Many lectin-containing foods
- Many saponin/glycoalkaloid–containing foods
- Capsaicin-containing chili peppers
- Alcohol
- NSAIDS (non-steroidal anti-inflammatory drugs: aspirin, ibuprofen, naproxen)
- Oral contraceptives
- Antacids that contain aluminum hydroxide

Lectin-Containing Foods

At first glance, the previous list doesn't seem remarkable, as you may be unfamiliar with all of the common foods that contain lectins, saponins, glycoalkaloids, and capsaicin. Let me be a little more blunt and point out the problematic foods. Let's first start with lectins. Almost all grains and legumes contain lectins, most of which promote a leaky gut. We are beginning to understand why the Paleo Diet, a grain- and legume-free diet, has such potent healing effects in autoimmune patients—it is virtually free of the lectins that may increase intestinal permeability. By eliminating grains and legumes from our diets, intestinal function returns to normal, and toxins within our guts can no longer cross the gut barrier and interact with our immune systems to elicit autoimmune diseases.

Lectin-containing foods that autoimmune patients should avoid are

1. All commonly consumed cereal grains, including wheat, rye, barley, oats, corn, and rice—note that rice is probably the least damaging grain.
2. All beans and legumes.

3. Potatoes and tomatoes.
4. All pseudo grains, including amaranth, quinoa, buckwheat, and chia seeds.

Almost all plant foods contain lectins, but most seem to be benign when it comes to our health, except for lectins in grains, legumes, and a few other foods that may enter our bloodstream and interact with most cells in our bodies, including those in our immune systems.

Saponins and Leaky Gut

My current insight into how the Paleo Diet may prove to be therapeutic for autoimmune disease patients involves saponins—toxic compounds found in many plants that ward off microbial and insect attacks. A specific subcategory of saponins found in nightshade plants such as tomatoes and potatoes are called glycoalkaloids, which I will discuss later in the chapter. Unfortunately, saponins are noxious not only for insects and microbes that eat plants containing these compounds, but also for humans. As I pointed out, if we eat saponins in high enough amounts, they can become lethally toxic. Even at low doses, they may cause a leaky gut. Beans, legumes, potatoes, and soy products are concentrated sources of gut-permeating saponins. This is why the Paleo Diet is such a good remedy for autoimmune patients, as these foods are not on the menu.

When I first wrote *The Paleo Diet*, I counseled you not to eat potatoes, chiefly because of their high glycemic load, which may impair blood sugar and insulin levels. In retrospect, this recommendation is also good advice for autoimmune patients. I now know that potatoes contain two specific saponins called glycoalkaloids, α-solanine and α-chaconine, which may increase intestinal permeability. By purging potatoes from your diet, you not only prevent blood glucose and insulin surges, but also prevent a leaky gut and autoimmune diseases and allergies.

A couple of other saponin-containing foods you should definitely avoid if you suffer from an autoimmune disease are alfalfa sprouts and quillaja extract. In the 1970s, I remember visiting my local co-op in Eugene, Oregon, and purchasing alfalfa seeds, along with a kit to sprout them. What could be healthier than home-grown alfalfa sprouts eaten fresh from my own kitchen? Back in the day, except for a few obscure scientific papers, there was virtually no data suggesting that dietary saponins were harmful.

We now know better. Alfalfa sprouts contain some of the highest concentrations of saponins (8,000 mg/kg) found in any food, along with another antinutrient called L-canavanine that is known to cause lupus (a systemic autoimmune disease) in monkeys and perhaps humans.

Quillaja (sometime called quillaia) extract is probably unknown to everyone who reads this book, except for the most vigilant label reader of processed foods or to immunologists. Quillaja is a saponin that is derived from the bark of a South American tree and used by the food-processing industry to cause beverages to foam. Who wants to drink root beer without a good head of foam? Many commercial root beers and soft drinks contain significant amounts of quillaja extract, which is limited by the USDA to 100 mg per liter of beverage. Even at these low concentrations, quillaja is known to be one of the most potent saponins ever discovered because it powerfully stimulates the immune system. So much so, that tiny amounts of this compound are routinely added to vaccines to boost their effectiveness. The last thing in the world that autoimmune patients want is for their immune systems to become even more agitated. If you have an autoimmune disease, definitely cross off quillaja-containing root beer and soft drinks from your menu.

The list of saponin-containing foods to be avoided by people with autoimmune diseases is similar to the list of lectin-containing foods:

1. All beans and legumes
2. Potatoes and tomatoes
3. All pseudo grains, including amaranth, quinoa, buckwheat, and chia seeds

Besides contributing to a leaky gut, certain dietary saponins agitate the immune system in a manner that makes it much more likely to cause an autoimmune disease. The bottom line is, if you have an autoimmune disease, you should avoid foods that are concentrated sources of saponins.

Nightshades and Autoimmune Disease

Potatoes are concentrated sources of saponins, but these starchy tubers are just one of many commonly consumed foods that belong to the nightshade family of plants. Some notorious inedible night-shades include tobacco, petunias, jimson weed, mandrake, and deadly nightshade.

The nightshade family comprises plant foods most of us eat every day, such as potatoes, tomatoes, green peppers, chili peppers, eggplants, and tomatillos. Tomatoes, particularly when consumed unripe or green, are a significant source of saponins, which can increase intestinal permeability. Virtually all chili peppers contain a chemical called capsaicin, which compromises intestinal func-tion, causing it to become leaky. Note that chili peppers include all varieties, such as bell peppers, jalapeño, wax, cayenne, habañero, Anaheim, Thai, Tabasco, cherry, pepperoncini, and serrano, among others. We frequently eat chili peppers as dried spices such as paprika, chili powder, and cayenne and also as key ingredients in salsas, hot sauces, and Tabasco sauces. The table on page 174 shows the per capita consumption of commonly consumed nightshades in the U.S. diet.

You can see that nightshades are a staple food, almost univer-sally consumed in our diets. Are there any health hazards associ-ated with eating almost 230 pounds of nightshades on a yearly basis?

There are *huge* problems with eating more than 200 pounds of nightshades per year. Potatoes are nightshades that represent a major contributor to the high glycemic load in the U.S. diet and to diseases associated with high-glycemic-index foods. More important,

U.S. per Capita Consumption
of Nightshades

Item	Pounds
Potatoes (total)	126
Frozen	53
Fresh	44
Chips	16
Dehydrated	13
Fresh Tomatoes	18.5
Processed Tomatoes (total)	67.2
Tomato sauces	23.5
Tomato paste	12.1
Canned whole tomatoes	11.4
Ketchup	10.1
Tomato juice	10.1
Bell peppers	9.1
Chili peppers	6.4
Eggplant	0.8
Total	**228**

for people with autoimmune diseases, these starchy foods increase intestinal permeability—one of the key events suspected in triggering these illnesses.

I believe that nightshade plants represent a significant risk for anybody suffering from autoimmune diseases or allergies. Nevertheless, except for potatoes, these foods pose little or no danger for most healthy people and in fact may contribute numerous vitamins, minerals, and phytochemicals that have a positive effect on our health and well-being. Yet if you are afflicted with one of the hundred or more known autoimmune diseases, you need to proceed cautiously with these foods. Here's why.

Tomatoes

In addition to potatoes, tomatoes represent another nightshade food that increases intestinal permeability. The primary saponin in tomatoes that causes a leaky gut is called α-tomatine. The next table shows the concentration of α-tomatine in a variety of tomatoes and tomato food products.

Note that smaller and unripe tomatoes have markedly increased levels of α-tomatine, whereas this compound is barely detectable in a standard ripe, red tomato. By contrast, ketchup, green salsa,

α-Tomatine Concentrations (mg/kg) in Tomatoes and Tomato Food Products

Item	α-tomatine (mg/kg)
Unripe, small immature green	548
Unripe, medium immature green	169
Pickled green tomatoes (Brand A)	71.5
Unripe, pickled green	28
Pickled green tomatoes (Brand B)	28
Green salsa	27.5
Sun-dried red tomatoes	21
Unripe, green large	16
Unripe, large immature green	10
Sungold cherry tomatoes	11
Fried green tomatoes	11
Microwaved green tomatoes	11
Yellow cherry tomatoes	9.7
Ketchup	8.6
Red sauce	5.7
Yellow pear cherry tomatoes	4.5
Tomato juice	2.8
Red cherry tomatoes	2.7
Condensed tomato soup	2.2
Red pear cherry tomatoes	1.3
Medium yellow tomatoes	1.3
Large yellow tomatoes	1.1
Stewed canned tomatoes	1.1
Ripe red beefsteak tomato	0.9
Green zebra tomatoes	0.6
Roma	0.4
Standard red ripe tomato	0.3

pickled green tomatoes, and cherry tomatoes are all potent sources of α-tomatine. Although tomatoes typically have lower concentrations of α-tomatine than potatoes have α-solanine and α-chaconine, α-tomatine in tomatoes is more effective than potato glycoalkaloids in disrupting the intestinal membrane and promoting a leaky gut. The adverse effects of α-tomatine are dose dependent—the more tomato foods you eat, the worse are the effects. A few slices of ripe red tomato in a salad probably will have minimal or no adverse effects on your intestinal or immune system function, but a diet high in unripe, green tomatoes, salsa, and ketchup should be avoided.

In addition to α-tomatine, tomatoes contain another antinutrient called tomato lectin, which rapidly crosses the gut barrier and enters our bloodstream, compromising intestinal function and promoting a leaky gut. Leaky gut is a serious health problem that we are just beginning to recognize and understand; to date, no scientific studies have been performed regarding the Paleo Diet and leaky gut.

Additionally, a convincing body of literature from animal studies shows that α-tomatine from tomatoes is also a powerful stimulator of the immune response—so much so, that it is employed in vaccines as an adjuvant, a substance that increases the potency of the vaccine. The crucial issue is how much α-tomatine you consume. At low dietary concentrations, this tomato chemical probably has little or no effect in most healthy people. I cannot say the same for autoimmune disease patients.

Chili Peppers

Chili peppers are members of the nightshade family of plants and are among the most heavily consumed spices throughout the world. The following table shows the five most common species of chili peppers and lists a few of the more familiar varieties within each species.

Chili peppers are popular spices all over the world because of their pungent or hot taste and aroma. The heat from chili peppers comes from a group of compounds called capsaicinoids or capsaicins. The greater the concentration of capsaicins in the chili pepper, the

Common and Scientific Names for Five Chili Peppers

Common Name	Scientific Name
Bell pepper, cayenne pepper, cherry pepper, chili pepper, paprika, jalapeño pepper, pimento, serrano pepper	*Capsicum annuum*
Aji, Brown's Pepper, Peruvian pepper	*Capsicum baccatum*
habañero chili, bonnet pepper	*Capsicum chinense*
Tabasco pepper	*Capsicum frutescens*
Rocoto pepper	*Capsicum pubescens*

hotter it tastes. More than twenty capsaicins are found in chili peppers; their total concentrations range from 0 percent to more than 2 percent by weight. Daily per capita consumption of capsaicins in the United States and Europe is around 1.5 mg, whereas in India, Mexico, and Thailand, it ranges from 25 to 200 mg. The table below shows the concentrations of total capsaicins in a variety of chili peppers and foods.

Chili peppers seem to have both beneficial and harmful health effects. They have long been used in Mayan and Ayurvedic healing remedies and more recently have found therapeutic application in modern medicine regarding pain relief.

Concentrations of Total Capsaicins in Chili Peppers and Chili Pepper–Containing Foods

Pepper/Food Product	Total Capsaicin Content (microgram/g)
McCormick ground cayenne pepper	3,588
Habañero pepper, fresh	2,261
Thai pepper, fresh	1,333
McCormick original chili seasonings	830
McIlhenny hot habañero sauce	547
Hungarian hot paprika	439
La Costena Chipotle, whole, canned	416
McCormick hot taco seasoning	394
Mezzetta hot chili, canned	306

(continued)

Concentrations of Total Capsaicins in Chili Peppers and Chili Pepper–Containing Foods (*continued*)

Pepper/Food Product	Total Capsaicin Content (microgram/g)
La Costena jalapeño, green, whole, pickled, canned	210
Lawry Choula hot sauce	201
McIlhenny Tabasco original hot sauce	195
McCormick mild taco seasoning	186
Lawry Crystal hot sauce, extra hot	174
La Costena serrano, green, whole, pickled, canned	164
Star Foods pepperoncini, canned	82
Serrano, fresh	77
Green jalapeño, fresh	76
Red jalapeno, fresh	46
Safeway hot pepper sauce	45
Mezzetta sliced jalapeño, canned	19
Green, red, and yellow bell peppers, fresh	0
Roasted red, canned	0
Roasted green, canned	0
Whole canned peppers	0

One of the potential shortcomings of chili peppers is their ability to increase intestinal permeability, and perhaps that is their greatest threat to human health. In 1998, it was suggested by Dr. Jensen-Jarolim that chili peppers, because of their capsaicins, "may modulate the absorption of low molecular weight food constituents that are involved in the pathogenesis of food allergy and intolerance." This means that chili pepper capsaicins increase intestinal permeability and therefore allow gut microorganisms and food proteins access to our immune systems, which in turn may promote allergies and autoimmune diseases.

When the gut becomes leaky, it is not a good thing, as the intestinal contents may then interact with our immune systems, which in turn become activated, thereby causing a chronic low-level systemic inflammation known as *endotoxemia* that may promote cardiovascular disease and diseases of insulin resistance. To date, this chain of events has not yet been demonstrated in human studies. I believe, though, that anyone suffering from an autoimmune disease should remove suspect foods from their diet for an extended period and then monitor their symptoms. If your conditions get worse after you reintroduce the food, this particular food should not be part of your lifelong diet.

In the United States, we consume almost 230 pounds of nightshades per person on a yearly basis. These common foods, such as potatoes, tomatoes, chili peppers, and eggplants, have become such staples in our diets that few people rarely or ever consider that they are very recent additions to worldwide human nutrition. Prior to 1492 and Columbus's "discovery" of the New World, no Europeans, Middle Easterners, Africans, or Asians had access to these foods because they are indigenous to Central and South America. Humanity has had very little evolutionary experience with these recently introduced foods from North and South America, which contain multiple toxins such as saponins and lectins that may cause numerous adverse health effects.

For Paleo Dieters, my advice would to be to eliminate or drastically reduce potato consumption and for autoimmune and allergy patients to be cautious with the consumption of tomatoes, chili peppers, and eggplants.

Paleo Bottom Line

If you are an autoimmune or allergy patient, be cautious with your consumption of tomatoes, chili peppers, and eggplants. Everyone should eliminate or drastically reduce your consumption of potatoes.

PART THREE

Maximum Paleo Living

I've been on the Paleo Diet since May, and I'm down 30 pounds (most of it lost in the first two months) and have never been leaner in my life. I can't stop talking about it when I'm with my friends and family when they say how good I look. I've been evangelizing my Wall Street buddies every time we enjoy a steak house dinner. My acid reflux, IBS, allergies, attitude, and complexion have never been better, and I never go into a food coma any more. I wish your book had been around in the 1980s when I was a teenager.

—Rudy

10

The Paleo Answer
7-Day Diet Plan

I strictly followed your diet, and in the first two weeks, I lost 10 pounds! I did not exercise during this time, and I felt rather light-headed at times, but I was never hungry. I imagine that it was quite a shock for my body to stop living on sugar. I started to feel energized as my body began to learn to live on protein without sugar, and during the course of the next three months, I lost another 15 pounds. I'm now down to a normal weight of 125 pounds (I'm 5'6"). Not only am I happy with how I look, I'm ecstatic about how I feel. I'm no longer tired in the afternoons, I have a new energy, and I don't catch every head cold that goes around.

I have relaxed in my eating habits a bit in the last few months, and I watch the scale carefully, so that if I start to gain weight, I can tighten the reins on my eating habits.

What you have given me and countless others is not a diet but new knowledge of how our bodies function and what we can do to lay down habits that are essential for good health for the rest of our lives.

Thank you, thank you, thank you!

—Jennifer

In *The Paleo Diet Cookbook*, Lorrie, Nell, and I outlined virtually all of the practical aspects of Paleo dieting, including recipes, food choices, meal preparation, necessary kitchen utensils, and a two-week meal plan. In this chapter, for both newbies to the Paleo Diet and veterans, I want to summarize some of the practical dietary advice from the previous chapters by giving you a one-week prescriptive plan. Furthermore, I'll add a few tidbits of wisdom involving health and lifestyle issues.

Meal plans: In general, three daily meals plus snacks are included in this prescriptive plan. As I mentioned earlier, though, hunter-gatherers typically did not eat three meals per day. After nearly twenty years of personal experience with contemporary Stone Age diets, I find that lunch is unnecessary for me, and I rarely eat it. On the other hand, Lorrie seldom misses it. Some Paleo Dieters fast for a few days each month—others don't. As always, the bottom line is to listen to your body when it comes to the number of daily meals and snacks you require and their timing.

Supplements: Supplements other than vitamin D3 and fish oils are unnecessary because meats, fish, fruits, and veggies are such nutrient-dense foods. On days that you don't eat fatty fish (salmon, mackerel, sardines, herring, and so on), I recommend that you take fish oil capsules or bottled fish oil. Try to consume at least 500 to 1,800 milligrams of EPA + DHA per day. If you have cardiovascular disease, you should include at least 1 gram (1,000 milligrams) of DHA + EPA in your supplement.

I personally prefer bottled fish oil because it goes down easier and you can smell whether it has become spoiled. Except for an increased susceptibility to nose bleeds, no adverse health effects have ever been identified with fish oil supplementation—even at extremely high doses. If you are currently not eating fatty fish on a regular basis or are not supplementing your diet with fish oil capsules, perhaps the best overall health strategy you can take is to do so.

Most of us have indoor jobs and don't get regular daily sun exposure. If this is your situation, I recommend that you supplement your diet with at least 2,000 I.U. of vitamin D3 per day. In the summertime, fifteen to twenty minutes of sunshine exposure during midday on your face and arms will give most of you sufficient and healthful vitamin D levels in your bloodstream. If you live above 40 degrees north latitude (e.g., in cities such as Boston, New York, and elsewhere), fifteen to twenty minutes of sunlight on your face and arms during the winter months will have little or no positive effects on your blood concentrations of vitamin D. Consequently, daily supplementation with at least 2,000 I.U. of vitamin D3 becomes a necessity for most of us, except for during the summer months.

I am a university professor, and my wife, Lorrie, is an elementary school teacher, so we both are pretty much locked into indoor jobs from September until June. Accordingly, our sunlight exposure is minimal for nine months, making vitamin D3 supplementation essential for us throughout most of the year. During our summer beach vacations at Tahoe, we completely forget about vitamin D3 capsules. It is ironic that in our modern world, these three simple environmental elements—the outdoors, sunshine, and fresh air—which were originally the birthright of all human beings, have increasingly become either a luxury of the privileged or, alternatively, an obligation of the disadvantaged.

Exercise: As with sunlight and fresh air, exercise is also a luxury in our modern world. Most of us have occupations in which little strenuous physical activity is required to get through the day. Consequently, as a modern-day Paleo Dieter, try to take every opportunity to get into the open air to partake in physical activity outdoors. It may only be walking or gardening a few times a week—even eating lunch or walking outdoors at noon will help.

Any exercise is better than no exercise. Standing is better than sitting. Walking is better than standing. Uphill walking is better than horizontal walking. You get the picture—whenever you have the opportunity to use your muscles or move—do it. Take the stairs—always! Park your car a half mile from the office, and walk the rest of the way in to your office. View physical work not as labor, but rather as an escape from your sedentary prison in front of the computer or your stationary workplace. Any time and every time you can stretch your legs, walk, climb stairs, or go outside—do it!

Unfortunately, as good as these job-related efforts are to help you become more active, you will still have to do much more to catch up with the activity patterns of our hunter-gatherer ancestors. Our scientific analysis of forager-movement behavior shows that a hunter-gatherer mom normally hiked four miles with a child on her hip or shoulder. Double this distance, and we get into the activity levels of hunter-gatherer men when they left camp for a hunt and returned. Few of us have two to six hours per day to hike for four to ten miles with a load on our backs. Nevertheless, these kinds of activity patterns and energy outputs are typical for our species and tend to improve almost all health parameters, particularly if we observe a Paleo Diet.

Exercise alone is a powerful panacea to restore health. A few years back, one of my departmental coworkers applied for a sabbatical leave to hike the Appalachian Trail for the fall semester. Forty-nine-year-old Dale started out weighing a flabby 188 pounds, but after 118 days of trekking from dawn until dusk—typically, ten-hour days—with a 40-pound pack, he ended up at a lean and fit 163 pounds. More important, his total blood cholesterol fell from 276 to 196 and his triglycerides dropped from 319 to an amazing 79 (a 75 percent reduction). I barely recognized Dale when this former fat man walked into the office as a slim, fit man restored to his high school weight.

During Dale's 118-day hike, he didn't eat Paleo but rather consumed hikers' dried and concentrated trail foods (gorp, refined sugars, dried fruit, nuts, and processed dehydrated foods). His notable changes in body weight (a 25-pound loss) and health occurred despite his eating a diet consisting mainly of processed trail foods. Had he the chance to eat real foods (fresh meats, fish, and fresh fruits and veggies) during his 118-day journey, I suspect that his weight loss and health gains would have improved even more.

You don't have to walk ten hours a day for 118 days with a 40-pound pack, as Dale did, to lose weight or experience dramatic improvements in your health. Rather, the Paleo Diet allows you to produce these therapeutic body and blood chemistry changes almost entirely through diet alone. Clearly, any regular exercise program on top of a modern-day Paleo Diet will accelerate your fitness and health gains.

As I outlined in *The Paleo Diet* and in *The Paleo Diet for Athletes*, your conditioning program should include all types of exercise. Try to regularly mix aerobic and strength-training activities, along with stretching. If we heed the example of our hunter-gatherer ancestors, hard workouts should be followed by easy or rest days. I also support the nationwide CrossFit movement and know that it dovetails nicely with the Paleo Diet. You may want to visit the owners of your local CrossFit Gym and see the type of fitness program they have to offer.

The 7-Day Plan

The starred items (*) are recipes in *The Paleo Diet Cookbook*.

Sunday

Breakfast	Omega 3 eggs scrambled in olive oil with chopped parsley
	Grapefruit
	Herbal tea
Snack	Sliced lean beef
	Fresh apricots or seasonal fruit
Lunch	Caesar Salad with chicken (olive oil and lemon dressing)
	Herbal tea
Snack	Apple slices
	Raw walnuts
Dinner	Tomato and avocado slices
	Grilled skinless turkey breast
	Steamed broccoli, carrots, and artichoke
	Bowl of fresh blueberries, raisins, and almonds
	1 glass white wine or mineral water (Clearly, wine would never have been available to our ancestors, but don't forget the 85/15 rule, which allows you to consume three non-Paleo meals per week.)

Supplements: Fish oil and vitamin D3 (if you don't get sufficient sun exposure).

Exercise and Relaxation: If you have a sandy beach nearby, try walking or running barefoot at an intensity and duration that are appropriate for your fitness level. Get your feet wet, and let the sand naturally massage your soles.

Health tip: Peaceful sleep is absolutely essential to our health and well-being. Two dietary elements that can impair restful sleep are alcohol and salt. Try eliminating both of these substances for a few days and see how you do.

Monday

BREAKFAST	Banana Blast Smoothie*
	Hard-boiled omega 3–enriched eggs
SNACK	Apple with ¼ cup raw walnuts
LUNCH	Grilled halibut steak on a bed of spinach with mandarin orange slices and slivered almonds
	Herbal tea
SNACK	Sliced lean flank steak
	Melon balls
DINNER	Cucumber with avocado dip
	Cold peel-and-eat shrimp
	Steamed carrot and celery slices with parsley
	Bowl of fresh boysenberries, raisins, and hazelnuts
	Mineral water

Supplements: Fish oil and vitamin D3 (if you don't get sufficient sun exposure). Try to eat your lunch outside if the weather permits.

Exercise and Relaxation: Try to give yourself a least an hour a day alone for relaxation (meditation, quiet reading, listening to music, walking the dog, sewing, wood working, or fishing).

Health Tip: Following a hot shower, turn the water to cold and stand under the spray for about a minute. The invigorating cold water will improve your circulation and increase substances called heat shock proteins, which improve long-term health and resistance to chronic disease.

Tuesday

BREAKFAST   So Cal Omelet*
            Kiwi fruit
            Herbal tea

SNACK   Steamed broccoli, drizzled with olive oil, topped
            with shredded chicken (use last night's leftovers)

LUNCH   Lean turkey breast on mache lettuce, drizzled with
            flaxseed oil and lemon
            Fresh pear slices
            Spa Water*

SNACK   Mixed fresh berries
            Lean beef jerky
            Celery sticks

DINNER   Paleo Tuna Niçoise Salad*
            Steamed cauliflower
            1 cup red or green grapes
            Baked Apples*
            Herbal tea

Supplements: Fish oil and vitamin D3 (if you don't get sufficient sun exposure).

Exercise and Relaxation: Improvements in long-term physical fitness occur due to three variables: exercise intensity, frequency, and duration. Of these three, the intensity of the exercise bout is most important to fitness improvement. Whether you are a novice or a seasoned athlete, try to step up the intensity of your workout as you become more fit. You will find that brief, intense bouts of exercise will ultimately make you stronger and fitter more rapidly than will lower-intensity exercise of a longer duration.

Health Tip: If you have recently adopted the Paleo Diet, you may want to take two tablespoons of psyllium (such as Metamucil) once or twice a week to help normalize bowel function and reduce intestinal permeability as you transition from a typical low-fiber Western diet to a high-fiber Paleo Diet. After a few months on the Paleo Diet, this recommendation will no longer be needed, as you gradually change your intestinal flora to a healthier, less inflammatory pattern.

Wednesday

BREAKFAST   Bowl of diced apples, shredded carrots, and raisins
Poached omega 3 eggs
Cup of decaffeinated coffee

SNACK   Cucumber, carrot, and apple, chopped and tossed in
olive oil, lemon juice, and mint leaves

DINNER   Caramelized Broccoli with Orange Zest*
Bison-Stuffed Bell Peppers*
Sliced tomatoes and cucumbers with olive oil and
freshly ground pepper
Half a cantaloupe stuffed with sliced strawberries
and mint
1 glass red wine or mineral water

Supplements: Both omega 3 enriched eggs and grass-fed bison are moderate sources of the healthy omega 3 fatty acids (EPA and DHA). To obtain sufficient amounts of these healthy nutrients, you need to either eat fatty fish (salmon, mackerel, sardines, herring, and so on) or supplement with fish oil. If you didn't get into the sun today, you will also need to take vitamin D3 capsules. Your body stores the vitamin D it makes from sunlight, so if you were able to sunbathe for a while on the weekend, then you wouldn't require supplements during the week.

Exercise and Relaxation: I favor exercise in which we minimize machines and maximize our bodies' natural movements. Lifting free weights appears to have certain advantages over machine-generated workloads, because it stresses muscles more naturally throughout their entire range of motion and prevents overuse injuries. Lifting free weights, climbing rope, doing pull-ups and pushups, and tossing medicine balls around sounds archaic in this day and age of computerized ergometers and stair-step and lifting machines, but it is precisely these tried-and-true exercises that are being successfully used in CrossFit Gyms throughout the country.

Health Tip: In dry climates, some otherwise very healthy people experience recurrent nose bleeds that are difficult to stop—even following cauterization by their physicians. A surefire cure, known to few health professionals, is to coat the inside of the nostrils with zinc oxide ointment (I recommend Desitin) for a few days. The healing power of this ointment stems from zinc that potently stimulates the growth of new tissues.

Thursday

BREAKFAST   Salmon, green onion, and mushroom omelet
              Tangerine segments
              Herbal tea
SNACK   Apple mixed with raw almonds
LUNCH   Mixed green salad with Salad Dressing Starter*
              Sliced lean beef, topped with blueberries
              Steamed artichoke
              Herbal tea
SNACK   Paleo Warrior's Jerky* (homemade beef jerky)
              Sliced avocado, drizzled with lime juice and cilantro
DINNER   Greek Salata à la Paleo*
              Baked haddock
              Steamed asparagus
              Almonds, raisins, and peaches
              1 glass white wine or mineral water

Supplements: Because salmon was on the menu today, no fish oil supplementation is necessary. If you were unable to get a minimum of 15 to 20 minutes of sunlight exposure during the day or an extended bout of sunbathing earlier in the week, supplement with 2,000 IU of vitamin D3.

Exercise and Relaxation: One of the most recent developments in footwear is more natural shoes that mimic bare feet and let our feet do the walking without fancy "scientific" insoles, stiff uppers, computer-designed heel cups, and other fallible human-designed tweaks. Our feet are incredible engineering feats designed by the wisdom of evolution through natural selection over millions of years. We are perfectly suited to walk and run barefoot across all terrains that our ancestors crossed without protective foot gear. No human beings wore shoes until perhaps fifty thousand years ago, and those primitive soft leather pieces, similar to modern shoes that were designed to simulate being barefoot, provided only warmth and slight protection from mechanical footstep injury.

Our modern, style-conscious shoes force our toes, ankles, and legs into unnatural positions and don't allow our feet to have natural contact with the earth. Because of these features, our feet are forced to become narrower and weaker; our toes grow shorter, and we lack the foot sensitivity our hunter-gatherer ancestors had throughout their lives. When we come home from a long day at work, our first response it to kick off our shoes and relax. If we take just a little bit of time to examine our suffering shod feet, they are hot, red, and swollen, and they smell bad.

The elixir for our feet, as is that of our bodies with diet, is to be restored to the environment for which they were designed. We need to walk barefoot whenever possible. I am on board with modern shoe designs that allow our feet the freedom to support our bodies with their ligaments, tendons, bones, and muscles as they were naturally designed to do.

Health Tip: As you adopt a milk-, grain-, potato-, and legume-free diet most of you will notice that your sinuses become remarkably clear. You will wake up in the morning clear-headed, with little phlegm or nasal stuffiness, and your joints will be loose, pain free, and ready for the day.

As with my recommendation for psyllium and gastrointestinal tract health, you can accelerate nasal clearances by sniffing salt water. Put a tablespoon or less of salt into a cup or neti pot of tap water, stir well, pinch off a nostril, and sniff the solution into your nose. Hold it and then release. Repeat a few times, and you have effectively cleansed your nostrils because of the hypertonic effect of salt water. This measure will clear your nostrils of all obstructions that may impair your breathing. After a few weeks on the Paleo Diet, this practice will become unnecessary.

Friday

BREAKFAST   Roast turkey breast, drizzled with olive oil and basil
              Sliced apples
              Water with freshly squeezed lemon juice

SNACK	Cold peel-and-eat shrimp
	Fresh orange
LUNCH	Spinach salad with tomatoes, walnuts, olive oil, and
	lemon juice
	Carne Asada*
	Raspberries
	Spa Water*
SNACK	Pear slices
	Raw pecans
DINNER	Steamed crab legs
	Sandy Point Spinach Sauté*
	Tossed green salad with purple onions, tomatoes,
	parsley, and dressed with olive oil and lemon juice
	Iced herbal tea

Supplements: Note that this menu is rich in shrimp, crab, and spinach (which contain moderate to high concentrations of omega 3 fatty acids), but it still does not contain sufficient long chain (> 20 carbon) omega 3 fatty acids to completely protect you from cancer or cardiovascular or autoimmune disease. I recommend that you supplement with either fish oil capsules or liquid fish oil.

Supplement with 2,000 IU of vitamin D3 (if you don't get sufficient sunlight exposure).

Exercise and Relaxation: Although clearly not an option available to our ancestors, modern technology has given our bodies an incredible relaxation tool. It's called a sauna, and alternated with a cooling bath or shower, you can almost guarantee yourself a long and restful night's sleep.

Health Tip: One of the most therapeutic nonpharmacological remedies you can treat yourself to is a full body massage lasting for thirty to sixty minutes. Do this weekly, and you will feel like a million dollars.

Saturday

BREAKFAST	Melon Mania Smoothie*
	Cold broiled halibut
SNACK	Shredded kale, tossed with lime juice, olive oil, and

	minced red onion, topped with chopped turkey breast
Lunch	Salmon Caesar Salad* (use leftover salmon from an earlier meal)
	Sliced tomatoes
	Fresh pineapple
	Water with freshly squeezed lemon juice
Snack	Grapes
	Cold steamed oysters
Dinner	Spaghetti Squash Italiano*
	Grilled lamb chops
	Sliced peaches covered with chopped walnuts and liqueur (optional)
	French Country Salad*
	1 glass red wine or mineral water

Supplements: If you eat Paleo (fresh fruits, veggies, meats, seafood, nuts, and healthful oils), the only supplements you will need are fish oil and/or vitamin D3. If you eat fatty fish (salmon, mackerel, sardines, or herring) a few times a week and get out into the summer sun, fish oil and vitamin D3 supplementation are unnecessary.

Exercise and Relaxation: I have one recommendation—whenever and wherever you can use your body instead of machines to get the job done, do it! Preferably, exercise outdoors and in the sunshine—this is our species' genetic heritage and represents the conditions under which our health flourishes.

11

Paleo Supplements and Sunshine

I promote the Paleo Diet every second I get. In my private practice, it has cured more patients than any other supplement or medication I have prescribed.

—Brooks Rice, M.D.

Paleo Miracles: George's Story

I have been on a strict Paleo diet for six weeks, and I now believe in miracles. Five years ago, at the age of sixty-four, I stopped playing golf because I had too many aches and pains in my muscles, joints, and bones, and my energy level was very low. At that time, I thought it was old age! Now, within six weeks I play golf, and I work and/or exercise ten hours a day.

As a lifelong skeptic, this is hard for me to believe. And now I'm telling my flabbergasted friends that I'm going for one hundred. The only supplements I take are omega 3 and vitamin D.

When you start eating Paleo, you simply won't require most vitamins and supplements. In fact, except for fish oil and vitamin D, if you take antioxidants and/or B vitamins, you will increase your risk of cancer, heart disease and dying from all causes.

One of my first jobs after high school was with the U.S. Forest Service on a wildfire crew in Markleville, California. During the summer of 1969, I bunked with eight other firefighters in a rustic shack where we shared a communal kitchen and bathroom. As an eighteen-year-old barely out of my parents' house, I had to buy groceries to last a week before my days off. I managed to purchase a box of Total cereal, thinking this was a sensible food to help me obtain 100 percent of my daily vitamins and minerals.

Forty years later, I realize that my naïve food choice reflected a global perspective on diet that has emerged since World War II. Instead of focusing on natural, healthy foods in my diet, I was suckered into focusing on micronutrients. Until only recently this perspective has dominated scientific, as well as lay, thought on nutritious diets. I quote a recent study by Drs. Lichtenstein and Russell from Tufts University that appeared in the prestigious *Journal of the American Medical Association*:

> The most promising data in the area of nutrition and positive health outcomes relate to dietary patterns, not nutrient supplements. These data suggest that other factors in food or the relative presence of some foods and the absence of other foods are more important than the level of individual nutrients consumed.

No amount of vitamins, minerals, or supplements added to breakfast cereals will ever make them a healthful food. Similarly, athletic drinks boasting vitamins, amino acids, and additives are nothing more than liquid candy. The food-processing industry "fortifies" highly processed foods such as breakfast cereals, soft drinks, designer yogurts, granola, mayonnaise, and orange juice with various nutrients and then recharacterizes them as "nutritious" or "heart healthy." These marketing ploys not only cause widespread adverse health effects, they also propagate the misleading idea that micronutrients (vitamins and minerals) are more important than foods.

We need to get back to healthy eating patterns characterized by a diet of traditional foods such as fresh fruits, vegetables, seafood, and grass-produced meats that have nourished and sustained our species from the very beginning. When we eat real, living foods, there is little or no need to supplement our diet with any single nutrient that is thought to be protective against disease.

The mentality that has dominated nutritional thought in the post–World War II era, since vitamins and supplements became widely available, was that if a little bit is good, more must be better. Let's take a look at the Dietary Reference Intake (DRI), which used to be called the Recommended Dietary Allowance (RDA), for the B vitamins in the table below.

Notice that we actually need only tiny amounts of these essential nutrients. For instance, the daily DRI for vitamin B1 is 1.2 milligrams. A milligram is just one-thousandth (1/1,000) of a gram, and a microgram (mcg) is just one-millionth of a gram (1/1,000,000). When I first started buying multivitamins back in the late 1960s and the early 1970s, about the only brand available was One-A-Days. Back then, these vitamins contained precisely the DRI—no more and no less.

These days, if you go down to your local pharmacy or health food store and decide to buy a mixed B-vitamin formula or a multivitamin, you are immediately met with a staggering number of choices. Do you want the 10-milligram version, the 50 mg form,

Vitamin	DRI
Thiamine (vitamin B1)	1.2 mg
Riboflavin (vitamin B2)	1.3 mg
Niacin (vitamin B3)	16 mg
Pantothenic acid (vitamin B5)	5 mg
Pyrodoxine (vitamin B6)	1.3 mg
Cyanocobalamin (vitamin B12)	2.4 mcg
Folate	400 mcg
Biotin	30 mcg

or the 100 mg variety? You go with the 100 mg version because you're getting more vitamins for your buck. We all know that B vitamins are water soluble, so what you don't use will simply be excreted in your urine. Once again, let's allow the evolutionary template to give us guidance. Foraging human beings have always consumed vitamins, minerals, and phytochemicals in a range of concentration that was available through diet alone. Processed foods were not on the menu, nor were vitamin supplements or fortified foods. Our ancestral vitamin, mineral, and nutrient intake always fell within a narrow range—not too low and not too high.

The relative levels of one B vitamin to another or any single nutrient to another fell within a range determined by the types of unprocessed plant and animal foods that were consumed. It would have been impossible for any hunter-gatherer ever to obtain ten times the DRI for any B vitamin, much less one hundred times this value. In addition, the natural ratio of one B vitamin to the next or any nutrient to another would never have been exactly one to one, as it is in most modern vitamin formulations.

Paracelsus, one of the greatest Renaissance physicians of sixteenth-century Europe, is credited with the quote *"Dose makes the poison."* Indeed, this ancient wisdom is now coming back to haunt us in the twenty-first century as we indiscriminately lace our food supply with artificially produced vitamins and minerals that we perceive to enhance our health and prevent disease. On page 199 is a graph that shows how dosages of vitamin and mineral supplements can relate to your health and well-being. Notice that when a nutrient intake is low, it increases our risk for disease—this really isn't news to most of us. What may surprise you is that an excessive intake of many so-called safe vitamins and minerals has increasingly been shown to be harmful and to actually cause illness.

Our hunter-gatherer ancestors rarely or never would have ingested too few or too many nutrients that caused disease by landing on either the left- or the right-hand extremes of the curve. Prior to the agricultural revolution, it would have been difficult or nearly impossible for any forager to develop a vitamin or nutrient deficiency by falling on the left-hand side of the curve. Wild plant and animal foods are rich sources of all known nutrients required

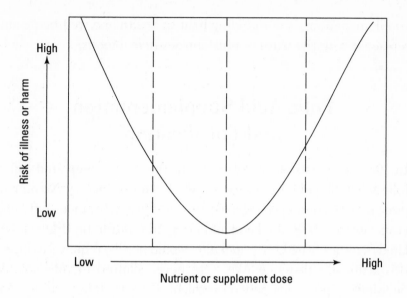

for optimal human health. When these foods or their modern counterparts are regularly consumed, nutrient deficiencies never develop. Only in the postagricultural period could people have wound up on the left side of the curve.

Vitamin and mineral deficiencies became commonplace in early farmers as nutrient-poor cereal grains replaced wild meats, fish, fruits, and vegetables. With the Industrial Revolution and the introduction of refined grains, sugars, vegetable oils, canned foods, and eventually processed and junk food, the consumption of nutrient-depleted foods became the norm. It's high time that we return to the foods to which our species is genetically adapted. By doing so, you will never have to worry about landing on the left side of the curve.

Probably more alarming to you is not the left side of the curve but rather the right. I realize that you may be taking high doses of B and antioxidant vitamins because you think they provide protection from cancer and heart disease. Nothing could be further from the truth, and in fact this practice will increase your risk of dying from cancer, heart disease, and all causes combined. Except for fish oil and vitamin D, supplementation is a total waste of your time and money. It's high time to dismantle the myth of nutrient supplementation as our guiding light to health and well-being and replace it with the truth of nutrient-dense real foods.

Folic Acid Supplementation and Fortification

In 1947, scientists at Lederle Labs synthesized a compound called folic acid that had never previously existed on our planet. No human prior to 1947 had ever ingested this artificial substance. Fifty-one years later, in 1998, the Food and Drug Administration (FDA) legislated that the entire U.S. population would now be required to ingest this artificial substance. We were never allowed to vote on this decision; it simply happened overnight. One day folic acid was not part of our food supply, and the next day every man, woman, and child in the United States was forced to ingest folic acid, whether they wanted to or not. This unilateral decision has turned into one of the worst health fiascos in the history of our country. In the thirteen years since its inception, this mandatory legislation has resulted in untold deaths, diseases, and disabilities.

If you are currently a Paleo Dieter, you probably don't have to worry about ingesting folic acid, provided that you are not taking any vitamin supplements that contain this compound. In 1998, the FDA mandated that all enriched wheat flour was to be fortified with folic acid. Because most commercial wheat products—breakfast cereals, bread, cookies, cakes, crackers, doughnuts, pizza crust, hamburger and hot dog buns, wheat tortillas, and so on—are made with enriched wheat flour, essentially the entire U.S. population began to consume folic acid in 1998. At the time, this national mandate seemed like a pretty good idea because convincing data existed to show that low *folate* status caused neural tube birth defects such as spina bifida. *Folate* is an entirely different compound than folic acid. In our bodies, folate and folic acid are metabolized in completely different ways. Folate is a natural vitamin found in leafy green vegetables, organ meats, and some nuts. Folic acid is a manmade substance that can be converted to folate in the liver. The problem is that folic acid is not efficiently converted to folate, thereby causing an excess pool of both folic acid and folate to build up in our bodies. It creates this pool even at doses as low as 200 mcg, half the RDA. And that's the problem.

I would be the first person to congratulate the FDA for mandating a national policy that could reduce or eliminate birth defects. Unfortunately, its shotgun approach to curing neural tube birth defects put the entire U.S population at risk for death and disability from other more serious diseases. In a six-year period (1990–1996) before mandatory folic acid fortification, the average number of neural tube defects per year in the United States was 1,582. In the first year (1998–1999) following fortification, neural tube defects dropped to 1,337, so 245 cases of these diseases were prevented.

A much better strategy would be to selectively supplement pregnant women with folate—not with folic acid. Only fetuses, not the entire U.S. population, are at risk for neural tube defects.

Folic Acid and Breast, Prostate, and Colorectal Cancers

In the last decade, an accumulating body of scientific evidence now makes it clear that the FDA's mandatory folic acid fortification program represents one of the worst blunders in the history of U.S. public health. An alarming number of human clinical trials, animal experiments, and epidemiological studies convincingly show that excess folate via folic acid fortification has resulted in population-wide increases in the risk for breast, prostate, and colorectal cancers.

A 2010 meta analysis at Bristol University demonstrated that high levels of blood folate were associated with an increased prostate cancer risk. Even more convincing evidence comes from a clinical trial by Dr. Figueiredo at the University of Southern California. In this experiment, 643 men were randomly assigned to either a folic acid supplementation group or a placebo group. After nearly eleven years, the percentage of men who developed prostate cancer in the folic acid treatment group was 9.7 percent, whereas only 3.3 percent of the men in the placebo group were diagnosed with prostate cancer.

Higher blood concentrations of folate from folic acid supplementation also cause a faster progression of this often fatal disease. Although scientists aren't completely sure how excess folate and folic acid promote cancer, animal experiments indicate that these compounds induce a cancer-causing reaction called hypermethylation in the DNA of cancer cells.

An alarming number of recent population studies have also suggested that high folate intake, largely from folic acid in supplements and fortified foods, may increase breast cancer risk. In a study of 70,656 postmenopausal women who were followed from 1992 until 2005, dietary folate intake from both folic acid and folate was positively associated with breast cancer risk.

I'd like to make it clear that folate and folic acid are not one and the same compound. Folate is the natural, healthful B vitamin that is found in leafy green veggies, organ meats, and some nuts. Folic acid is an artificial chemical that can be converted to folate in the liver. Because folic acid builds up and forms pools of this manmade chemical in our bodies at doses as low as 200 mcg (half the DRI), it is known to disrupt normal folate metabolism. Dietary folate from natural food sources does not produce harmful health effects, whereas folic acid does. A recent animal experiment by Dr. Ly at the University of Toronto demonstrated that folic acid supplementation led to an increased risk of mammary cancer in rats. It is notable that the equivalent (around 800 mcg) dietary levels of folic acid necessary to produce breast cancer in the rats could easily be achieved in humans by eating fortified foods and taking folic acid supplements.

The situation with colorectal cancers and folic acid supplementation/fortification is nearly identical to those for breast and prostate cancers. Animal, tissue, epidemiological, and human dietary trials all reveal that folic acid increases the risk for colorectal cancers. The most powerful type of research design in human supplementation experiments is called a double-blind, placebo-controlled, randomized trial. With these types of experiments, scientists can be relatively sure that a certain treatment causes a specific outcome. Such a study of 1,021 men and women was carried out during a ten-year period. I quote the authors of this study, "Folic acid was associated with higher risks of having 3 or more adenomas [cancers] and of noncolorectal cancers." A similar double-blind, placebo-controlled, randomized trial from Norway came up with similar conclusions: "Treatment with folic acid plus vitamin B12 was associated with increased cancer outcomes, and all-cause mortality in patients with ischemic heart disease in Norway, where there is no folic acid fortification of foods." Indeed, many European nations, including the United Kingdom, have taken a more cautious approach and have decided not to fortify their food supplies with folic acid.

Folic Acid Fortification/Supplementation and Autism

A disturbing development involving folic acid fortification/supplementation has recently arisen. A number of scientists now believe that excessive folic acid may play an important role in the autism spectrum disorder (ASD), which includes autism, Asperger's syndrome, and other developmental problems. The most recent epidemiological studies of autism show that the increasing prevalence of ASD in the United States coincides with the same time period that mandatory folic acid fortification began. It is known that excessive folic acid during the embryonic period may adversely affect normal brain development.

Unlike the folic acid/cancer story, the data for ASD is still preliminary. Large population studies will be required to determine whether the mandatory folic acid fortification program is responsible for the disturbing recent increase in ASD.

Antioxidant Supplements Do More Harm than Good

Of all of the supplements people take, antioxidants are one of the most popular, particularly with seniors and cancer patients. The most commonly supplemented antioxidants are beta carotene, vitamin A, vitamin C, vitamin E, and selenium. About 11 percent of the U.S. population supplement their diets with antioxidants on a daily basis; this number rises to almost 20 percent in adults fifty-five years of age and older. The perception with most antioxidant consumers is that these nutrients increase longevity and may prevent cancer, heart disease, and whatever else ails them. More is almost always thought to be better.

Let's examine the U-shaped curve once again. If people are deficient in these nutrients, there is little doubt that health will suffer. On the other hand, more is definitely not better. Our bodies operate optimally when nutrients are supplied to them in the ranges for which they were designed. If you underinflate a tire, your car performs poorly—if you overinflate it, the tire ruptures. Just like tires, our bodies' natural defenses against disease, as well as the rate at which we age, is dependent on just the right amount of antioxidants from our diets—not too little, but also not too much.

The idea behind antioxidant supplements is that they capture and inactivate free radicals. These are highly reactive particles formed within our tissues as by-products of metabolism. Excessive free radicals may damage cells and tissues in many ways. In animal experiments, high free radical production can promote cancer, heart disease, and premature aging. Our bodies use dietary antioxidants to disarm free radicals and prevent damage to cells. We also manufacture antioxidants within our bodies that work together with dietary antioxidants to keep free radicals at bay.

An often overlooked fact when it comes to free radicals is that they are necessary components of normal body function and a healthy immune system. Free radicals are used by the immune system to destroy cancer cells, kill invading microorganisms, and detoxify cells. If we overload our bodies with massive doses of antioxidants, these essential functions are impaired as normal free radical activity is suppressed. Alternatively, supranormal doses of antioxidant vitamins upset other delicate aspects of cellular machinery, which can actually turn antioxidants into pro-oxidants and ultimately increase free radical activity.

In 1994, one of the first realizations that high doses of antioxidants may be harmful arose with the ATBC study, a randomized, placebo-controlled experiment of 29,133 male smokers. The experiment wanted to determine whether beta carotene or vitamin E supplementation could reduce lung cancer incidence in this group of heavy smokers. Following five to eight years of supplementation, the researchers were shocked—treatment with beta carotene actually increased lung cancer rates by 16 to 18 percent and overall death rates by 8 percent. Furthermore, the men who took vitamin E suffered more hemorrhagic strokes than did those taking placebo pills. A similar trial known as the CARET study had been ongoing concurrently with the ATBC study. In the CARET trial, smokers and former smokers received beta carotene (20 mg) in combination with high doses of vitamin A (25,000 I.U.) for an average of five years. The men who received the antioxidants experienced a 28 percent greater incidence in lung cancer and a 17 percent higher death rate than those taking an inert placebo pill. The CARET trial was immediately stopped when the results of the ATBC trial were reported.

In the years since those studies, more convincing data has verified the harmful effects of antioxidant supplementation. A 2007 meta analysis of sixty-seven randomized, controlled trials studies involving 232,606 participants showed that supplementation with vitamin E, beta carotene, or vitamin A increased overall death rates. In 2008, a large randomized controlled trial, the SELECT study of vitamin E and selenium supplementation in 35,533 men, was prematurely halted when it was discovered that these two antioxidants increased the risk for prostate cancer and type 2 diabetes. In addition, a large meta analysis involving twenty randomized controlled trials and 211,818 subjects revealed that antioxidant supplementation (beta carotene, vitamin A, vitamin C, vitamin E, and selenium) did not protect against gastrointestinal cancer and increased overall death rates.

A series of recent meta analyses show that high vitamin E intake may be particularly dangerous. Dr. Miller at Johns Hopkins analyzed nineteen randomized trials that included more than 136,000 subjects and stated, "High-dosage (more than or equal to 400 IU a day) vitamin E supplements may increase all-cause mortality and should be avoided." In a meta analysis of 118,765 people and nine randomized, controlled trials evaluating the effects of vitamin E on stroke, Dr. Schürks and coworkers at Harvard Medical School concluded, "In this meta analysis, vitamin E increased the risk for haemorrhagic stroke by 22 percent . . . indiscriminate widespread use of vitamin E should be cautioned against."

Even the once-acclaimed vitamin C may have little therapeutic value for cancer or heart disease. In the Physicians' Health Study, a randomized, placebo-controlled trial of vitamins E and C in 14,641 male doctors, the authors summarized, "Neither vitamin E nor C supplementation reduced the risk of prostate or total cancer. These data provide no support for the use of these supplements for the prevention of cancer in middle-aged and older men."

The situation for cardiovascular disease and vitamin C and other antioxidants appears to be the same as for cancer—they are a waste of your money. Dr. Bleys demonstrated in a meta analysis of eleven randomized, controlled trials: "Our meta-analysis showed no evidence of a protective effect of antioxidant vitamin-mineral or B vitamin supplementation on the progression of atherosclerosis. Our findings add to recent skepticism about the presumed beneficial effects of vitamin-mineral supplementation on clinical cardiovascular endpoints."

If you are an athlete, a series of recent human and animal experiments suggest that mega doses of vitamin C may have detrimental effects on your performance. Surprisingly, supplementation with vitamin C may decrease training efficiency, cancel the beneficial effects of exercise on insulin sensitivity, and delay healing after exercise. In addition, vitamin C supplementation did not decrease free radical damage to DNA that may occur following exercise.

These kinds of studies further cement the notion that fitness, vitality, and well-being can never be achieved by single isolated nutrients, supplements, or fortified foods. The available evidence conclusively shows that these compounds are harmful by causing nutritional imbalances within our bodies. The Paleo Diet has never been about supplements but rather about real, wholesome living foods.

I'm thirty-six years old, and 5 feet, 8.5 inches tall. I started the Paleo Diet about four months ago. Since then, I've lost almost 25 pounds, bringing me down to my ideal weight of 150. My blood pressure went from 115/70 to 92/56. I decided to try the Paleo Diet because I read (on About.com) that it may help alleviate depression and anxiety. To my delight, it worked—my depression and anxiety have disappeared. My energy levels are much higher than before. I'm no longer tired throughout the day. My mind is clearer—I can focus much more easily, and my short-term memory has improved greatly. My skin is much smoother and less dry. Another improvement that I've found, which is kind of strange to me because I never expected it, is that my shinbones are no longer really sensitive. It used to be that if I barely bumped my shinbones against something, the pain was quite bad. Now they're hardly sensitive at all. Thanks much!
—Scott

Sunshine

Starting in the summer of 1974, I worked as a lifeguard at Sand Harbor Beach on Lake Tahoe's pristine North Shore for the next twenty consecutive summers. Besides experiencing some of the greatest times of my life, I took in a lot of sunshine—to say the least! Back in the 1970s, there were only two brands of "sun tan lotions" (Coppertone and Sea & Ski) because "sunscreens" had yet to be invented. There were no sun-blocking agents in either lotion, and we used them mainly to moisturize our skin. No one on our lifeguarding crew worried about skin cancer, and if anybody got too much sun, he or she simply sat beneath an umbrella on the lifeguard tower. We wore short shorts and Vuarnet sunglasses. In the day, our goal was not to avoid the sun but rather to get the deepest, darkest tan possible.

Times and styles have changed considerably since then (thank God), but one big difference today that may produce adverse health effects is the universal application of sunscreen lotions.

I still spend my summers at Sand Harbor but no longer as a lifeguard. Very few beachgoers have deep tans the way they did back in the 1970s, and sunscreens are to be found in every beach bag because "everyone knows that sunscreens prevent skin cancer."

Just as the milk industry campaigned to convince us that milk drinking prevents osteoporosis, sunscreen manufacturers have promoted the myth that sunscreens prevent cancer. In a recent paper, Dr. Berwick from the University of New Mexico Cancer Center, summarized the most recent scientific findings on sunscreens: "Sunscreens protect against sunburn. . . . Thus far, no rigorous human evidence has shown that sunscreens prevent the major types of skin cancer: cutaneous melanoma and basal cell carcinoma." If the truth be known, melanoma risk is actually increased with the use of sunscreens because they allow you longer exposure to the sun without burning.

The part of sunlight that causes damage to our skin is ultraviolet (UV) radiation, a spectrum that is divided into two categories: UVA and UVB. Most of the sunlight that reddens our skin, causing sunburn, is UVB. Consequently, almost all sunscreens employ one or more ingredients in their formula to block UVB to various degrees. Until recently, few sunscreens blocked UVA. Although it hasn't been completely settled, a consensus in the scientific community now indicates that UVA sunlight is the chief cause of melanoma. If your sunscreen blocks only UVB and not UVA, it most likely increases the risk for melanoma.

You might think that the best sunscreen would be one that blocks both UVB and UVA equally, but this conclusion is erroneous and would actually end up increasing your risk of dying from numerous cancers. Sunlight exposure has a paradoxical effect that is both good and bad. Chronic, long-term exposure to the sun, such as what lifeguards and other outdoor workers experience, is protective from melanomas and many other cancers, whereas intermittent, infrequent intense burning, followed by little sun exposure, may promote this deadly form of skin cancer and many other cancers.

Blocking UVB sunlight turns out to be very poor idea because this spectrum of light stimulates vitamin D production in our skin.

Sunscreens that block UVB suppress the synthesis of vitamin D, one of the most powerful anticancer substances our bodies produce. In the last twenty years, compelling evidence reveals that low vitamin D blood status increases the risk for sixteen cancers, many autoimmune diseases, cardiovascular disease, type 2 diabetes, hypertension, mental illness, osteoporosis, and susceptibility to infectious diseases. So what is the solution? How can you and your children enjoy a nice sunny summer day outdoors and not get sunburned but still benefit from the sun's healthy vitamin D–boosting effects?

If we look to the evolutionary template and use a little common sense and some modern technology, we can easily overcome this problem. The first thing you've got to do is change your mind-set—sunlight is not harmful but rather is incredibly healthy, providing that we get it in the same U-shaped dose that we get of other nutrients.

Lorrie and I have been taking our boys to the beach every summer of their lives. None has ever had a severe sunburn, and each of them gets very dark tan by summer's end. Here's our strategy. At the beginning of summer, we apply lotion liberally for the first few days, preferably with sunscreens containing both UVA and UVB blockers and a moderate SPF value—8 to 15. As the boys gradually tan, we simultaneously reduce the sunscreen quantity and the SPF value.

After a week to ten days, when they are tan, we pay little attention to sunscreens anymore, although we encourage them to sit under beach umbrellas or put on their shirts if they are hot or have had too much sun. A similar strategy will work for adults, depending on your skin color and initial tan. The key here is moderation and to gradually increase your exposure. The best protection from excessive sunlight is not a sunscreen, but rather shade, hats, and light clothing.

Regular sunlight exposure is one of the most healthy habits we can get into because it increases our blood levels of vitamin D, which in turn reduces our risk for developing most diseases and illnesses in the Western world. But how much sun do we need? This depends on your skin color. Very-dark-skinned people need almost twice the time in the sun as light-skinned people do to achieve similar blood concentrations of vitamin D. The following table shows blood levels of vitamin D and their classification.

Vitamin D Levels in the Blood

Blood Levels of Vitamin D	Category
Less than 20 ng/ml	Deficiency
21 to 29 ng/ml	Insufficiency
Greater than 30 ng/ml	Sufficiency
60 ng/ml	Maximal with sunlight exposure

Lifeguards and other outdoor workers can achieve blood concentrations that top out at about 60 ng/ml, but you don't need values this high. Most experts agree that values higher than 30 ng/ml will significantly reduce your risk for developing cancer and all of the other diseases associated with low vitamin D status. The good news is that daily sunlight exposure in the summertime for short periods of fifteen to thirty minutes will rapidly boost your blood levels of vitamin D above 30 ng/ml. The bad news is that it is virtually impossible to do this with diet alone because almost all real foods that we commonly eat contain little or no vitamin D.

Vitamin D Supplementation

For most of us, regular sunlight exposure is a luxury that is difficult or impossible to come by on a year-round basis. Obviously, our hunter-gatherer ancestors did not have this problem. Consequently, you will need to supplement your diet with vitamin D3 capsules. If we look at the official governmental recommendation for vitamin D intake—between 400 and 600 IU—it is woefully inadequate. This DRI, like the folic acid supplementation fiasco, represents a failure in public health policy. The most recent human experiments show that blood levels of 30 ng/ml could never be achieved with vitamin intakes between 400 and 600 IU. In fact, 400 IU does not raise insufficient blood concentrations of vitamin D at all.

The majority of Americans maintain blood levels of vitamin D that are either deficient or insufficient. One of the best strategies you can take with adopting the Paleo Diet is to supplement daily with vitamin D3 if you are unable to get sunshine on a regular basis. Most vitamin D experts agree that daily supplementation of at least 2,000 IU of vitamin D3 is necessary to achieve blood levels of 30 ng/ml or greater. People who have never supplemented with vitamin D and/or who have had little sunlight exposure for years may need 5,000 IU per day.

Fish Oil Supplementation

One of the absolutely essential elements of the Paleo Diet is to increase your consumption of foods containing the long-chain omega 3 fatty acids known as EPA and DHA. Your best sources of these vital nutrients come from fatty fish such as salmon, mackerel, sardines, and herring. A 4-ounce serving of salmon contains around 1,200 milligrams of EPA + DHA. If you're like most Americans, your normal daily diet provides only from 100 to 200 milligrams of these healthy fatty acids.

Try to consume at least 500 to 1,800 milligrams of EPA + DHA per day, either by eating fish or taking fish oil supplements. If you have cardiovascular disease, you should include at least 1.0 gram of EPA + DHA in your diet. Patients with high blood triglycerides can lower their blood values by as much as 40 percent by taking 2 to 4 grams of EPA + DHA daily.

The problem with the typical American diet is that it contains insufficient EPA and DHA and excessive omega 6 fatty acids from vegetable oils. Today vegetable oils used in cooking, salad oils, margarine, shortening, and processed foods supply 17.6 percent of the total daily calories in the U.S. diet. This massive infusion of vegetable oils into our food supply, starting in the early 1900s, is to blame for elevating the ratio of dietary omega 6 to omega 3 to its current and damaging value of 10 to 1. In hunter-gatherer diets, the ratio of omega 6 to omega 3 was closer to 2 to 1.

Numerous diseases associated with this imbalance of omega 3 and omega 6 fatty acids include heart disease, cancer, autoimmune diseases, the metabolic syndrome, and almost all inflammatory diseases that end with "-itis." If we use the evolutionary model exclusively, vegetable oils should make up a minimal part of contemporary Paleo diets. By using this strategy and regularly eating fatty fish or supplementing with fish oil, you will reduce your risk of developing almost all of the diseases of Western civilization.

To increase your intake of the long-chain omega 3 fatty acids,

- Eat fatty fish such as salmon, mackerel, sardines, or herring two to three times per week.
- Consume grass-fed fed meats, rather than feedlot-produced meats.
- Eat omega 3–enriched eggs.
- Enjoy shellfish, such as crab, lobster, oysters, and clams.
- Eat almost any fish, as even lean fish are moderate sources of EPA and DHA.
- Eat organ meats.
- Supplement with fish oil or fish oil capsules.

Paleo Bottom Line

Get more sun in your life and more fish in your diet. If you can't or don't get enough, take vitamin D and fish oil supplements. You don't need or want any other supplements.

12

Paleo Water

I am a lifelong sufferer of depression. I have long exercised five or six days a week, and I was still depressed. When I stumbled upon your website, I decided to start eating the Paleo way and have found that I have had no depressive episodes since. Even the mood swings are not evident. It feels great not to be battling depression every day. Thank you so much for the Paleo Diet.

—Sam

Multiple Sclerosis (MS) in Remission: Elizabeth's Story

I was diagnosed in August 2003, eight months and three severe MS episodes later. I was sixteen at the time, fifteen when symptoms first appeared. Postdiagnosis, I was told by the medical team to be aware of information claiming to aid MS, especially dietary. So I was a good, quiet patient and went onto Rebif, subcutaneously [Rebif is an interferon, to aid in reducing MS relapses]. I felt awful on these injections and was in the middle of school exams. I then decided it was time to research other therapies to aid MS.

Several months later, after lots of research I told my medical team I was coming off the Rebif. They were unsupportive and told me how shortsighted my decision was. I was committed to feeling better, however, not just staying clear of MS relapses. I haven't touched a medication—any—since 2004. The combination of these therapies (as well as a certain optimistic mind-set) has served me well. Despite a grim diagnosis and prognosis, here I am as an above-average twenty-one-year-old. I'm studying for a tough university degree (in nutrition), I play college basketball, and I am virtually symptom free, though I have a slight balance and coordination problem, tracing back to my first MS attack. The power of nutrition in MS, autoimmune diseases, health, and longevity is so underrated.

During my halcyon days of youth as a lifeguard on Tahoe's pristine North Shore in the 1970s, one of the brilliant ideas my fellow guards and I came up with was the notion that we should all be drinking pure water. As we sat in our lifeguard towers and sweltered all day long underneath the hot summer sun, the question arose—how should we replace the water we lost from our sweat? In those days, commercial bottled water in individual plastic containers didn't exist and was at least ten years or more in the future. Even if such products were available, none of us, as underpaid young lifeguards, would have ever bought bottled water when we could have quenched our thirst for free from the tap.

A better idea surfaced. Why not drink Tahoe's crystal-clear, immaculate waters? In those days, contamination of Sierra Nevada mountain lakes and streams by bacterial pathogens such as *Giardia* was negligible, so we all bought into the idea. We all saw how Tahoe's waters close to the shoreline were clouded with pollen, insects, driftwood, crawdad carcasses, silt, and whatever, but moving out another hundred yards into deeper water was a completely different story. Tahoe's pristine waters at this depth were breathtakingly clear. From my lifeguard rescue board on the lake's surface, I remember staring down into incredibly clear images of granite boulders lying far below me, as if no water existed. I took a deep breath, fastened my goggles, and dove almost twenty feet down into Tahoe's exhilarating icy waters. When I reached bottom, I opened the nozzle of my water bottle and filled it.

This is how my fellow lifeguards and I regularly drank water during that magical summer of 1974. I drank deeply from Tahoe's clear, unpolluted waters, but at the time, I was unaware of what I was ingesting or what I wasn't ingesting. All I knew was that this product of the High Sierra snowmelt tasted crisp and pure and better than any tap water I had ever drunk. I now know why. It was not contaminated with chlorine, fluoride, heavy metals, pesticides, solvents, fertilizers, sewer runoff, or other toxic elements. To me, Tahoe's pristine waters were a refreshing elixir that not only quenched my thirst but also cleansed my body as I swam in this unspoiled alpine lake.

Except for the air we breathe, perhaps the single most crucial element in maintaining our day-to-day health is water. Without a regular source of uncontaminated drinking water, we simply could not exist for more than a few days. Although our kidneys and immune systems are remarkably efficient at removing toxic compounds found in any polluted waters we may ingest, we are a lot better off by drinking fresh, clear waters unadulterated by added chemicals, heavy metals, herbicides, toxic compounds, hormones, and pesticides.

The Problems with Tap Water

If I had to rate the most important achievements modern technology has made in public health, there is little doubt in my mind that uncontaminated drinking water and waste-water treatment would be at the top of my list. Prior to the advent of community-based water-treatment plants, infectious diseases such as cholera and typhoid fever caused death tolls as high as 1 per 1,000 in many major American cities. We can be thankful for the chlorination of our drinking waters, which first occurred in 1908 in Chicago and rapidly spread to the rest of the country and worldwide. Death from infectious diseases borne by contaminated water has been effectively eliminated since our water supply has been treated with chlorine.

Unfortunately, we unknowingly traded a huge problem—death by infectious disease—for a lesser predicament. It is now convincingly known that the chlorination process produces compounds that increase our risk for developing a variety of cancers. Although municipal water works regulate the maximal concentrations of these compounds that can be present in our drinking water, they cannot eliminate them.

In the 1970s, scientists discovered that when chlorine was added to our drinking water, it combined with naturally occurring organic matter such as vegetation and algae to produce toxic compounds called trihalomethanes. Since the discovery of these chemicals, epidemiological (population) studies have consistently demonstrated that trihalomethanes increase our risk for developing bladder and colorectal cancers. Additionally, trihalomethanes in our drinking water may impair normal menstrual function, increase the risk for spontaneous abortion, and produce other undesirable reproductive effects in women.

When we think about the adverse health effects associated with tap water, most of us assume that they originate only from the water we drink from our faucets. Unfortunately, this is not the case. A ten-minute shower increases our blood chloroform (a chlorine by-product) levels almost 100 percent from the chlorine compounds we breathe in from the vaporized water. Hence, our chlorinated water supply hits us with a double whammy—we drink this noxious compound, and we also breathe it when we shower. Not all cities and municipalities employ chlorination to sanitize their water supplies, but alternative procedures such as ozone gas and ultraviolet light, which are used at a few hundred water treatment plants in the United States, are not without their own problems.

Given this scenario, how can we possibly find fresh, clean, unadulterated water to drink and shower with? Is plastic bottled water a viable solution for our daily drinking water? Our local municipal water-treatment plants have eliminated disease-causing microorganisms from our water supply, but unfortunately, most of these plants add chlorine and fluoride back into our water. They also frequently use outdated filtering technology that fails to remove known toxins and contaminants.

The Problem with Plastic Bottled Water

As with the milk mustache, you should just say no to plastic bottled water. This product has been labeled one of the greatest cons of the twentieth century, and I would totally agree. Compared to tap water, the cost of bottled water is staggering. A gallon of bottled water can run you from one to ten dollars, whereas water from your tap costs less than a penny per gallon. The environmental impact of bottled water is worse still. It takes three times as much water to produce the plastic bottle as it does to fill it. An estimated sixty million plastic bottles are produced, filled, and bought daily in the United States, requiring seventeen million barrels of oil, which represents enough energy to fuel one million cars for a year. Only one in five bottles is recycled—meaning that we dump three billion pounds of plastic into the environment each year.

The bottled-water middlemen with their slick advertising hype would make us think that we are getting higher-quality water when we buy their products. In reality, 40 percent of all bottled water is simply taken from municipal tap water. Almost 22 percent of bottled water brands contain chemical contaminants at higher concentrations than stipulated by governmental limits. Municipal water supplies are not allowed to have any fecal bacteria, whereas no such limitations are required for bottled water. Similarly, governmental regulations impose limits for bisphenol A (BPA) and phthalates in tap water, but no such rules exist for producers of bottled water.

The Problem with Plastics

As a Paleo Dieter, you realize that the closer we can mimic the beneficial aspects of our ancestral lifestyles, the better off we will be in the twenty-first century. We live in a world that is vastly different from that of our hunter-gatherer ancestors and is even very much different from the world of our grandparents and great grandparents. One of the more important environmental pollutants that didn't exist two hundred years ago is plastics. Plastics and plastic materials dominate our twenty-first-century world, whereas prior to World War II, most Americans rarely encountered these manmade compounds. It would be nearly impossible for any of us to get through a single day without touching, breathing, or ingesting plastic compounds. These materials are everywhere—from our cell phones to our computers, our cars, our food, and our clothing. We live in a "plastic, fantastic" world, to quote a lyric from one of my favorite sixties rock groups.

Only recently did we discover that tiny plastic particles pollute our world and may impair our health and well-being. Plastic chemicals are present in the dust we breathe in our homes and offices, and they contaminate our food, water supply, and medicines. In an earlier era, it was assumed that plastics were inert and had no harmful effects, but nothing could be further from the truth. We now know that at least two plastic compounds, bisphenol A (BPA) and phthalates, are injurious to our health and should be avoided whenever possible. Unfortunately, our contemporary world makes it difficult to escape these toxins.

As a modern-day hunter-gatherer, one of the best strategies you can take to reduce your BPA and phthalate load is to forgo any processed food item that comes in a can, a plastic container, or a plastic bottle—including water. Another unexpected source of BPA is from the thermally printed receipts you receive at many retail outlets. If you simply touch the printed label, BPA can permeate your skin. In the scientific community, BPA and phthalates are officially known as endocrine disruptors, meaning that these chemicals interfere with our bodies' normal hormonal functions, providing that they reach a high-enough concentration in our bloodstream.

It had always been assumed that we couldn't achieve harmful blood levels of BPA or phthalates while living, breathing, and eating in the normal Western environment. Regrettably, this assumption has turned out to be wrong. A 2008 study published by Dr. Lang and colleagues in the *Journal of the American Medical Association* demonstrated that even low blood levels of BPA increased the risk for cardiovascular disease, diabetes, and liver enzyme abnormalities in 1,455 adults. Although the mechanisms are not completely known, ingested BPA seems to act like one of the body's own female hormones and may bind hormonal receptors in various tissues, thereby producing its harmful effects.

Another reason why you should avoid processed foods packaged in plastics is the presence of phthalates. Like BPA, these chemicals can leach into our foods from their surrounding plastic containers and promote cancers, allergies, and infertility, among other health problems. Phthalates are found in adhesives, detergents, floorings, cosmetics, shampoos, fragrances, plastic bags, garden hoses, cleaning materials, toys, food packaging, and insecticides. As was the case with BPA, phthalates seem to initiate their harmful effects by mimicking the female hormone estrogen.

You can take a number of precautions to reduce your exposure to both BPA and phthalates. First, avoid foods sold in plastic containers and preferentially buy condiments, oils, or manufactured goods packaged in glass containers only. Canned goods are generally not part of the Paleo Diet—another good reason to avoid them is because cans are lined with a plastic spray that contains BPA.

Another effective strategy to reduce your intake of these plastic compounds is to thoroughly rinse your fruits and produce before eating. Also, try to purchase cosmetics and deodorants that are free of these chemicals—read your labels carefully. Phthalates come in at least ten different versions and are frequently abbreviated as MiBP, MnBP, DIBP, DNPB, MEP, and so on. Any time you see the word "phthalate" in the ingredient list, choose another product.

If you have the luxury, being outdoors is almost always better than being indoors, as we breathe in fewer plastic particles outside. We live in a plastic-polluted world, and there is no way that we can completely eliminate BPA, phthalates, and other plastics from our environments, but by adopting a modern-day Paleo diet filled with fresh fruits, veggies, lean meats, seafood, and unprocessed foods, we can significantly lower our intake of these toxic chemicals.

Water for the Paleo Diet

I have spent a lot of time discussing the health problems associated with drinking tap or bottled water, but I haven't yet provided you with much of an alternative. Part of the problem is that it is difficult or impossible for municipal water-treatment plants to deliver to our doorsteps a chlorine-free product devoid of all major contaminants. And once treated water arrives at our homes, it can be further polluted by the lead, copper, and polyvinyl chloride pipes within our own household plumbing systems.

Our water supply is not immune to political decisions for which we have little or no input. For instance, fluoride is routinely added to about 70 percent of America's municipal water supplies with the intent of reducing dental cavities. Yet this practice is controversial within the scientific community and may have a number of unexpected harmful health effects that we are only beginning to understand. The best protection against cavities is not fluoride but rather a Paleo diet devoid of refined sugars and processed foods, along with regular flossing and brushing.

The evolutionary template contraindicates chlorine, fluoride, heavy metals, pesticides, solvents, fertilizers, hormones, plastics, sewer runoff, and any other toxic element in our drinking water. Analyses of the few remaining pristine lakes and streams worldwide show these waterways to be generally free of bacterial contamination because their rain water or snow sources are naturally filtered through sand and gravel as they make their way to lower ground. Additionally, healthful minerals such as magnesium and calcium leached from earthen sources infiltrate free-flowing streams, rivers, and lakes, giving these waters the sweet taste I experienced when I drank of Tahoe's waters as a young man.

The evolutionary formula for our drinking water is obvious. What we should strive for with our contemporary water supply is the pristine quality our ancestors most frequently enjoyed. We need pure, clean water devoid of chlorine, fluoride, and all of the other toxic compounds detected in municipal water sources. To partially accomplish this, you will need to purchase a home filtration system that can elevate your tap water to the next level. A variety of commercial products are available. Most will improve the quality of your tap water but cannot guarantee absolute purity from all environmental contaminants. My recommendation is to make sure the filtration system you purchase removes chlorine, chloroform, trihalomethanes, fluoride, heavy metals (lead, copper, arsenic, rust), nitrates, volatile organic chemicals (industrial solvents, pesticides, herbicides, etc), sediments, and chlorine-resistant parasites (*Giardia* and *Cryptosporidium*).

When you purchase a home water filter, you will have two choices for its location: point of entry or point of use. Point-of-entry systems filter water as it comes into your house from the municipal water supply and consequently purify every tap in your entire house. Point-of-use devices filter water only at a single location— so if you want to filter one faucet for drinking water and another for showering, you obviously will have to buy a filter for each tap you want to treat. The highest-quality water is obtained from point-of-use filters because nothing stands between you and the purified water. The downside to point-of-entry (whole house) filters is that the filtered water must travel throughout your home plumbing system, where it may become contaminated from materials leaching in from the pipes in your house.

Most of us don't have a clue about the plumbing in our homes, much less the types of materials found in the pipes through which our home drinking water flows. Modern houses and apartments are most frequently plumbed with copper pipes, but plastic pipes made from polyvinyl chloride (PVC), chlorinated polyvinylchloride (CPVC), or cross-linked polyethylene (PEX) are becoming more popular. All of these materials are not ideal—they all may leak toxic compounds into our home water supplies that potentially affect our health and well-being.

Although copper pipes have served us for more than a hundred years, a number of problems remain. If you live in an area where the water is soft or acidic, your in-house copper pipes can become corroded as they age. If excessive copper finds its way into your drinking water, numerous serious health problems can arise, including anemia, nausea, diarrhea, kidney and liver damage, and an increased risk for developing Alzheimer's disease.

If your house was built before 1987 and contains copper plumbing, your drinking water may also contain excessive lead. Prior to the passage of the Safe Drinking Water Act on June 19, 1986, lead was routinely used in plumbing fixtures, pipes, and the solder that joined pipes. Even such seemingly miniscule amounts of lead in copper pipe solder joints represent a powerful poison known to cause irreversible learning disabilities in young children and health problems in adults. If you live in an older home, another potential source of lead poisoning comes from the service line that connects your house to the water main in the street. Prior to the passage of the Safe Drinking Water Act, lead pipes were routinely used to bring water into your home from their municipal supply. These pipes are well-recognized sources of lead poisoning. Do yourself and your family a favor and examine the water pipe leading into your house. If it is light gray in color and can be easily scraped with a pen knife, it is probably made of lead. Contact officials at your city's water department and have them immediately replace this pipe.

In recent years, copper plumbing systems have been replaced with plastics. I cannot recommend either PVC or CPVC, as residual toxic chemicals from these pipes are known to leak into our in-house water supplies and increase our risk for developing numerous cancers. Both PVC and CPVC are sources of BPA. The most recent darling of the plastics industry for plumbing houses is cross-linked polyethylene, more commonly known as PEX. Initial reports suggest that PEX does not contain BPA, but it does harbor other compounds, such as ETBE, which make their way into our water and give it an unpleasant odor.

The Bottom Line for In-Home Water-Purification Systems

To date, the safest plumbing material for your house appears to be copper, unless you live in areas of the country where the water is acidic and/or soft. These types of waters cause copper in your plumbing to dissolve in your drinking water, and this situation is definitely is not a good thing. By employing high-quality point-of-use filtration systems, you can minimize copper contamination for everyone in your home, along with most other municipal water pollutants.

If money is not an issue, the best way to decontaminate your in-house water supply is to employ both point-of-entry and point-of-use filters. Point-of-entry filtration systems will entirely eliminate chlorine and chloroform compounds for everybody who showers or bathes at every location in your home. Point-of-use filters then become necessary only where drinking or cooking water is drawn. Typically, the kitchen faucet would be the most likely location for an additional point-of-use filter.

Drinking Water Storage

Glass bottles are always best for storing your filtered water; stainless steel bottles come in a close second. Both of these containers are virtually inert, and the water you put into them will remain pure and free of chemicals. Although polycarbonate plastic bottles are sometimes viewed as the next-best alternative to glass and stainless steel, the most recent experiments don't support this assumption. Experiments from Dr. Amiridou's laboratory at Aristotle University in Greece show that polycarbonate containers leaked the most BPA into bottled waters. Hence, I believe it is best that you entirely avoid plastic bottles and containers for water and food storage. One final thought: make sure that you refrigerate your stored filtered water, as it no longer contains chlorine and consequently can become contaminated with bacteria if opened and left at room temperature.

Paleo Bottom Line

Try to drink and use the purest natural water you can.

PART FOUR

The Paleo Answer for Everyone

The Paleo Diet Works: Carolyn's Story

I visited my seventy-three-year-old father last year for three weeks. I said, "Sorry, Dad. No more pizza for me." He said, "Fine. You cook. I'll eat." After three days, he woke up and said, "Gee whiz—I haven't slept this well in years." The next day, "Gee whiz—my sinuses are free." The next day, "Gee whiz—there's no pressure behind my eyes." By the end of my stay, he was so revitalized that he decided to continue with the diet.

Two months later, he had a checkup, and his critical sugar level was absolutely fine. His HDL/LDL ratio had swung from bad to great. His blood pressure had lowered so much that he was able to stop taking his medication.

A few months after that, he called me and said that his gout had not acted up in weeks—no more medication was necessary. The icing on the cake was his visit to the eye doctor, who was astounded that my father's glaucoma had receded.

13

The Paleo Diet for Women

Feeling Better: Liz's Story

I am a sixty-one-year-old woman. I started the Paleo Diet in November 2005 and have been on it ever since. I do indulge in some of the forbidden foods, such coffee with half-and-half, a habit seemingly impossible for me to break. It gives me the energy to do the things I want to do, and unless you can give me a formula for getting more energy otherwise, I may be in trouble on that one. Also, after experimenting without or with drastically less salt, I have added back my habitual amounts of salt again. But it is a lot, lot less than in the typical American diet, I assure you. Other than that, I stick to meat, vegetables, and fruit. No dairy, no grains, no legumes, no potatoes. I don't miss any of it.

I found an organic farmer in Marin County near where I live and got a hog, a quarter steer, and chickens from them. The meat is lean and outstanding. I get fresh-caught fish and vegetables from the farmer's market, as well as organic eggs. My trips to the supermarket are now limited to bananas, half-and-half, and a few other things occasionally.

I feel good. Some friends say I am the picture of health. At the start of the diet, I weighed 145 pounds; now I weigh 130 pounds and have stayed there for months.

I never suffer from indigestion now. My husband, who is also on this diet, eats toast and butter and jam for breakfast, a gourmet lunch with his colleagues, and what I cook for dinner. Even so, he has gone from having a hiatal hernia, with daily doses of Mylanta and Prilosec, to no problems at all. And he has lost at least 30 pounds. I would like to see him eat better; maybe he'll come around.

For a while I did experience daily leg cramps. Once I read one of Dr. Cordain's papers on potassium and what contained the most potassium. I try to get those vegetables and throw mushrooms into everything when I have them.

Since I have been on the diet, I have been virtually free of almost weekly, random, very debilitating headaches. I feel so free and at this point take it for granted! There used to be days when I just would have to stay in bed because the headaches were so bad, and the doctor always said they were tension headaches.

Bottom line—I like eating the way I do, and I will never change.

The Paleo Diet is a lifetime way of eating that has been adopted by hundreds of thousands, perhaps millions, of people worldwide. Men, women, and children of all ages and from all walks of life have decided to replicate the diets of their hunter-gatherer ancestors but with foods commonly available at their local supermarkets. There are many ways to approach the Paleo Diet—many different Paleo diets, so to speak. People can fine-tune this nutritional plan to their individual needs, and I have always felt that this is the correct approach.

We should use the Paleo Diet as a starting point for optimal nutrition, but we should always listen to our own bodies, as we adjust our diets to our specific nutritional and lifestyle requirements. For instance, I view freshly steamed crab legs with pleasure and consider it a favorite food, whereas others may have allergies to shellfish that would obviously exclude this nutritious food. Some people seem to do better on higher-fat versions of the Paleo Diet, whereas others prefer less meat and more fruit and veggies.

Protein and Pregnancy

It is increasingly becoming clear that one size doesn't necessarily fit all. A modern-day Paleo Diet may be one of the best strategies for you and your partner to become pregnant. Once women have a successful conception, however, it is important for them to reduce their protein intake during pregnancy.

There is no doubt that contemporary Paleo diets will provide you with considerably more protein than the amount consumed in the typical U.S. diet. The average protein intake in the U.S. diet is 98.6 grams per day (15.5 percent of the total calories) for men and 67.5 grams per day (15.1 percent of the total calories) for women. Animal products provide approximately 75 percent of the protein in the U.S. food supply, followed by dairy, cereals, eggs, legumes, fruits, and vegetables. Because dairy, cereals, and legumes are not part of the Paleo Diet, you will be obtaining nearly all of your protein from animal foods. Diets that contain 20 percent or more protein have been labeled high-protein diets, and those that contain 30 percent or more protein have been dubbed very-high-protein diets. Accordingly, a high-protein diet (20 to 30 percent protein) for the average U.S. man would contain between 125 and 186 grams of protein per day and for the average woman from 89 to 133 grams of protein per day. Most contemporary Paleo Dieters follow high-protein diets because their protein intake falls between 20 and 30 percent of their daily calories.

I need to point out that there is a physiological limit to the amount of protein you can ingest before it becomes toxic. A by-product of dietary protein metabolism is nitrogen, which in turn is converted into urea by your liver and then excreted by the kidneys into your urine. The upper limit of protein ingestion is determined by your liver's ability to synthesize urea. When nitrogen intake from dietary protein exceeds the ability of the liver to synthesize urea, excessive nitrogen (as ammonia) and amino acids spill into the bloodstream, causing toxicity. For most people, the dietary protein ceiling occurs when protein exceeds 35 to 40 percent of their normal daily caloric intake. Consequently, very-high-protein diets for the average U.S. man could range from 187 to 270 grams per day and for women, 134 to 246 grams per day.

Our hunter-gatherer ancestors knew that they could get too much of a good thing and avoided eating very lean, fat-depleted animals. Excess consumption of protein from the lean meats of wild animals leads to a condition referred to by early American explorers as "rabbit starvation," which resulted in nausea, then diarrhea, and eventually death. Anthropologists, including my colleague John Speth at the University of Michigan, have documented that hunter-gatherer women have a lower tolerance for protein when they become pregnant. The medical literature has recently substantiated the anthropological observations, and it is now known that during pregnancy, women have a reduced ability to metabolize dietary protein. High maternal protein intake increases the risk for low-birth-weight babies and overall fetal mortality. During pregnancy, the estimated safe upper limit for dietary protein is about 25 percent of the daily calories. Here's a breakdown of protein content in the average American diet.

- Average protein intake in the United States: 15 percent of caloric intake
- Diets considered to be high protein: 20–30 percent of average caloric intake
- Diets considered very high protein: 30–40 percent of average caloric intake

Most modern-day Paleo Dieters eat high-protein diets that contain between 20 and 30 percent protein. If you are pregnant, a 25 percent protein limit would amount to no more than 110 grams of protein per day. This goal can easily be achieved by eating fattier cuts of meat; fatty fish such as salmon, mackerel, and herring; and more nuts, avocadoes, and eggs, along with using more olive oil in your salads and cooking. Besides including more fat in your diet, you should also displace lean proteins with more carbohydrates. Yams, sweet potatoes, bananas, and other fresh fruits are a great starting point.

Eating Paleo is perhaps the best strategy you can take in becoming pregnant, and by slightly lowering your protein intake during pregnancy, you can help assure yourself of an easy delivery and a healthy baby.

Paleo Diets and Gestational Diabetes Mellitus

One of the greatest risks for pregnant women and their fetuses is the development of diabetes during pregnancy. This condition is known as gestational diabetes mellitus (GDM) and is present in 4 to 7 percent of all pregnancies in the United States. GDM heightens the risk for premature births, birth defects, and still births. For the mother-to-be, GDM increases her chances of developing preeclampsia, a blood pressure condition that can be life threatening to the mother and the child. The chief metabolic problem with GDM is that maternal blood sugar levels remain elevated during pregnancy; this condition is largely responsible for the health risks in both mother and fetus.

GDM is definitely bad news, but the good news is that low-glycemic-index/load diets are known to improve pregnancy outcomes if they are started from the first trimester onward. My colleague Jennie Brand-Miller from the University of Sydney has recently demonstrated that low-glycemic-index diets effectively halved the number of women who required medication to control their high blood sugar levels during pregnancy. And a recent study from David Ludwig's group at Harvard Medical School showed that a low-glycemic-load diet resulted in longer pregnancy duration, greater infant head circumferences, and improved maternal cardiovascular risk factors.

Because the Paleo Diet is a low-glycemic-index nutritional plan, it represents one of the best steps pregnant women can adopt to prevent GDM and improve their own health and that of their children.

The Paleo Diet, Omega 3 Fatty Acids, and Pregnancy

One of the most therapeutic aspects of the Paleo Diet for virtually all chronic Western diseases is its high omega 3 fatty acid content, particularly EPA and DHA. So it should not surprise you that these essential nutrients will also help ensure a successful pregnancy and a healthy baby. Adequate maternal intake of EPA and DHA during pregnancy can improve your infant's cognitive and visual performance because these fatty acids represent the building blocks of fetal brain and retinal tissues. Omega 3 fatty acids play a key role in determining the length of gestation and may reduce the incidence of preterm birth. Some studies also suggest that sufficient consumption of fish (high sources of EPA and DHA) during pregnancy may be effective in preventing postpartum depression. Unfortunately, many pregnant women avoid fish because of concerns about adverse effects of mercury and other contaminants.

The Paleo Diet is an extraordinarily rich source of omega 3 fatty acids, particularly if you consume fatty fish such as salmon, mackerel, herring, or sardines a few times a week. Shellfish and leaner fish are good sources of EPA and DHA; grass-fed meats and omega 3–enriched eggs contain moderate amounts of these health-promoting fatty acids. Pregnant women should strive for a minimum of 200 mg of DHA per day. Note that a 100 gram serving, around 4 ounces, of Atlantic salmon gives you 300 mg of EPA and 900 mg of DHA. If you don't like to eat fish or seafood or have worries about mercury and other toxins in fish, I recommend that you supplement with fish oil, either capsules or liquid, during your pregnancy.

The Paleo Diet and Polycystic Ovary Syndrome

Polycystic ovary syndrome (PCOS) is the most common hormonal disease in females, afflicting between 5 and 10 percent of all women of childbearing age; it is a major cause of infertility. Common symptoms include menstrual irregularities, ovarian cysts, and high levels of male hormones, producing acne, excessive body hair, and hair loss. The majority of women with PCOS have insulin resistance and frequently are obese. They maintain a ten times greater incidence of type 2 diabetes than healthy normal women and are at a much greater risk of dying from premature cardiovascular disease.

The good news is that diet is known to be a major player underlying this syndrome. Weight-loss programs seem to reduce disease symptoms, but more important, so may low-glycemic-index diets. A new study by Dr. Jennie Brand-Miller has shown that a low-glycemic-index diet could improve PCOS symptoms by preventing menstrual irregularities. Two other new studies have demonstrated that supplementation with omega 3 fatty acids may also be therapeutic in PCOS patients. The Paleo Diet is just what the doctor ordered if you have PCOS. Because our ancestral diet is a high-protein, low-glycemic nutritional plan, rich in omega 3 fats, it will help you to lose weight, normalize your hormones, and reduce your risk for developing diabetes and cardiovascular disease.

Relieving Menstrual Problems: Phyllis's Story

I have not read of any other women talking about relief from period pain on a Paleo diet, but if only I'd known about it years earlier!

I have always had extremely severe cramps in the first few hours of my period. I spoke to many women but have met only a few who seemed to experience the same degree of pain as me. If I didn't take medication in time, I always repeatedly vomited, even after my stomach was empty. I had diarrhea and terrible cramps. I just could not believe how painful they were. My hair was usually wet within minutes, due to my sweating from the pain, and I could see the sweat bead down my arms, too. I could not even sit upright; mostly, I just curled into a ball. I lived in terror of being caught away from home, without medication, when my cramps started.

Although being on the pill solved the problem for a couple of years in my twenties, I did not want to be on the pill long term. No other solution worked, and even referrals to gynecologists did not help. Yet for the two years I lived in Japan in my midtwenties, I was free of all pain. I put this down to a diet high in seaweed, tofu, and fish and was frustrated that I never managed to replicate the benefits at home in Australia, despite trying hard to achieve a similar diet.

It seems odd now that I didn't realize that the solution lay in what I was not eating in Japan: I was eating very little dairy and wheat. A doctor who specialized in nutritional medicine made this clear to me. After one week on a Paleo diet, I had my first period in eleven years that did not require medication. I was astonished and jubilant.

I have experienced most of the other benefits that people have talked so much about, such as weight loss, increased energy, and no colds. My premenstrual tension is almost entirely gone after months of getting progressively worse. My favorite thing is not having an afternoon slump during my workday.

The Paleo Diet and Breast and Other Cancers

Although many women fear breast cancer—and rightly so—the greatest risk to health for both men and women comes not from cancer but rather from cardiovascular disease.

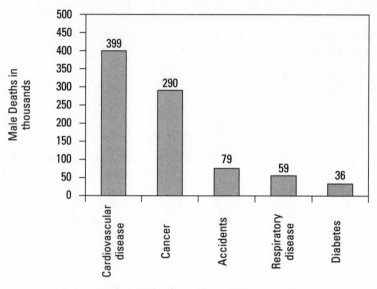

Male Deaths from Various Causes

The leading cause of death in the United States is cardiovascular disease, followed by cancer. In both men and women, cardiovascular disease plus cancer are responsible for a little more than 60 percent of all deaths from all causes combined. The Paleo Diet

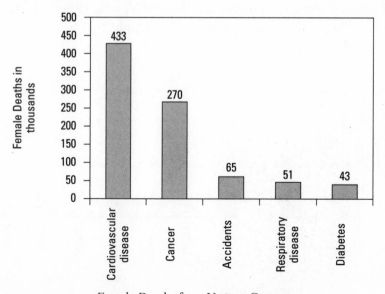

Female Deaths from Various Causes

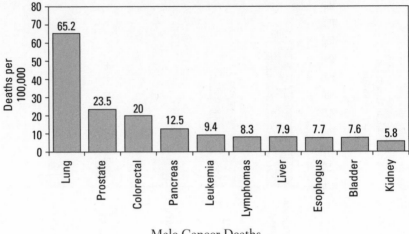

Male Cancer Deaths

contains many nutritional elements that can greatly reduce your risk of contracting both of these diseases.

There is no doubt that breast cancer is a serious illness that in many cases can be life threatening. The graphs on this page show the top ten causes of cancer deaths in the United States in 2007. Note that for both men and women, lung cancer is responsible for nearly twice as many fatalities as the next leading cancer deaths—breast for women and prostate for men. Almost all lung cancer is caused by smoking and consequently is preventable by eliminating this nasty habit.

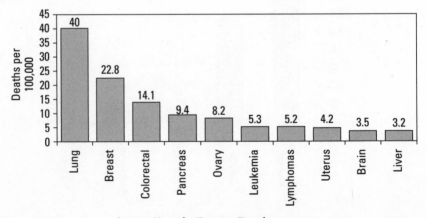

Female Cancer Deaths

Breast cancer was rare or nonexistent in historically studied hunter-gatherers and other less-Westernized peoples. Similar observations have been consistently noted for almost all of the other common modern cancers: prostate, colorectal, pancreatic, leukemia, and ovarian. Some of the most convincing evidence demonstrating that cancer is a disease of modern civilization comes from studies of the Inuit (Eskimo) people as they made the transition from their Stone Age way of life to the Space Age in less than two generations.

Here is a quote from an article on Eskimo health that appeared in the *Canadian Medical Association Journal* in 1936: "In the Western Arctic Dr. Urquhart has as yet not met with a single case of cancer in the seven years of his practice. Cancer must be extremely rare in the Eastern Arctic also." Similar observations come from yet another frontier physician, Dr. Samuel Hutton, who treated non-Westernized Inuit people in Labrador from 1902 to 1913: "Some diseases common in Europe have not come under my notice during a prolonged and careful survey of the health of the Eskimos. Of these diseases the most striking is cancer. I have not seen or heard of a case of malignant new growth in an Eskimo." As the Inuit people became more and more Westernized and began to replace their traditional foods with processed foods, their relative immunity to cancer diminished. In a paper published in 1984, Drs. Hildes and Schaefer examined cancer rates in the Inuit from 1950 to 1980 and noted, "The most frequent tumours in the most recent period studied were lung, cervical and colorectal cancers. Breast cancer was absent before 1966 and was found in only 2 of 107 Canadian Inuit women stricken with cancer from 1967 to 1980, whereas the recent rates in the longer-acculturated Inuit of Alaska and Greenland have approached those prevailing in modern Western women."

The virtual absence of breast cancer and other common Western cancers is not entirely restricted to the Inuit. The Nobel prize–winning physician Dr. Albert Schweitzer commented, "On my arrival in Gabon, in 1913, I was astonished to encounter no case of cancer . . . I cannot, of course, say positively that there was no cancer at all, but, like other frontier doctors, I can only say that if any cases existed they must have been quite rare. This absence of cancer seemed to me due to the difference in nutrition of the natives as compared with the Europeans. . . . In the course of the years, we have seen cases of cancer in growing numbers in our region. My observations incline me to attribute this to the fact that the natives were living more and more after the manner of the whites." Dr. Schweitzer got it right. The virtual absence of breast, prostate, colorectal, and other common Western cancers in the hunter-gatherers of Gabon had everything to do with their diet.

The Paleo Diet maintains multiple nutritional characteristics that will help protect you against breast and other common Western cancers. The Paleo Diet is a low-glycemic-index, low-glycemic-load diet. A recent meta analysis involving ten studies and more than 575,000 subjects by Drs. Dong and Qin clearly show that high-glycemic-index diets increase the risk for developing breast cancer. Similar results were observed in an even larger meta analysis by Dr. Barclay and colleagues from the University of Sydney.

It is not only the Paleo Diet's low glycemic index and load that will protect you from breast cancer but also its rich omega 3 fatty acid content and low levels of high omega 6 vegetable oils. In tissue and animal models of breast cancer, omega 6 fatty acids from vegetable oils stimulate cancer growth, whereas omega 3 fatty acids inhibit it. A large meta analysis by Dr. Saadatian-Elahi showed a significant protective effect of omega 3 fatty acids on breast cancer risk.

The Paleo Diet is a milk- and dairy-free diet. As discussed earlier, milk drinking boosts your blood concentrations of female hormones, whether you are a man or a woman. If you are a woman, elevated blood estrogen and its metabolites increase your lifetime risk for breast and ovarian cancers. For men, milk's added estrogen may heighten your risk for prostate and testicular cancer.

The Paleo Diet is also exceedingly rich in fresh fruits and veggies. These foods are Mother Nature's best medicine; meta analyses of population studies confirm that fresh fruits and vegetables protect women from breast and many other cancers.

However you look at it, the Paleo Diet is a good natural way to prevent cancer.

Surviving Breast Cancer: Debbie's Story

I am a breast cancer survivor. I was first diagnosed with breast cancer on May 25, 2001: T1, Node Negative, Her 2 positive and nuclear grade 3. I had a lumpectomy, aggressive chemotherapy, and radiation. On March 26, 2004, my breast cancer returned to my L-1 disk in my spine. I had six months of weekly chemotherapy and radiation. By December 15, 2004, I was declared in remission.

Herceptin was part of the chemo protocol that I had received in 2004, and I have been receiving it every three weeks since the beginning of January 2005. Tumor marker tests are also conducted every other month. Unfortunately, my tumor markers started rising, and by the end-of-May tests, the upward trend was disturbing.

On May 28, I shared this news with my pharmacist, who is also a certified nutritionist. He recommended that I immediately eliminate sugar and grains from my diet. I found the Paleo Diet and started to eliminate sugar, grains, and dairy from my diet that day.

The results have been astonishing, to say the least. On May 24, 2005, my CA 27 29 marker was 43 and as of October 24, 2005, is 24. My CA 15 3 marker was 28.6 on May 24, 2005 and is now 22.9. I am 100 percent convinced that it is a result of my being a very compliant follower of the Paleo Diet. Cancer likes sugar. Sugar is not my friend and is an enemy to my health.

I am very thankful to an astute pharmacist/certified nutritionist who is on top of the current diets and their effects on one's health. We are what we eat. I do not miss any of the sweets that I craved so, and I love the fact that I have finally lost the 25 pounds of chemo/radiation weight that I could not lose, no matter how much exercise or dieting I did since 2002. Fresh fruits, fresh vegetables, and lean meats and fish are the mainstay of my current good health.

I will continue to spread the message to my support group and other women I meet who have breast cancer. Mind, body, and soul—keeping each healthy is essential to survive this terrible disease. The diet recommended to me on May 28, 2005, empowered me to continue to do everything possible to win this battle.

The Paleo Diet and Osteoporosis

One of the greatest fears many women have when they first adopt the Paleo Diet is how—without drinking milk or eating dairy products—they will get enough calcium to build strong bones to prevent osteoporosis. As I mentioned, large meta analyses (combined population studies) clearly show that neither calcium supplementation nor increased milk drinking reduces the risk for osteoporotic fractures. The current obsession with calcium *intake* as the single and most important factor involved with bone health is misguided. What the dairy lobbyists don't tell us is that bone mineral content is determined not only by calcium *intake* but rather by *calcium balance*.

The calcium stores in your bones are like your checkbook. If you spend more money than you earn, your checking account will have a negative balance. Similarly, if we lose more calcium in our urine than we ingest, we will be in negative calcium balance. This phenomenon helps explain why U.S. women maintain one of the worst rates of osteoporosis in the world, despite having one of the highest calcium intakes.

When we talk about calcium balance, calcium loss in the urine is just as important as the calcium we ingest from our diets. Urinary calcium losses are primarily dependent on dietary acid/base balance. After digestion, all foods ultimately report to the kidneys as either acid or base. If our diet is net acid producing, the acid must be buffered by the alkaline stores of base in our bones. Acid-producing foods are hard cheeses, cereal grains, salted foods, and almost all processed foods, meats, fish, and eggs. The only alkaline base–producing foods are fruits and vegetables. Because the average

American diet is overloaded with grains, cheeses, and salty processed foods at the expense of fruits and vegetables, virtually everyone in the United States has an acid-yielding diet that leaches calcium from his or her bones.

Because Paleo Dieters consume anywhere from a third to half of their daily calories as fresh fruits and veggies, their diets are net alkaline yielding—reducing urinary calcium losses and restoring a positive calcium balance. High-protein diets such as the Paleo Diet are also bone healthy because protein increases calcium absorption and stimulates production of a hormone (IGF-1) that promotes new bone formation. Besides yielding a net alkaline load to the kidneys, most fresh veggies are rich sources of calcium, particularly leafy green vegetables—think broccoli, kale, cabbage, Brussels sprouts, cauliflower, kohlrabi, and mustard greens.

Vitamin C from fresh fruits and veggies, like protein from meats and fish, increases calcium absorption, further promoting a net positive calcium balance. Vitamin D is also one of our best allies in ensuring strong, fracture-resistant bones. Elsewhere in this book, I show you some simple dietary and lifestyle strategies you can adopt to ensure adequate blood levels of vitamin D.

Rest assured, evolution via natural selection has engineered successful biological systems that build strong, fracture-resistant bones for every species of mammal on the planet—including us. Without drinking cow's milk.

14

The Paleo Diet
for Children

Treating Type 1 Diabetes:
JoAnne's Story

On September 10, 2009, I took my six-year-old daughter
to the pediatrician for what I thought was a urinary tract
infection. She had been very thirsty and going to the bathroom
excessively. Little did I know that these were symptoms of
hyperglycemia. Her blood glucose was tested at 542 in the
doctor's office, and she spent two days in the hospital.
During that time, she was diagnosed with type 1 diabetes.
Her A1c [a long-term marker of glucose and insulin
metabolism] was 10.8. They sent us home to begin a regimen
of insulin injections: one basal in the evening, one before
each meal. We did what any parent would do: what the
doctors told us.

After a week or so, however, we realized that we were
counting carbohydrates in foods such as Pop-Tarts. It
seemed absurd. We decided that all of us needed to clean

up our diets. Since we worked out in a CrossFit gym, the diet that came to mind was the Paleo Diet.

What happened next was amazing! My daughter's insulin needs plummeted. During the next week, we made numerous calls to the endocrinologist to adjust her dosages downward. After about two weeks, she was completely off insulin. That was October 1, 2009. She has continued with BG testing, endocrinologist visits, and the Paleo Diet, and as of this day, January 31, 2010, she has close-to-normal BG and requires no insulin. My challenge is to make a believer out of the endocrinologist. He believes she is in remission and that it will surely wear off. Yet as more time goes by, I can see his curiosity beginning to awaken. He said that there are some cases of remission lasting this long, but if she makes it to a year, he will have to write a paper.

A few months later

I wanted to give you an update on my daughter. She had her quarterly checkup with the endocrinologist today. Her A1C was 5.7! She has been eating around 100 or 125 grams of carbohydrates a day, mostly in the form of fruit and some vegetables and tree nuts. We have been about 95 percent faithful to the diet. She eats eggs every other morning for breakfast, and occasionally she has a treat, which is a diet soda or a gluten-free cookie made of rice flour. I have found those are best eaten either right after a meal or with some other fat or protein food, or else it spikes her blood sugar.

We now have a solid six months of total remission under our belts.

With the growing popularity of the Paleo Diet, many people have asked me for more information about adapting the Paleo Diet to the growth and nutritional needs of infants and young children. With a little modification, the Paleo Diet can meet your children's nutritional requirements, help them escape the rising childhood obesity epidemic, and build lifelong eating habits to lower their risk of disease and ensure them long and healthy lives.

Paleo Diets during Infancy

The best model we have for infant nutrition comes from the example given to us by our hunter-gatherer ancestors. Obviously, we cannot precisely duplicate their nutritional patterns, nor would it be practical. Yet we can certainly do better than the typical diets most infants in the United States must tolerate.

Hunter-gatherer children were generally introduced to solid food later than what is considered normal in the United States and the Western world. Studies of foraging societies show that the average age of weaning was 2.9 years. Hunter-gatherer infants were highly dependent on their mother's milk for most of their daily nutrition. Obviously, it would be impractical or nearly impossible for most Western women to nurse for such an extended period, but there are some important lessons to be learned.

First, hunter-gatherer diets were rich in omega 3 fatty acids, compared to typical Western diets. Mother's milk contained more of these essential fats than milk from Western mothers does. This difference is crucial because numerous studies have revealed the importance of sufficient omega 3 fatty acids during pregnancy and nursing for proper brain and cognitive development of your child. By eating fatty fish two or three times a week or by taking fish oil capsules (EPA plus DHA), you can be guaranteed that your milk will contain ample amounts of omega 3 fatty acids for your infant's normal development.

Although weaning at age 3 may be impractical, you should delay weaning as long as possible—preferably until 1 to 1.5 years of age. After weaning, I recommend that you give your infant formula that is enriched with both docosahexaenoic acid (DHA) and arachidonic acid (AA). Also, try to stay away from soy-based formulas. Do not give your infant either fish oil or fish oil capsules in any form because they contain an omega 3 fatty acid, EPA, that competes with AA metabolism and can result in impaired motor nerve development.

Human milk contains very little iron; nonetheless, infants are born with sufficient iron stores to last for about nine to twelve months. Hunter-gatherer mothers introduced their infants to solid foods by thoroughly chewing meat, marrow, nuts, seeds, fruits, and so on, and then giving these premasticated foods to their infants. Obviously, you don't have to go to these extremes. Pediatricians typically recommend that infants' first solid foods be iron-fortified cereals to restore depleted iron supplies in their little bodies. I completely disagree with this recommendation. I suggest that you consider commercial baby meats, such as beef, pork, and chicken, as better alternatives to cereals. Processed baby meats are good sources of iron with high bioavailability. Make sure that these meats don't contain added cereal fillers or other additives. Baby cereals should be avoided for all of the same reasons that adults should steer clear of these second-class foods.

Lorrie and I fed all three of our infant sons commercial baby meats because of the difficulty of mincing and pureeing fresh meat into a consistency that could be easily swallowed without the risk of choking. Scrambled omega 3 eggs are easy to swallow and are good sources of protein for your infant's first solid foods. With our three boys, we mainly tried to feed them fresh fruits and veggies that we prepared ourselves rather than giving them processed commercial versions of these foods. It's easy to make homemade applesauce, pureed carrots, mashed sweet potatoes, pureed fruits, and pureed veggies. Simply cook your veggies until soft and then puree them in a blender. Be creative and try to give your infant variety. Also be sensitive to your baby's tastes. Don't force foods on your baby—when he or she spits out your homemade creations, it is a pretty good sign that your child may not like a certain food.

Virtually all pediatricians recommend that cow's milk and other dairy products, such as yogurt and cheese, be excluded from infant diets during their first year of life. Early exposure to dairy products has been implicated in an increased risk of developing allergies and autoimmune diseases, particularly type 1 diabetes. I believe this recommendation is not stringent enough. I suggest that dairy products should be excluded for an even greater period, lasting until at least age two or beyond. With all three of our boys, we never gave any of them milk during their infant years or even during their childhood. We simply do not stock it in our home. To this day, as young men and teenagers, they don't drink milk. By the way, all three boys grew up to be tall, lean, and athletic. None wears glasses, and dental cavities have been few and far between in our family. Eliminating milk from your child's diet inadvertently eliminates another problem—breakfast cereals. Without milk, breakfast cereals taste about as good as dried cardboard. In our household, we occasionally stock cheese, but rarely do ice cream or frozen yogurt find their way into our refrigerator. As they became teens, all three boys quickly discovered the connection between ice cream and acne flair-ups.

Paleo Diets during Childhood

When you switch your infant to solid foods after weaning, I recommend that you focus on the same basic food types that I recommend for adults: fresh fruits, vegetables, nuts, seeds, fresh meats, fish, shellfish, and eggs.

There is evidence that children's livers are less able to deal with high intakes of protein—around 30 to 40 percent of total calories—than adults' livers are. Fattier meats and fish should not be restricted in your child's diet because giving them fattier meats will help lower their protein intake. Fresh lamb and pork are delicious fattier cuts of meat that most children relish. High-fat plant foods, such as nuts, olives, avocados, and healthful oils, are also useful, but monitor your child for nut allergies. Omega 3–enriched eggs should be the eggs of choice, as they are good sources of brain-healthy EPA and DHA.

I also believe that you should supply your children with as much dried fruits (dates, raisins, and figs) as they want. Healthy, normal-weight, active children have exquisitely tuned insulin and glucose metabolisms, so these foods present few health problems. Dried fruits will not promote obesity and represent some of the healthiest natural sweets you can give your child. Trail mix and gorp without added candy make delicious snacks for active children. Other good concentrated carbohydrate sources include bananas, yams, and sweet potatoes.

I don't advocate completely restricting processed foods from children because eating involves multiple behavioral issues that go far beyond the mere nutritional aspects of diet. The best way to get a child to eat junk food is to completely forbid it. In our home, we serve Paleo foods at every meal. We also stock very few processed foods in our refrigerator and pantry, so if our children are hungry, their choices are primarily healthy foods. We don't allow unlimited access to TV, computers, or electronic games, but we do encourage outdoor play.

For active children who exercise outdoors, I don't believe that processed high-glycemic-index foods are harmful on an occasional basis. Built into the Paleo Diet is the 85/15 rule, which allows you and your children to cheat and eat three non-Paleo meals per week if you decide to do so. Birthday parties are part of being a kid, and your child should have the option of eating pizza or cake once in a blue moon. Yet even though we allowed our boys to eat these foods occasionally, our oldest son who is now in college is strictly Paleo and wouldn't even consider pizza or cake. We have always given our children the choice to make their own decisions, and this policy seems to have worked.

While most people in nearly all Western countries view tall children and adults positively, height has a downside, particularly from a lifelong health perspective. Scientists have known for decades that tall adults and children maintain an increased risk for developing many cancers, myopia (nearsightedness), and acne. Although the nature of this relationship remains somewhat obscure, it is becoming increasingly clear that diet represents a powerful environmental factor underlying these conditions and illnesses.

Milk drinking during childhood is known to increase adult stature because it elevates a hormone (IGF-1) that promotes growth and height. As I discussed, milk and dairy consumption also raise the risk for breast and prostate cancer from the same hormonal mechanism

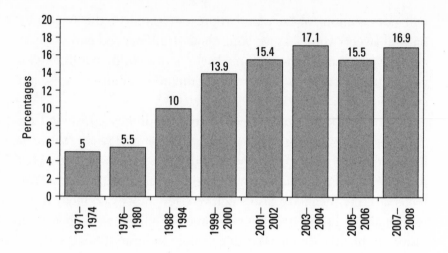

that increases stature. The typical U.S. diet not only contains loads of milk and dairy products but also high-glycemic carbohydrates that elevate IGF-1. Milk, dairy, and high-glycemic-index carbohydrates make up about half of the calories in the normal U.S. diet, so it is not surprising that our nation produces some of the tallest, heaviest people in the world whose risk of dying from cancer is second only to heart disease.

Before I move on to Paleo diets for teenagers, there's one more topic about nutrition and your child's health that I need to address—overweight children. Every few months, we hear about yet another study showing that Americans are the fattest people on the planet and that we keep getting fatter. More alarming are the studies showing that our children are following in our footsteps. In the chart above you can see that the percentage of obese children and teenagers between the ages of two and nineteen has more than tripled since 1971.

The Obesity Epidemic

In 2002, when I wrote the first edition of *The Paleo Diet*, the most effective type of weight-loss diet was still being hotly debated within scientific circles. It was thought that low-fat, high-carb diets were the way to go, although the first well-controlled scientific studies of low-carb, high-fat diets, such as Atkins, were being tested. At the time, just a trickle of studies had suggested that a more effective strategy to get weight off and keep it off was a high-protein, low-glycemic-index diet. These are just the recommendations I made in *The Paleo Diet*, recommendations that have been validated by a great deal of scientific research since the publication of my first book.

A 2010 randomized trial involving 773 subjects and published in the *New England Journal of Medicine* confirmed once again that high-protein, low-glycemic-index diets were the most effective strategy to keep weight off. More important, the same beneficial effects of high-protein, low-glycemic-index diets were dramatically demonstrated in the largest nutritional trial, the DiOGenes Study, ever conducted in children, with a sample of 827 subject. Children assigned to low-protein, high-glycemic diets became significantly fatter during the six-month experiment, whereas those overweight and obese children assigned to the high-protein, low-glycemic nutritional plan lost significant amounts of weight.

I find it curious that the National Institutes of Health spends hundreds of millions of dollars on research attempting to determine the causes of the obesity epidemic sweeping our country, when the simple answer lies before their very eyes. If you don't want your children to become part of the obesity epidemic, start them early on the Paleo Diet.

Paleo Diets during the Teenage Years

As a father of three teenage boys, I have personally experienced the trials and tribulations parents go through with this age group. Remarkably, Lorrie and I have enjoyed this time of life with our children, and I believe that diet, along with parental compassion, love, and consistency, guide children toward healthy, productive lives. It's important to realize that proper diet eliminates environmental elements that may contribute to or worsen the stresses of this pivotal stage of your child's life. The same dietary characteristics that help you optimize your health will also do the same for your children as they grow and develop during their teen years. A high-protein, low-glycemic-index diet with minimal processed foods, no cereal grains, few dairy products, and lots of fresh fruits and veggies represents the ideal diet not only for adults, but also for teenagers.

Making the transition from childhood to adulthood is not easy, as hormones affect every tissue in a teen's rapidly growing body—including the brain. Lorrie and I have noticed that the Paleo Diet has had a calming effect on all three of our sons' behavior, compared to typical adolescents'. Both dairy and wheat contain psychoactive substances called exorphins that enter the bloodstream and bind opioid (pain) receptors in the brain. Dr. Dohan has shown that wheat- and dairy-free diets have proven healing value in schizophrenic patients under clinical settings. In perhaps the most comprehensive review examining cereals and schizophrenia, Dr. Lorenz from Colorado State University concluded, "In populations eating little or no wheat, rye, and barley, the prevalence of schizophrenia is quite low and about the same regardless of type of acculturating influence."

Wheat- and dairy-free diets such as the Paleo Diet also appear to have therapeutic potential in other mental disorders, such as attention deficit disorder (ADHD), depression, and autism. Few well-controlled experiments have been carried out to examine the efficacy of wheat- and dairy-free diets in children or adults with these mental conditions. Nevertheless, the preliminary evidence is encouraging. In a review of the seven trials that eliminated either wheat or dairy, or both, from the diets of autistic children, Drs. Christison and Ivany summarized, "All [trials] reported efficacy in reducing some autism symptoms, and 2 groups of investigators also reported improvement in nonverbal cognition."

In a study of 132 celiac patients, Drs. Niederhofer and Pittschieler reported that "ADHD-like symptomatology is markedly overrepresented among untreated celiac disease patients and that a gluten-free diet may improve symptoms significantly within a short period of time." Similar beneficial results with gluten-free diets have been reported for celiac patients with chronic depression.

Paleo Helped My Son at School: Suzanne's Story

I tried the diet out on my ten-year-old son. I noticed an immediate improvement in his concentration, problem-solving skills, and ability to deal with stressful situations. When he "falls off the wagon" at his grandmother's house or with his dad, who thinks this diet philosophy is a lot of baloney, my son becomes cranky, difficult, and indecisive. He makes mistakes on his homework, and his test grades slip.

Acne is a huge health issue that targets most teens. Metabolically, we know that acne develops during this time of life because adolescence is a period of natural insulin resistance, which aggravates acne. When high-glycemic-load carbohydrates, refined sugars, and dairy products are added into this mix, it becomes a perfect formula for producing adolescent acne. No wonder 90 percent of all U.S. teenagers get acne, as processed foods are staples in their diets. In sharp contrast, my research team and I found absolutely no acne in more than three hundred non-Westernized adolescents living on the remote island of Kitava.

Sometimes it may prove difficult to convince your teens to forgo pizza and soda, but if they know that their complexions will clear up, this decision may become much easier.

Healing Acne: Lara's Story

Our fifteen-year-old son is a competitive swimmer and has had acne for several years. A few weeks ago, we decided it was time to help him follow the Paleo Diet. His acne has cleared up. Last weekend, he had a big invitational meet. He swam like never before in his six years of competition. Everyone who saw his times was amazed.

He is already lean, anyway, but in these last few weeks he is looking more fit than ever. His muscles are more obvious, especially in his back. Now he trains under a college coach six days a week. His training is quite intensive. He realized after this last swim meet, and as his acne has cleared, that there is something to the Paleo Diet.

My daughters also eat the Paleo way at home. They are ages eleven and eight and are competitive gymnasts. We started on the Paleo Diet a couple of years ago, and it was fascinating to watch my oldest daughter's body change. She became extraordinarily strong and muscular, and her stamina far exceeds that of the other girls on the team.

I always insist that she have a protein snack before she goes to gymnastics practice. One day she left for gymnastics practice from a teammate's house. The other mom gave the girls a cookie and lemonade for a snack. My daughter was shocked to discover that she couldn't make it through practice. She found herself sitting on the side, tired like the other girls on the team. She was used to being the girl who always had enough energy for another rep.

Acknowledgments

For me, popular book writing represents a labor of love that came unexpectedly and later in life. Were it not for my wife Lorrie's gentle prodding to make my message available to a wider audience, I suspect that my literary efforts would have been exclusively limited to my scientific writings. Consequently, Lorrie's initial encouragement is the impetus for all of my popular books dealing with the Paleo Diet, including this one. Many thanks are due to Tom Miller, my editor, for his meticulous care in bringing this manuscript into its final form and for his continual support of the Paleo Diet concept over the past decade. I am especially indebted to Channa Taub, my agent, for her friendship, patience, and literary guidance over the years. It goes without saying that my popular writings have been influenced by mentors, colleagues, students, family, and friends whom I have previously acknowledged.

References

Preface and 1. Paleo 2.0

Abrams HL. A dischronic perview of wheat in hominid nutrition. *J Appl Nutr* 1978;30:41–43.

Abrams HL. The relevance of Paleolithic diet in determining contemporary nutritional needs. *J Applied Nutr* 1979;31:43–59.

Chaitow L. *Stone Age Diet*. London: Macdonald & Co. (Publishers) Ltd., 1987.

Cordain L, Lindeberg S, Hurtado M, Hill K, Eaton SB, Brand-Miller J. Acne vulgaris: a disease of Western civilization. *Arch Dermatol* 2002 Dec;138(12):1584–1590.

DeVries A. *Primitive Man and His Food*. Chicago: Chandler Book Company, 1952.

Dobzhansky T. *Am Biol Teacher* 1973 March;35:125–129.

Eaton SB, et al. Stone agers in the fast lane: chronic degenerative diseases in evolutionary perspective. *Am J Med* 1988;84:739–749.

Eaton SB, Konner M. Paleolithic nutrition. A consideration of its nature and current implications. *N Engl J Med* 1985;312:283–289.

Eaton SB, Shostak M, Konner M. *The Paleolithic Prescription*. New York: Harper & Row, 1988.

Frassetto LA, Schloetter M, Mietus-Synder M, Morris RC Jr., Sebastian A. Metabolic and physiologic improvements from consuming a Paleolithic, hunter-gatherer type diet. *Eur J Clin Nutr* 2009.

Ho-Pham LT, Nguyen ND, Nguyen TT, Nguyen DH, Bui PK, Nguyen VN, Nguyen TV. Association between vitamin D insufficiency and tuberculosis in a Vietnamese population. *BMC Infect Dis* 2010 Oct 25;10:306.

Jönsson T, Ahren B, Pacini G, Sundler F, Wierup N, Steen S, Sjoberg T, Ugander M, Frostegard J, Goransson, Lindeberg S: A Paleolithic diet confers higher insulin sensitivity, lower C-reactive protein and lower blood pressure than a cereal-based diet in domestic pigs. *Nutr Metab* (Lond) 2006;3:39.

Jönsson T, Granfeldt Y, Ahrén B, Branell UC, Pålsson G, Hansson A, Söderström M, Lindeberg S. Beneficial effects of a Paleolithic diet on cardiovascular risk factors in type 2 diabetes: a randomized cross-over pilot study. *Cardiovasc Diabetol* 2009;8:35.

Jönsson T, Granfeldt Y, Erlanson-Albertsson C, Ahren B, Lindeberg S. A Paleolithic diet is more satiating per calorie than a Mediterranean-like diet in individuals with ischemic heart disease. *Nutr Metab* (Lond) 2010 Nov 30;7(1):85.

Lindeberg S, Lundh B. Apparent absence of stroke and ischaemic heart disease in a traditional Melanesian island: a clinical study in Kitava. *J Intern Med* 1993, 233(3):269–275.

Lindeberg S, Nilsson-Ehle P, Terént A, Vessby B, Scherstén B.Cardiovascular risk factors in a Melanesian population apparently free from stroke and ischaemic heart disease: the Kitava study. *J Intern Med* 1994 Sep;236(3):331–340.

Lindeberg S, Berntorp E, Carlsson R, Eliasson M, Marckmann P. Haemostatic variables in Pacific Islanders apparently free from stroke and ischaemic heart disease—the Kitava Study. *Thromb Haemost* 1997 Jan;77(1):94–98.

Lindeberg S, Eliasson M, Lindahl B, Ahrén B. Low serum insulin in traditional Pacific Islanders—the Kitava Study. *Metabolism* 1999;48(10):1216–1219.

Lindeberg S, Jonsson T, Granfeldt Y, Borgstrand E, Soffman J, Sjostrom K, Ahren B. A Palaeolithic diet improves glucose tolerance more than a Mediterranean-like diet in individuals with ischaemic heart disease. *Diabetologia* 2007;50(9):1795–1807.

Nnoaham KE, Clarke A. Low serum vitamin D levels and tuberculosis: a systematic review and meta-analysis. *Int J Epidemiol* 2008 Feb;37(1):113–119.

Nesse RM, Stearns SC, Omenn GS. Medicine needs evolution. *Science* 2006;311:1071.

O'Dea K. Marked improvement in carbohydrate and lipid metabolism in diabetic Australian aborigines after temporary reversion to traditional lifestyle. *Diabetes* 1984;33(6):596–603.

Osterdahl M, Kocturk T, Koochek A, Wandell PE. Effects of a short-term intervention with a Paleolithic diet in healthy volunteers. *Eur J Clin Nutr* 2008;62(5):682–685.

Price WA. *Nutrition and Pphysical Degeneration: A Comparison of Primitive and Modern Diets and Their Effects*. New York: P.B. Hoeber, Inc., 1939.

Pritchard JK. How we are evolving. *Sci Am*. 2010 Oct;303(4):40–47.

Shatin R. Man and his cultigens. *Scientific Australian* 1964;1:34–39.

Shatin R. The transition from food-gathering to food-production in evolution and disease. *Vitalstoffe Zivilisationskrankheitein* 1967;12:104–107.

Talat N, Perry S, Parsonnet J, Dawood G, Hussain R. Vitamin D deficiency and tuberculosis progression. *Emerg Infect Dis* 2010 May;16(5):853–855.

Truswell AS. Diet and nutrition of hunter-gatherers. In: *Health and disease in tribal societies*. New York: Elsevier, 1977:213–221.

Truswell AS. Human Nutritional Problems at Four Stages of Technical Development. Reprint. Queen Elizabeth College (University of London), Inaugural Lecture, May, 1972.

Voegtlin WL. *The Stone Age Diet*. New York: Vantage Press, 1975.

Yamshchikov AV, Kurbatova EV, Kumari M, Blumberg HM, Ziegler TR, Ray SM, Tangpricha V. Vitamin D status and antimicrobial peptide cathelicidin (LL-37) concentrations in patients with active pulmonary tuberculosis. *Am J Clin Nutr* 2010 Sep;92(3):603–611.

Yudkin J. Archaeology and the nutritionist. In: *The Domestication and Exploitation of Plants and Animals*, PJ Ucko, GW Dimbleby (Eds.), Chicago: Aldine Publishing Co., 1969, pp. 547–552.

Williams GC, Nesse RM. The dawn of Darwinian medicine. *Q Rev Biol* 1991 Mar;66(1):1–22.

2. The Truth about Saturated Fat

Appel LJ, Sacks FM, Carey VJ, Obarzanek E, Swain JF, Miller ER 3rd, Conlin PR, Erlinger TP, Rosner BA, Laranjo NM, Charleston J, McCarron P, Bishop LM, OmniHeart Collaborative Research Group. Effects of protein, monounsaturated fat, and carbohydrate intake on blood pressure and serum lipids: results of the OmniHeart randomized trial. *JAMA* 2005 Nov 16;294(19):2455–2464.

Astrup A, Dyerberg J, Elwood P, Hermansen K, Hu FB, Jakobsen MU, Kok FJ, Krauss RM, Lecerf JM, Legrand P, Nestel P, Risérus U, Sanders T, Sinclair A, Stender S, Tholstrup T, Willett W. The role of reducing intakes of saturated fat in the prevention of cardiovascular disease: where does the evidence stand in 2010? *Am J Clin Nutr* 2011 Jan 26.

Aude YW, Agatston AS, Lopez-Jimenez F, Lieberman EH, Marie Almon, Hansen M, Rojas G, Lamas GA, Hennekens CH. The national cholesterol education program diet vs a diet lower in carbohydrates and higher in protein and monounsaturated fat: a randomized trial. *Arch Intern Med* 2004 Oct 25;164(19):2141–2146.

Boaz N.T. *Evolving Health: The Origins of Illness and How the Modern World Is Making Us Sick.* New York: John Wiley & Sons, Inc., 2002.

Campbell TC, Junshi C. Diet and chronic degenerative diseases: perspectives from China. *Am J Clin Nutr* 1994 May;59(5 Suppl):1153S–1161S.

Campbell TC, Parpia B, Chen J. Diet, lifestyle, and the etiology of coronary artery disease: the Cornell China study. *Am J Cardiol* 1998 Nov 26;82(10B):18T–21T.

Clarke R, Frost C, Collins R, Appleby P, Peto R. Dietary lipids and blood cholesterol: quantitative meta-analysis of metabolic ward studies. *BMJ* 1997 Jan 11;314(7074):112–117.

Cordain L, Miller JB, Eaton SB, Mann N, Holt SH, Speth JD. Plant-animal subsistence ratios and macronutrient energy estimations in worldwide hunter-gatherer diets. *Am J Clin Nutr* 2000 Mar;71(3):682–692.

Cordain L. Saturated fat consumption in ancestral human diets: implications for contemporary intakes. In: *Phytochemicals, Nutrient-Gene Interactions*, Meskin MS, Bidlack WR, Randolph RK (eds.), CRC Press (Taylor & Francis Group), 2006, pp. 115–126.

Farnsworth E, Luscombe ND, Noakes M, Wittert G, Argyiou E, Clifton PM. Effect of a high-protein, energy-restricted diet on body composition, glycemic control, and lipid concentrations in overweight and obese hyperinsulinemic men and women. *Am J Clin Nutr* 2003 Jul;78(1):31–39.

Flegal KM. Evaluating epidemiologic evidence of the effects of food and nutrient exposures. *Am J Clin Nutr* 1999 Jun;69(6):1339S–1344S.

Fraser GE. A search for truth in dietary epidemiology. *Am J Clin Nutr* 2003 Sep;78 (3 Suppl):521S–525S.

Freudenheim JL. Study design and hypothesis testing: issues in the evaluation of evidence from research in nutritional epidemiology. *Am J Clin Nutr* 1999 Jun; 69(6): 1315S–1321S.

German JB, Dillard CJ. Saturated fats: what dietary intake? *Am J Clin Nutr* 2004;80: 550.

Hegsted DM, Ausman LM, Johnson JA, Dallal GE. Dietary fat and serum lipids: an evaluation of the experimental data. *Am J Clin Nutr* 1993 Jun;57(6):875–883.

Hegsted DM, McGandy RB, Myers ML Stare FJ. Quantitative effects of dietary fat on serum cholesterol in man. *Am J Clin Nutr* 1965;17:281–295.

Howell WH, McNamara DJ, Tosca MA, Smith BT, Gaines JA. Plasma lipid and lipoprotein responses to dietary fat and cholesterol: a meta-analysis. *Am J Clin Nutr* 1997 Jun;65(6):1747–1764.

Hu FB, Stampfer MJ, Manson JE, Rimm E, Colditz GA, Speizer FE, Hennekens CH, Willett WC. Dietary protein and risk of ischemic heart disease in women. *Am J Clin Nutr* 1999 Aug;70(2):221–227.

Keys A, Anderson IT, Grande F. Prediction of serum-cholesterol responses of man to changes in fats in the diet. *Lancet* 1957;2:959–966.

Layman DK, Boileau RA, Erickson DJ, Painter JE, Shiue H, Sather C, Christou DD. A reduced ratio of dietary carbohydrate to protein improves body composition and blood lipid profiles during weight loss in adult women. *J Nutr* 2003 Feb;133(2):411–417.

Luscombe-Marsh ND, Noakes M, Wittert GA, Keogh JB, Foster P, Clifton PM. Carbohydrate-restricted diets high in either monounsaturated fat or protein are equally effective at promoting fat loss and improving blood lipids. *Am J Clin Nutr* 2005 Apr;81(4):762–772.

McAuley KA, Hopkins CM, Smith KJ, McLay RT, Williams SM, Taylor RW, Mann JI. Comparison of high-fat and high-protein diets with a high-carbohydrate diet in insulin-resistant obese women. *Diabetologia* 2005 Jan;48(1):8–16.

McDowell M, Briefel R, Alaimo K, et al. Energy and macronutrient intakes of persons ages 2 months and over in the United States. *Third National Health and Nutrition Examination Survey, Phase 1, 1988–91.* Washington, DC: US Government Printing Office, Vital and Health Statistics, 1994. CDC publication No. 255.

Mensink RP, Zock PL, Kester AD, Katan MB. Effects of dietary fatty acids and carbohydrates on the ratio of serum total to HDL cholesterol and on serum lipids and apolipoproteins: a meta-analysis of 60 controlled trials. *Am J Clin Nutr* 2003 May;77(5):1146–1155.

Micha R, Mozaffarian D. Saturated fat and cardiometabolic risk factors, coronary heart disease, stroke, and diabetes: a fresh look at the evidence. *Lipids* 2010 Oct;45(10):893–905. Epub 2010 Mar 31.

Micha R, Wallace SK, Mozaffarian D. Red and processed meat consumption and risk of incident coronary heart disease, stroke, and diabetes mellitus: a systematic review and meta-analysis. *Circulation* 2010 Jun 1;121(21):2271–2283.

Mozaffarian D, Micha R, Wallace S. Effects on coronary heart disease of increasing polyunsaturated fat in place of saturated fat: a systematic review and meta-analysis of randomized controlled trials. *PLoS Med* 2010 Mar 23;7(3):e1000252.

National Academy of Sciences, Institute of Medicine. Letter Report on Dietary Reference Intakes for Trans Fatty Acids, 2002 http://www.iom.edu/CMS/5410.aspx.

Nelson GJ. Dietary fat, trans fatty acids, and risk of coronary heart disease. *Nutr Rev* 1998 Aug;56(8):250–252.

Nesse RM, Williams GC. *Why We Get Sick: The New Science of Darwinian Medicine.* New York: *Times Books*, 1994.

Noakes M, Keogh JB, Foster PR, Clifton PM. Effect of an energy-restricted, high-protein, low-fat diet relative to a conventional high-carbohydrate, low-fat diet on weight loss, body composition, nutritional status, and markers of cardiovascular health in obese women. *Am J Clin Nutr* 2005 Jun;81(6):1298–1306.

No authors listed. Position paper on trans fatty acids. ASCN/AIN Task Force on Trans Fatty Acids. American Society for Clinical Nutrition and American Institute of Nutrition. *Am J Clin Nutr* 1996 May;63(5):663–670.

O'Dea K, Traianedes K, Chisholm K, Leyden H, Sinclair AJ. Cholesterol-lowering effect of a low-fat diet containing lean beef is reversed by the addition of beef fat. *Am J Clin Nutr* 1990 Sep;52(3):491–494.

Popkin BM. Where's the fat? Trends in U.S. Diets 1965–1996. *Prev Med* 2001; 32:245–254.

Potischman N, Weed DL. Causal criteria in nutritional epidemiology. *Am J Clin Nutr* 1999 Jun;69(6):1309S–1314S.

Ravnskov U. The fallacies of the lipid hypothesis. *Scand Cardiovasc J* 2008 Aug;42(4): 236–239.

Ravnskov U. The questionable role of saturated and polyunsaturated fatty acids in cardiovascular disease. *J Clin Epidemiol* 1998 Jun;51(6):443–460.

Ravnskov U, Allen C, Atrens D, Enig MG, Groves B, Kauffman JM, Kroneld R, Rosch PJ, Rosenman R, Werkö L, Nielsen JV, Wilske J, Worm N. Studies of dietary fat and heart disease. *Science* 2002 Feb 22;295(5559):1464–1466.

Sempos CT, Liu K, Ernst ND. Food and nutrient exposures: what to consider when evaluating epidemiologic evidence. *Am J Clin Nutr* 1999 Jun;69(6):1330S–1338S.

Siri-Tarino PW, Sun Q, Hu FB, Krauss RM. Saturated fatty acids and risk of coronary heart disease: modulation by replacement nutrients. *Curr Atheroscler Rep* 2010 Nov;12(6):384–390.

Siri-Tarino PW, Sun Q, Hu FB, Krauss RM. Saturated fat, carbohydrate, and cardiovascular disease. *Am J Clin Nutr* 2010 Mar;91(3):502–509.

Siri-Tarino PW, Sun Q, Hu FB, Krauss RM. Meta-analysis of prospective cohort studies evaluating the association of saturated fat with cardiovascular disease. *Am J Clin Nutr* 2010 Mar;91(3):535–546.

Stamler J. Diet-heart: a problematic revisit. *Am J Clin Nutr* 2010; 91:497–499.

Taubes G. Nutrition: The soft science of dietary fat. *Science* 2001 Mar 30;291(5513):2536–2545.

Weigle DS, Breen PA, Matthys CC, Callahan HS, Meeuws KE, Burden VR, Purnell JQ. A high-protein diet induces sustained reductions in appetite, ad libitum caloric intake, and body weight despite compensatory changes in diurnal plasma leptin and ghrelin concentrations. *Am J Clin Nutr* 2005 Jul;82(1):41–48.

3. Your Own Paleo Diet

http://www.ams.usda.gov/nop/NationalList/TAPReviews/shellac.pdf

http://www.ams.usda.gov/nop/NationalList/TAPReviews/morpholine.pdf

http://www.hc-sc.gc.ca/fn-an/securit/facts-faits/morpholine/exec_summary-resume_exec_e.html

Abegaz EG, Bursey RG. Formaldehyde, aspartame, migraines: a possible connection. *Dermatitis* 2009 May-Jun;20(3):176–177; author reply 177–179.

Alexiou P, Chatzopoulou M, Pegklidou K, Demopoulos VJ. RAGE: a multi-ligand receptor unveiling novel insights in health and disease. *Curr Med Chem* 2010;17(21):2232–2252.

Bai J, Hagenmaier RD, Baldwin EA. Volatile response of four apple varieties with different coatings during marketing at room temperature. *J Agric Food Chem* 2002 Dec 18;50(26):7660–7668.

Bandyopadhyay A, Ghoshal S, Mukherjee A. Genotoxicity testing of low-calorie sweeteners: aspartame, acesulfame-K, and saccharin. *Drug Chem Toxicol* 2008;31(4):447–457.

Baker BP, Benbrook CM, Groth E 3rd, Lutz Benbrook K. Pesticide residues in conventional, integrated pest management (IPM)-grown and organic foods: insights from three US data sets. *Food Addit Contam* 2002 May;19(5):427–446.

Baldwin EA. Edible coatings for fresh fruits and vegetables: past, present, and future. In *Edible Coatings and Films to Improve Food Quality*, Krochta, JM, Baldwin, EA, Nisperos-Carriedo, MO (eds). Lancaster, PA: Technomic Publishing Co., 1994: 25–64.

Barlovic DP, Thomas MC, Jandeleit-Dahm K. Cardiovascular disease: what's all the AGE/RAGE about? *Cardiovasc Hematol Disord Drug Targets* 2010 Mar;10(1):7–15.

Belpoggi F, Soffritti M, Padovani M, Degli Esposti D, Lauriola M, Minardi F. Results of long-term carcinogenicity bioassay on Sprague-Dawley rats exposed to aspartame administered in feed. *Ann N Y Acad Sci* 2006 Sep;1076:559–577.

Bengmark S. Advanced glycation and lipoxidation end products—amplifiers of inflammation: the role of food. *JPEN J Parenter Enteral Nutr* 2007 Sep–Oct;31(5):430–440.

Berkey CS, Rockett HR, Gillman MW, Field AE, Colditz GA. Longitudinal study of skipping breakfast and weight change in adolescents. *Int J Obes Relat Metab Disord* 2003 Oct;27(10):1258–1266.

Bigal ME, Krymchantowski AV. Migraine triggered by sucralose—a case report. *Headache* 2006 Mar;46(3):515–517.

Bigard AX, Boussif M, Chalabi H, Guezennec CY. Alterations in muscular performance and orthostatic tolerance during Ramadan. *Aviat Space Environ Med* 1998 Apr;69(4):341–346.

Brand-Miller JC, Holt SHA. Australian Aboriginal plant foods: a consideration of their nutritional composition and health implications. *Nut Res Rev* 1998;11:5–23.

Brown RJ, de Banate MA, Rother KI. Artificial sweeteners: a systematic review of metabolic effects in youth. *Int J Pediatr Obes* 2010 Aug;5(4):305–312.

Brown RJ, Walter M, Rother KI. Ingestion of diet soda before a glucose load augments glucagon-like peptide-1 secretion. *Diabetes Care* 2009 Dec;32(12):2184–2186.

Bourne D, Prescott J. A comparison of the nutritional value, sensory qualities, and food safety of organically and conventionally produced foods. *Crit Rev Food Sci Nutr* 2002; 42:1–34.

Clastres P. The Guayaki. In: *Hunters and Gatherers Today*, Bicchieri MG (ed). New York: Holt, Rinehart and Winston, Inc., 1972: 151.

Correia M, Barroso Â, Barroso MF, Soares DB, Oliveira MBPP, and Delerue-Matos C. Contribution of different vegetable types to exogenous nitrate and nitrite exposure. *Food Chem* 2010;120: 960–968.

Crinnion WJ. Organic foods contain higher levels of certain nutrients, lower levels of pesticides, and may provide health benefits for the consumer. *Altern Med Rev* 2010 Apr;15(1):4–12.

Fedail SS, Murphy D, Salih SY, Bolton CH, Harvey RF. Changes in certain blood constituents during Ramadan. *Am J Clin Nutr* 1982 Aug;36(2):350–353.

Fontana L, Meyer TE, Klein S, Holloszy JO. Long-term calorie restriction is highly effective in reducing the risk for atherosclerosis in humans. *Proc Natl Acad Sci USA.* 2004 Apr 27;101(17):6659– 6663.

Halldorsson TI, Strøm M, Petersen SB, Olsen SF. Intake of artificially sweetened soft drinks and risk of preterm delivery: a prospective cohort study in 59,334 Danish pregnant women. *Am J Clin Nutr* 2010 Sep;92(3):626–633.

Heilbronn LK, Ravussin E. Calorie restriction and aging: review of the literature and implications for studies in humans. *Am J Clin Nutr* 2003 Sep;78(3):361–369.

Higami Y, Yamaza H, Shimokawa I. Laboratory findings of caloric restriction in rodents and primates. *Adv Clin Chem* 2005;39:211–237.

Husain R, Duncan MT, Cheah SH, Ch'ng SL. Effects of fasting in Ramadan on tropical Asiatic Moslems. *Br J Nutr* 1987 Jul;58(1):41–48.

Jacob SE, Stechschulte S. Formaldehyde, aspartame, and migraines: a possible connection. *Dermatitis* 2008 May–Jun;19(3):E10–1.

Keim NL, Van Loan MD, Horn WF, Barbieri TF, Mayclin PL.Weight loss is greater with consumption of large morning meals and fat-free mass is preserved with large evening meals in women on a controlled weight reduction regimen. *J Nutr* 1997 Jan;127(1):75–82.

Keski-Rahkonen A, Kaprio J, Rissanen A, Virkkunen M, Rose RJ. Breakfast skipping and health-compromising behaviors in adolescents and adults. *Eur J Clin Nutr* 2003 Jul;57(7):842–853.

Kirkwood TB, Shanley DP. Food restriction, evolution and ageing. *Mech Ageing Dev* 2005 Sep;126(9):1011–1016.

Knekt P, Jarvinen R, Dich J, Hakulinen T. Risk of colorectal and other gastro-intestinal cancers after exposure to nitrate, nitrite and N-nitroso compounds: a follow-up study. *Int J Cancer* 1999 Mar 15;80(6):852–856.

Lee RB. The !Kung Bushmen of Botswana. In: *Hunters and Gatherers Today*, Bicchieri MG. (ed). New York: Holt, Rinehart and Winston, Inc., 1972: 151.

Lipton RB, Newman LC, Cohen JS, Solomon S. Aspartame as a dietary trigger of headache. *Headache* 1989 Feb;29(2):90–92.

Magkos F, Arvaniti F, Zampelas A. Organic food: nutritious food or food for thought? A review of the evidence. *Int J Food Sci Nutr* 2003;54:357–371.

Malaisse WJ, Vanonderbergen A, Louchami K, Jijakli H, Malaisse-Lagae F. Effects of artificial sweeteners on insulin release and cationic fluxes in rat pancreatic islets. *Cell Signal* 1998 Nov;10(10):727–733.

Masoro EJ. Overview of caloric restriction and ageing. *Mech Ageing Dev* 2005 Sep;126(9):913–922.

Mattison JA, Lane MA, Roth GS, Ingram DK. Calorie restriction in rhesus monkeys. *Exp Gerontol* 2003 Jan–Feb;38(1–2):35–46.

Mattson MP. The need for controlled studies of the effects of meal frequency on health. *Lancet* 2005;365:1978–1980.

Mattson MP, Wan R. Beneficial effects of intermittent fasting and caloric restriction on the cardiovascular and cerebrovascular systems. *J Nutr Biochem* 2005 Mar;16(3):129–137.

Mensinga TT, Speijers GJ, Meulenbelt J. Health implications of exposure to environmental nitrogenous compounds. *Toxicol Rev* 2003;22(1):41–51.

Newman LC, Lipton RB. Migraine MLT-down: an unusual presentation of migraine in patients with aspartame-triggered headaches. *Headache* 2001 Oct;41(9):899–901.

Nin JW, Jorsal A, Ferreira I, Schalkwijk CG, Prins MH, Parving HH, Tarnow L, Rossing P, Stehouwer CD. Higher plasma levels of advanced glycation end products are associated with incident cardiovascular disease and all-cause mortality in type 1 diabetes: a 12-year follow-up study. *Diabetes Care* 2011 Feb;34(2):442–447.

Osgood C. *Ingalik Social Culture.* New Haven: Yale University Press, 1958: 166.

Schalkwijk CG, Stehouwer CD, van Hinsbergh VW. Fructose-mediated non-enzymatic glycation: sweet coupling or bad modification. *Diabetes Metab Res Rev* 2004 Sep–Oct;20(5):369–382.

Schlundt DG, Hill JO, Sbrocco T, Pope-Cordle J, Sharp T. The role of breakfast in the treatment of obesity: a randomized clinical trial. *Am J Clin Nutr* 1992 Mar;55(3):645–651.

Semba RD, Nicklett EJ, Ferrucci L. Does accumulation of advanced glycation end products contribute to the aging phenotype? *J Gerontol A Biol Sci Med Sci* 2010 Sep;65(9):963–975.

Sinclair DA. Toward a unified theory of caloric restriction and longevity regulation. *Mech Ageing Dev* 2005 Sep;126(9):987–1002.

Soffritti M, Belpoggi F, Tibaldi E, Esposti DD, Lauriola M. Life-span exposure to low doses of aspartame beginning during prenatal life increases cancer effects in rats. *Environ Health Perspect* 2007 Sep;115(9):1293–1297.

Song WO, Chun OK, Obayashi S, Cho S, Chung CE. Is consumption of breakfast associated with body mass index in US adults? *J Am Diet Assoc* 2005 Sep;105(9):1373–1382.

Spindler SR. Rapid and reversible induction of the longevity, anticancer and genomic effects of caloric restriction. *Mech Ageing Dev* 2005 Sep;126(9):960–966.

Sweileh N, Schnitzler A, Hunter GR, Davis B. Body composition and energy metabolism in resting and exercising Muslims during Ramadan fast. *J Sports Med Phys Fitness* 1992 Jun;32(2):156–163.

Swithers SE, Baker CR, Davidson TL. General and persistent effects of high-intensity sweeteners on body weight gain and caloric compensation in rats. *Behav Neurosci* 2009 Aug;123(4):772–780.

Swithers SE, Davidson TL. A role for sweet taste: calorie predictive relations in energy regulation by rats. *Behav Neurosci* 2008 Feb;122(1):161–173.

Swithers SE, Martin AA, Clark KM, Laboy AF, Davidson TL. Body weight gain in rats consuming sweetened liquids. Effects of caffeine and diet composition. *Appetite* 2010 Dec;55(3):528–533.

Swithers SE, Martin AA, Davidson TL. High-intensity sweeteners and energy balance. *Physiol Behav* 2010 Apr 26;100(1):55–62.

Takeuchi M, Iwaki M, Takino J, Shirai H, Kawakami M, Bucala R, Yamagishi S. Immunological detection of fructose-derived advanced glycation end-products. *Lab Invest* 2010 Jul;90(7):1117–1127.

Uribarri J, Woodruff S, Goodman S, Cai W, Chen X, Pyzik R, Yong A, Striker GE, Vlassara H. Advanced glycation end products in foods and a practical guide to their reduction in the diet. *J Am Diet Assoc* 2010 Jun;110(6):911–916.

Whitehouse CR, Boullata J, McCauley LA. The potential toxicity of artificial sweeteners. *AAOHN J* 2008 Jun;56(6):251–259.

Williams CM. Nutritional quality of organic food: shades of grey or shades of green? *Proc Nutr Soc* 2002;61:19–24.

Woese K, Lange D, Boess C, Bogl KW. A comparison of organically and conventionally grown foods—Results of a review of the relevant literature. *J Sci Food Agric* 1997;74:281–293.

Worthington V. Effect of agricultural methods on nutritional quality: a comparison of organic with conventional crops. *Alternative Therapies* 1998;4: 58–68.

Worthington V. Nutritional quality of organic versus conventional fruits, vegetables, and grains. *J Altern Complement Med* 2001;2:161–173.

Xu Q, Yin X, Wang M, Wang H, Zhang N, Shen Y, Xu S, Zhang L, Gu Z. Analysis of phthalate migration from plastic containers to packaged cooking oil and mineral water. *J Agric Food Chem* 2010 Oct 15.

Yan SF, Ramasamy R, Schmidt AM. The RAGE axis: a fundamental mechanism signaling danger to the vulnerable vasculature. *Circ Res* 2010 Mar 19;106(5):842–853.

Yang Q. Gain weight by "going diet?" Artificial sweeteners and the neurobiology of sugar cravings. Neuroscience 2010. *Yale J Biol Med* 2010 Jun;83(2):101–108.

Zahm SH, Ward MH. Pesticides and childhood cancer. *Environ Health Perspect* 1998 Jun;106 Suppl 3:893–908.

Zender R, Bachand AM, Reif JS. Exposure to tap water during pregnancy. *J Expo Anal Environ Epidemiol* 2001 May–Jun;11(3):224–230.

4. Vegetarianism Can Be Hazardous to Your Health

Alexander D, Ball MJ, Mann J. Nutrient intake and haematological status of vegetarians and age-sex matched omnivores. *Eur J Clin Nutr* 1994 Aug;48(8):538–546.

Appleby P, Roddam A, Allen N, Key T. Comparative fracture risk in vegetarians and nonvegetarians in EPIC-Oxford. *Eur J Clin Nutr* 2007 Dec;61(12):1400–1406.

Appleton KM, Rogers PJ, Ness AR. Updated systematic review and meta-analysis of the effects of n-3 long-chain polyunsaturated fatty acids on depressed mood. *Am J Clin Nutr* 2010 Mar;91(3):757–770.

Baines M, Kredan MB, Davison A, Higgins G, West C, Fraser WD, Ranganath LR. The association between cysteine, bone turnover, and low bone mass. *Calcif Tissue Int* 2007 Dec;81(6):450–454.

Baines S, Powers J, Brown WJ. How does the health and well-being of young Australian vegetarian and semi-vegetarian women compare with non-vegetarians? *Public Health Nutr* 2007 May;10(5):436–442.

Bhushan S, Pandey RC, Singh SP, Pandey DN, Seth P. Some observations on human semen analysis. *Indian J Physiol Pharmacol* 1978 Oct-Dec;22(4):393–396.

Bennett M. Vitamin B12 deficiency, infertility and recurrent fetal loss. *J Reprod Med* 2001 Mar;46(3):209–212.

Berker B, Kaya C, Aytac R, Satiroglu H. Homocysteine concentrations in follicular fluid are associated with poor oocyte and embryo qualities in polycystic ovary syndrome patients undergoing assisted reproduction. *Hum Reprod* 2009 Sep;24(9):2293–2302.

Bissoli L, Di Francesco V, Ballarin A, Mandragona R, Trespidi R, Brocco G, Caruso B, Bosello O, Zamboni M. Effect of vegetarian diet on homocysteine levels. *Ann Nutr Metab* 2002;46(2):73–79.

Bocherens H, Drucker DG, Billiou D, Patou-Mathis M, Vandermeersch B. Isotopic evidence for diet and subsistence pattern of the Saint-Cesaire I Neanderthal: review and use of a multi-source mixing model. *J Hum Evol* 2005 Jul;49(1):71–87.

Boivin J, Bunting L, Collins JA, Nygren KG. International estimates of infertility prevalence and treatment-seeking: potential need and demand for infertility medical care. *Hum Reprod* 2007 Jun;22(6):1506–1512.

Boxmeer JC, Brouns RM, Lindemans J, Steegers EA, Martini E, Macklon NS, Steegers-Theunissen RP. Preconception folic acid treatment affects the microenvironment of the maturing oocyte in humans. *Fertil Steril* 2008 Jun;89(6):1766–1770.

Boxmeer JC, Smit M, Utomo E, Romijn JC, Eijkemans MJ, Lindemans J, Laven JS, Macklon NS, Steegers EA, Steegers-Theunissen RP. Low folate in seminal plasma is associated with increased sperm DNA damage. *Fertil Steril* 2009 Aug;92(2):548–556.

Boxmeer JC, Smit M, Weber RF, Lindemans J, Romijn JC, Eijkemans MJ, Macklon NS, Steegers-Theunissen RP. Seminal plasma cobalamin significantly correlates with sperm concentration in men undergoing IVF or ICSI procedures. *J Androl* 2007 Jul–Aug;28(4):521–527.

Brenna JT, Salem N Jr, Sinclair AJ, Cunnane SC. alpha-Linolenic acid supplementation and conversion to n-3 long-chain polyunsaturated fatty acids in humans. *Prostaglandins Leukot Essent Fatty Acids* 2009 Feb–Mar;80(2–3):85–91.

Brown KH, Peerson JM, Baker SK, Hess SY. Preventive zinc supplementation among infants, preschoolers, and older prepubertal children. *Food Nutr Bull* 2009 Mar;30 (1 Suppl):S12–40.

Bucciarelli P, Martini G, Martinelli I, Ceccarelli E, Gennari L, Bader R, Valenti R, Franci B, Nuti R, Mannucci PM. The relationship between plasma homocysteine levels and bone mineral density in post-menopausal women. *Eur J Intern Med* 2010 Aug;21(4):301–305.

Bunn, HT, Kroll EM. Systematic butchery by Plio-Pleistocene hominids at Olduvai Gorge, Tanzania. *Curr Anthropol* 1986;20:365–398.

Calder PC, Yaqoob P. Omega-3 (n-3) fatty acids, cardiovascular disease and stability of atherosclerotic plaques. *Cell Mol Biol (Noisy-le-grand)* 2010 Feb 25;56(1):28–37.

Campbell-Brown M, Ward RJ, Haines AP, North WR, Abraham R, McFadyen IR, Turnlund JR, King JC. Zinc and copper in Asian pregnancies—is there evidence for a nutritional deficiency? *Br J Obstet Gynaecol* 1985 Sep;92(9):875–885.

Cappuccio FP, Bell R, Perry IJ, Gilg J, Ueland PM, Refsum H, Sagnella GA, Jeffery S, Cook DG. Homocysteine levels in men and women of different ethnic and cultural background living in England. *Atherosclerosis* 2002 Sep;164(1):95–102.

Clarke R. B-vitamins and prevention of dementia. *Proc Nutr Soc* 2008 Feb;67(1):75–81.

Clarke R, Birks J, Nexo E, Ueland PM, Schneede J, Scott J, Molloy A, Evans JG. Low vitamin B-12 status and risk of cognitive decline in older adults. *Am J Clin Nutr* 2007 Nov;86(5):1384–1391.

Clarke R, Sherliker P, Hin H, Nexo E, Hvas AM, Schneede J, Birks J, Ueland PM, Emmens K, Scott JM, Molloy AM, Evans JG. Detection of vitamin B12 deficiency in older people by measuring vitamin B12 or the active fraction of vitamin B12, holotranscobalamin. *Clin Chem* 2007 May;53(5):963–970.

Cogswell ME, Looker AC, Pfeiffer CM, Cook JD, Lacher DA, Beard JL, Lynch SR, Grummer-Strawn LM. Assessment of iron deficiency in US preschool children and nonpregnant females of childbearing age: National Health and Nutrition Examination Survey 2003–2006. *Am J Clin Nutr* 2009 May;89(5):1334–1342.

Cordain L, Campbell TC. The protein debate. *Catalyst Athletics*, March 19, 2008 http://www.cathletics.com/articles/article.php?articleID=50.

Cordain L, Miller JB, Eaton SB, Mann N, Holt SH, Speth JD. Plant-animal subsistence ratios and macronutrient energy estimations in worldwide hunter-gatherer diets. *Am J Clin Nutr* 2000 Mar;71(3):682–692.

Craig WJ, Mangels AR; American Dietetic Association. Position of the American Dietetic Association: vegetarian diets. *J Am Diet Assoc*. 2009 Jul;109(7):1266–1282.

Crowe FL, Steur M, Allen NE, Appleby PN, Travis RC, Key TJ. Plasma concentrations of 25-hydroxyvitamin D in meat eaters, fish eaters, vegetarians and vegans: results from the EPIC-Oxford study. *Public Health Nutr* 2011 Feb;14(2):340–346.

Dasarathy J, Gruca LL, Bennett C, Parimi PS, Duenas C, Marczewski S, Fierro JL, Kalhan SC. Methionine metabolism in human pregnancy. *Am J Clin Nutr* 2010 Feb;91(2):357–365.

Davey GK, Spencer EA, Appleby PN, Allen NE, Knox KH, Key TJ. EPIC-Oxford: lifestyle characteristics and nutrient intakes in a cohort of 33 883 meat-eaters and 31 546 non meat-eaters in the UK. *Public Health Nutr* 2003 May;6(3):259–269.

de Bortoli MC, Cozzolino SM. Zinc and selenium nutritional status in vegetarians. *Biol Trace Elem Res* 2009 Mar;127(3):228–233.

de Heinzelin J, Clark JD, White T, Hart W, Renne P, WoldeGabriel G, Beyene Y, Vrba E. Environment and behavior of 2.5-million-year-old Bouri hominids. *Science* 1999 Apr 23;284(5414):625–629.

Dhonukshe-Rutten RA, van Dusseldorp M, Schneede J, de Groot LC, van Staveren WA. Low bone mineral density and bone mineral content are associated with low cobalamin status in adolescents. *Eur J Nutr* 2005 Sep;44(6):341–347.

Dror DK, Allen LH. Effect of vitamin B12 deficiency on neurodevelopment in infants: current knowledge and possible mechanisms. *Nutr Rev* 2008 May;66(5):250–255.

Ebisch IM, Peters WH, Thomas CM, Wetzels AM, Peer PG, Steegers-Theunissen RP. Homocysteine, glutathione and related thiols affect fertility parameters in the (sub) fertile couple. *Hum Reprod* 2006 Jul;21(7):1725–1733.

Ebisch IM, Pierik FH, DE Jong FH, Thomas CM, Steegers-Theunissen RP. Does folic acid and zinc sulphate intervention affect endocrine parameters and sperm characteristics in men? *Int J Androl* 2006 Apr;29(2):339–345.

Elmadfa I, Singer I.Vitamin B-12 and homocysteine status among vegetarians: a global perspective. *Am J Clin Nutr* 2009 May;89(5):1693S–1698S.

Falkingham M, Abdelhamid A, Curtis P, Fairweather-Tait S, Dye L, Hooper L.The effects of oral iron supplementation on cognition in older children and adults: a systematic review and meta-analysis. *Nutr J* 2010 Jan 25;9:4.

Fields C, Dourson M, Borak J. Iodine-deficient vegetarians: a hypothetical perchlorate-susceptible population? *Regul Toxicol Pharmacol* 2005 Jun;42(1):37–46.

Fischer Walker CL, Ezzati M, Black RE. Global and regional child mortality and burden of disease attributable to zinc deficiency. *Eur J Clin Nutr* 2009 May;63(5):591–597.

Food habits of a nation. In: *The Hindu*, August 14, 2006 http://www.hinduonnet.com/2006/08/14/stories/2006081403771200.htm.

Fort P, Moses N, Fasano M, Goldberg T, Lifshitz F. Breast and soy-formula feedings in early infancy and the prevalence of autoimmune thyroid disease in children. *J Am Coll Nutr* 1990 Apr;9(2):164–167.

Freeland-Graves JH, Bodzy PW, Eppright MA. Zinc status of vegetarians. *J Am Diet Assoc* 1980 Dec;77(6):655–661.

Freeland-Graves JH, Ebangit ML, Hendrikson PJ. Alterations in zinc absorption and salivary sediment zinc after a lacto-ovo-vegetarian diet. *Am J Clin Nutr* 1980 Aug;33(8):1757–1766.

Gilsing AM, Crowe FL, Lloyd-Wright Z, Sanders TA, Appleby PN, Allen NE, Key TJ. Serum concentrations of vitamin B12 and folate in British male omnivores, vegetarians and vegans: results from a cross-sectional analysis of the EPIC-Oxford cohort study. *Eur J Clin Nutr* 2010 Sep;64(9):933–939.

Hansen CM, Leklem JE, Miller LT. Vitamin B-6 status indicators decrease in women consuming a diet high in pyridoxine glucoside. *J Nutr* 1996 Oct;126(10):2512–2518.

Harris WS, Kris-Etherton PM, Harris KA. Intakes of long-chain omega-3 fatty acid associated with reduced risk for death from coronary heart disease in healthy adults. *Curr Atheroscler Rep* 2008 Dec;10(6):503–509.

Herbert V. Staging vitamin B-12 (cobalamin) status in vegetarians. *Am J Clin Nutr* 1994 May;59(5 Suppl):1213S–1222S.

Herrmann M, Peter Schmidt J, Umanskaya N, Wagner A, Taban-Shomal O, Widmann T, Colaianni G, Wildemann B, Herrmann W. The role of hyperhomocysteinemia as well as folate, vitamin B(6) and B(12) deficiencies in osteoporosis: a systematic review. *Clin Chem Lab Med* 2007;45(12):1621–1632.

Herrmann M, Widmann T, Colaianni G, Colucci S, Zallone A, Herrmann W. Increased osteoclast activity in the presence of increased homocysteine concentrations. *Clin Chem* 2005 Dec;51(12):2348–2353.

Herrmann W, Obeid R, Schorr H, Geisel J. Functional vitamin B12 deficiency and determination of holotranscobalamin in populations at risk. *Clin Chem Lab Med* 2003 Nov;41(11):1478–1488.

Herrmann W, Obeid R, Schorr H, Hübner U, Geisel J, Sand-Hill M, Ali N, Herrmann M. Enhanced bone metabolism in vegetarians—the role of vitamin B12 deficiency. *Clin Chem Lab Med* 2009;47(11):1381–1387.

Herrmann W, Schorr H, Obeid R, Geisel J. Vitamin B-12 status, particularly holotranscobalamin II and methylmalonic acid concentrations, and hyperhomocysteinemia in vegetarians. *Am J Clin Nutr* 2003 Jul;78(1):131–136.

Heyland DK, Jones N, Cvijanovich NZ, Wong H. Zinc supplementation in critically ill patients: a key pharmaconutrient? *JPEN J Parenter Enteral Nutr* 2008 Sep–Oct;32(5):509–519.

Hinton PS, Sinclair LM. Iron supplementation maintains ventilatory threshold and improves energetic efficiency in iron-deficient nonanemic athletes. *Eur J Clin Nutr* 2007 Jan;61(1):30–39.

Hirwe R, Jathar VS, Desai S, Satoskar RS. Vitamin B12 and potential fertility in male lactovegetarians. *J Biosoc Sci* 1976 Jul;8(3):221–227.

Ho-Pham LT, Nguyen ND, Nguyen TV. Effect of vegetarian diets on bone mineral density: a Bayesian meta-analysis. *Am J Clin Nutr* 2009 Oct;90(4):943–950.

Hotz C. Dietary indicators for assessing the adequacy of population zinc intakes. *Food Nutr Bull* 2007 Sep;28(3 Suppl):S430–453.

Huang YC, Chang SJ, Chiu YT, Chang HH, Cheng CH. The status of plasma homocysteine and related B-vitamins in healthy young vegetarians and nonvegetarians. *Eur J Nutr* 2003 Apr;42(2):84–90.

Humphrey LL, Fu R, Rogers K, Freeman M, Helfand M. Homocysteine level and coronary heart disease incidence: a systematic review and meta-analysis. *Mayo Clin Proc* 2008 Nov;83(11):1203–1212.

Hunt JR, Matthys LA, Johnson LK. Zinc absorption, mineral balance, and blood lipids in women consuming controlled lactoovovegetarian and omnivorous diets for 8 wk. *Am J Clin Nutr* 1998 Mar;67(3):421–430.

Hunt JR, Roughead ZK. Nonheme-iron absorption, fecal ferritin excretion, and blood indexes of iron status in women consuming controlled lactoovovegetarian diets for 8 wk. *Am J Clin Nutr* 1999 May;69(5):944–952.

Hvas AM, Morkbak AL, Nexo E. Plasma holotranscobalamin compared with plasma cobalamins for assessment of vitamin B12 absorption; optimisation of a non-radioactive vitamin B12 absorption test (CobaSorb). *Clin Chim Acta* 2007 Feb;376(1–2):150–154.

Jathar VS, Hirwe R, Desai S, Satoskar RS. Dietetic habits and quality of semen in Indian subjects. *Andrologia* 1976;8(4):355–358.

Jenkins DJ, Kendall CW, Connelly PW, Jackson CJ, Parker T, Faulkner D, Vidgen E. Effects of high- and low-isoflavone (phytoestrogen) soy foods on inflammatory biomarkers and proinflammatory cytokines in middle-aged men and women. *Metabolism* 2002 Jul;51(7):919–924.

Karabudak E, Kiziltan G, Cigerim N. A comparison of some of the cardiovascular risk factors in vegetarian and omnivorous Turkish females. *J Hum Nutr Diet* 2008 Feb;21(1):13–22.

Katre P, Bhat D, Lubree H, Otiv S, Joshi S, Joglekar C, Rush E, Yajnik C. Vitamin B12 and folic acid supplementation and plasma total homocysteine concentrations in pregnant Indian women with low B12 and high folate status. *Asia Pac J Clin Nutr* 2010;19(3):335–343.

Key TJ, Appleby PN, Rosell MS. Health effects of vegetarian and vegan diets. *Proc Nutr Soc* 2006 Feb;65(1):35–41.

Key TJ, Appleby PN, Spencer EA, Travis RC, Roddam AW, Allen NE. Mortality in British vegetarians: results from the European Prospective Investigation into Cancer and Nutrition (EPIC-Oxford). *Am J Clin Nutr* 2009 May;89(5):1613S–1619S.

Key TJ, Appleby PN, Spencer EA, Travis RC, Roddam AW, Allen NE. Cancer incidence in vegetarians: results from the European Prospective Investigation into Cancer and Nutrition (EPIC-Oxford). *Am J Clin Nutr* 2009 May;89(5):1620S–1626S.

Key TJ, Fraser GE, Thorogood M, Appleby PN, Beral V, Reeves G, Burr ML, Chang-Claude J, Frentzel-Beyme R, Kuzma JW, Mann J, McPherson K. Mortality in vegetarians and nonvegetarians: detailed findings from a collaborative analysis of 5 prospective studies. *Am J Clin Nutr* 1999 Sep;70(3 Suppl):516S–524S.

Khedr E, Hamed SA, Elbeih E, El-Shereef H, Ahmad Y, Ahmed S. Iron states and cognitive abilities in young adults: neuropsychological and neurophysiological assessment. *Eur Arch Psychiatry Clin Neurosci* 2008 Dec;258(8):489–496. Epub 2008 Jun 20.

Koebnick C, Hoffmann I, Dagnelie PC, Heins UA, Wickramasinghe SN, Ratnayaka ID, Gruendel S, Lindemans J, Leitzmann C. Long-term ovo-lacto vegetarian diet impairs vitamin B-12 status in pregnant women. *J Nutr* 2004 Dec;134(12):3319–3326.

Knovich MA, Storey JA, Coffman LG, Torti SV, Torti FM. Ferritin for the clinician. *Blood Rev* 2009 May;23(3):95–104.

Kornsteiner M, Singer I, Elmadfa I. Very low n-3 long-chain polyunsaturated fatty acid status in Austrian vegetarians and vegans. *Ann Nutr Metab* 2008;52(1):37–47.

Krajcovicová-Kudláčková M, Bucková K, Klimes I, Seboková E. Iodine deficiency in vegetarians and vegans. *Ann Nutr Metab* 2003;47(5):183–185.

Krivosíková Z, Krajcovicová-Kudláčková M, Spustová V, Stefíková K, Valachovicová M, Blazícek P, Němcová T. The association between high plasma homocysteine levels and lower bone mineral density in Slovak women: the impact of vegetarian diet. *Eur J Nutr* 2010 Apr;49(3):147–153.

Kumar J, Garg G, Sundaramoorthy E, Prasad PV, Karthikeyan G, Ramakrishnan L, Ghosh S, Sengupta S. Vitamin B12 deficiency is associated with coronary artery disease in an Indian population. *Clin Chem Lab Med* 2009;47(3):334–338.

Laidlaw SA, Grosvenor M, Kopple JD. The taurine content of common foodstuffs. *JPEN J Parenter Enteral Nutr* 1990 Mar–Apr;14(2):183–188.

Laidlaw SA, Shultz TD, Cecchino JT, Kopple JD. Plasma and urine taurine levels in vegans. *Am J Clin Nutr* 1988 Apr;47(4):660–663.

Leboff MS, Narweker R, LaCroix A, Wu L, Jackson R, Lee J, Bauer DC, Cauley J, Kooperberg C, Lewis C, Thomas AM, Cummings S. Homocysteine levels and risk of hip fracture in postmenopausal women. *J Clin Endocrinol Metab* 2009 Apr;94(4):1207–1213.

Lee-Thorp J, Thackeray JF, van der Merwe N. The hunters and the hunted revisited. *J Hum Evol* 2000; 39: 565–576.

Lin PY, Huang SY, Su KP. A meta-analytic review of polyunsaturated fatty acid compositions in patients with depression. *Biol Psychiatry* 2010 Jul 15;68(2):140–147.

Mezzano D, Kosiel K, Martínez C, Cuevas A, Panes O, Aranda E, Strobel P, Pérez DD, Pereira J, Rozowski J, Leighton F. Cardiovascular risk factors in vegetarians. Normalization of hyperhomocysteinemia with vitamin B(12) and reduction of platelet aggregation with n-3 fatty acids. *Thromb Res* 2000 Nov 1;100(3):153–160.

Molloy AM, Kirke PN, Brody LC, Scott JM, Mills JL. Effects of folate and vitamin B12 deficiencies during pregnancy on fetal, infant, and child development. *Food Nutr Bull* 2008 Jun;29(2 Suppl):S101–111.

Molloy AM, Kirke PN, Troendle JF, Burke H, Sutton M, Brody LC, Scott JM, Mills JL. Maternal vitamin B12 status and risk of neural tube defects in a population with high neural tube defect prevalence and no folic acid fortification. *Pediatrics* 2009 Mar;123(3):917–923.

Mann N, Pirotta Y, O'Connell S, Li D, Kelly F, Sinclair A. Fatty acid composition of habitual omnivore and vegetarian diets. *Lipids* 2006 Jul;41(7):637–646.

Mariani A, Chalies S, Jeziorski E, Ludwig C, Lalande M, Rodière M. [Consequences of exclusive breast-feeding in vegan mother newborn—case report]. *Arch Pediatr* 2009 Nov;16(11):1461–1463.

McCann JC, Ames BN. An overview of evidence for a causal relation between iron deficiency during development and deficits in cognitive or behavioral function. *Am J Clin Nutr* 2007 Apr;85(4):931–945.

McCarty MF. Sub-optimal taurine status may promote platelet hyperaggregability in vegetarians. *Med Hypotheses* 2004;63(3):426–433.

McClung JP, Karl JP, Cable SJ, Williams KW, Nindl BC, Young AJ, Lieberman HR. Randomized, double-blind, placebo-controlled trial of iron supplementation in female soldiers during military training: effects on iron status, physical performance, and mood. *Am J Clin Nutr* 2009 Jul;90(1):124–131.

Michie CA, Chambers J, Abramsky L, Kooner JS. Folate deficiency, neural tube defects, and cardiac disease in UK Indians and Pakistanis. *Lancet* 1998 Apr 11;351(9109):1105.

Misra A, Vikram NK, Pandey RM, Dwivedi M, Ahmad FU, Luthra K, Jain K, Khanna N, Devi JR, Sharma R, Guleria R. Hyperhomocysteinemia, and low intakes of folic acid and vitamin B12 in urban North India. *Eur J Nutr* 2002 Apr;41(2):68–77.

Messina M, Redmond G. Effects of soy protein and soybean isoflavones on thyroid function in healthy adults and hypothyroid patients: a review of the relevant literature. *Thyroid* 2006 Mar;16(3):249–258.

Osendarp SJ, Murray-Kolb LE, Black MM. Case study on iron in mental development— in memory of John Beard (1947–2009). *Nutr Rev* 2010 Nov;68 Suppl 1:S48–52. doi: 10.1111/j.1753–4887.2010.00331.x.

Plourde M, Cunnane SC. Extremely limited synthesis of long chain polyunsaturates in adults: implications for their dietary essentiality and use as supplements. *Appl Physiol Nutr Metab* 2007 Aug;32(4):619–634.

Pront R, Margalioth EJ, Green R, Eldar-Geva T, Maimoni Z, Zimran A, Elstein D. Prevalence of low serum cobalamin in infertile couples. *Andrologia* 2009 Feb;41(1):46–50.

Proudman SM, Cleland LG, James MJ. Dietary omega-3 fats for treatment of inflammatory joint disease: efficacy and utility. *Rheum Dis Clin North Am* 2008 May;34(2):469–479.

Rana SK, Sanders TA. Taurine concentrations in the diet, plasma, urine and breast milk of vegans compared with omnivores. *Br J Nutr* 1986 Jul;56(1):17–27.

Refsum H, Yajnik CS, Gadkari M, Schneede J, Vollset SE, Orning L, Guttormsen AB, Joglekar A, Sayyad MG, Ulvik A, Ueland PM. Hyperhomocysteinemia and elevated methylmalonic acid indicate a high prevalence of cobalamin deficiency in Asian Indians. *Am J Clin Nutr* 2001 Aug;74(2):233–241.

Remer T, Neubert A, Manz F. Increased risk of iodine deficiency with vegetarian nutrition. *Br J Nutr* 1999 Jan;81(1):45–49.

Reynolds RD. Bioavailability of vitamin B-6 from plant foods. *Am J Clin Nutr* 1988;48: 863–67.

Richards MP, Pettitt PB, Trinkaus E, Smith FH, Paunovic M, Karavanic, I. Neanderthal diet at Vindija and Neanderthal predation: The evidence from stable isotopes. *Proc Natl Acad Sci* 2000;97: 7663–7666.

Richards MP, Hedges REM, Jacobi R, Current, A, Stringer C. Focus: Gough's Cave and Sun Hole Cave human stable isotope values indicate a high animal protein diet in the British Upper Palaeolithic. *J Archaeol Sci* 2000;27: 1–3.

Roe DA. History of promotion of vegetable cereal diets. *J Nutr* 1986;116:1355–1363.

Roed C, Skovby F, Lund AM. Severe vitamin B12 deficiency in infants breastfed by vegans. *Ugeskr Laeger* 2009 Oct 19;171(43):3099–3101.

Rosell MS, Lloyd-Wright Z, Appleby PN, Sanders TA, Allen NE, Key TJ. Long-chain n-3 polyunsaturated fatty acids in plasma in British meat-eating, vegetarian, and vegan men. *Am J Clin Nutr* 2005 Aug;82(2):327–334.

Rush EC, Chhichhia P, Hinckson E, Nabiryo C. Dietary patterns and vitamin B(12) status of migrant Indian preadolescent girls. *Eur J Clin Nutr* 2009 Apr;63(4):585–587. Epub 2007 Dec 19.

Sanders TA. DHA status of vegetarians. *Prostaglandins Leukot Essent Fatty Acids* 2009 Aug–Sep;81(2–3):137–41.

Sanders TA, Roshanai F. Platelet phospholipid fatty acid composition and function in vegans compared with age- and sex-matched omnivore controls. *Eur J Clin Nutr* 1992 Nov;46(11):823–831.

Sato Y, Honda Y, Iwamoto J, Kanoko T, Satoh K. Effect of folate and mecobalamin on hip fractures in patients with stroke: a randomized controlled trial. *JAMA* 2005 Mar 2;293(9):1082–1088.

Schneede J, Ueland PM. Novel and established markers of cobalamin deficiency: complementary or exclusive diagnostic strategies. *Semin Vasc Med* 2005 May;5(2):140–155.

Selhub J, Morris MS, Jacques PF. In vitamin B12 deficiency, higher serum folate is associated with increased total homocysteine and methylmalonic acid concentrations. *Proc Natl Acad Sci USA* 2007 Dec 11;104(50):19995–20000.

Shapin S. Vegetable love: the history of vegetarianism. *New Yorker* 2007 Jan 22:80–84.

Singh K, Singh SK, Sah R, Singh I, Raman R. Mutation C677T in the methylenetetrahy drofolate reductase gene is associated with male infertility in an Indian population. *Int J Androl* 2005 Apr;28(2):115–119.

Srikumar TS, Johansson GK, Ockerman PA, Gustafsson JA, Akesson B. Trace element status in healthy subjects switching from a mixed to a lactovegetarian diet for 12 mo. *Am J Clin Nutr* 1992 Apr;55(4):885–890.

Stabler SP, Allen RH. Vitamin B12 deficiency as a worldwide problem. *Annu Rev Nutr* 2004;24:299–326.

Stephen EH, Chandra A. Declining estimates of infertility in the United States: 1982–2002. *Fertil Steril* 2006 Sep;86(3):516–523.

Szymanski KM, Wheeler DC, Mucci LA. Fish consumption and prostate cancer risk: a review and meta-analysis. *Am J Clin Nutr* 2010 Nov;92(5):1223–1233.

Taneja S, Bhandari N, Strand TA, Sommerfelt H, Refsum H, Ueland PM, Schneede J, Bahl R, Bhan MK. Cobalamin and folate status in infants and young children in a low-to-middle income community in India. *Am J Clin Nutr* 2007 Nov;86(5):1302–1309.

te Velde E, Burdorf A, Nieschlag E, Eijkemans R, Kremer JA, Roeleveld N, Habbema D. Is human fecundity declining in Western countries? *Hum Reprod* 2010 Jun;25(6):1348–1353.

Tikkiwal M, Ajmera RL, Mathur NK. Effect of zinc administration on seminal zinc and fertility of oligospermic males. *Indian J Physiol Pharmacol* 1987 Jan-Mar;31(1):30–34.

van der Merwe NJ, Thackeray JF, Lee-Thorp JA, Luyt J. The carbon isotope ecology and diet of Australopithecus africanus at Sterkfontein, South Africa. *J Hum Evol* 2003;44:581–597.

van Meurs JB, Dhonukshe-Rutten RA, Pluijm SM, van der Klift M, de Jonge R, Lindemans J, de Groot LC, Hofman A, Witteman JC, van Leeuwen JP, Breteler MM, Lips P, Pols HA, Uitterlinden AG. Homocysteine levels and the risk of osteoporotic fracture. *N Engl J Med* 2004 May 13;350(20):2033–2041.

van Mil NH, Oosterbaan AM, Steegers-Theunissen RP. Teratogenicity and underlying mechanisms of homocysteine in animal models: a review. *Reprod Toxicol* 2010 Dec;30(4):520–531.

Vegetarianism in America. *Vegetarian Times Magazine*, 2008. http://www.vegetariantimes.com/features/archive_of_editorial/667.

Verkleij-Hagoort AC, Verlinde M, Ursem NT, Lindemans J, Helbing WA, Ottenkamp J, Siebel FM, Gittenberger-de Groot AC, de Jonge R, Bartelings MM, Steegers EA, Steegers-Theunissen RP. Maternal hyperhomocysteinaemia is a risk factor for congenital heart disease. *BJOG* 2006 Dec;113(12):1412–1418.

Vogel T, Dali-Youcef N, Kaltenbach G, Andrès E. Homocysteine, vitamin B12, folate and cognitive functions: a systematic and critical review of the literature. *Int J Clin Pract* 2009 Jul;63(7):1061–1067.

Wald DS, Law M, Morris JK. Homocysteine and cardiovascular disease: evidence on causality from a meta-analysis. *BMJ* 2002 Nov 23;325(7374):1202.

Waldmann A, Dörr B, Koschizke JW, Leitzmann C, Hahn A. Dietary intake of vitamin B6 and concentration of vitamin B6 in blood samples of German vegans. *Public Health Nutr* 2006 Sep;9(6):779–784.

Wang Q, Yu LG, Campbell BJ, Milton JD, Rhodes JM. Identification of intact peanut lectin in peripheral venous blood. *Lancet* 1998;352:1831–1832.

Werder SF. Cobalamin deficiency, hyperhomocysteinemia, and dementia. *Neuropsychiatr Dis Treat* 2010 May 6;6:159–195.

Whorton JC. Historical development of vegetarianism. *Am J Clin Nutr* 1994;59 (suppl) 1103S-1109S.

Wilson AK, Ball MJ. Nutrient intake and iron status of Australian male vegetarians. *Eur J Clin Nutr* 1999 Mar;53(3):189–194.

Wong WY, Merkus HM, Thomas CM, Menkveld R, Zielhuis GA, Steegers-Theunissen RP. Effects of folic acid and zinc sulfate on male factor subfertility: a double-blind, randomized, placebo-controlled trial. *Fertil Steril* 2002 Mar;77(3):491–498.

Xavier D, Pais P, Devereaux PJ, Xie C, Prabhakaran D, Reddy KS, Gupta R, Joshi P, Kerkar P, Thanikachalam S, Haridas KK, Jaison TM, Naik S, Maity AK, Yusuf S; CREATE registry investigators. Treatment and outcomes of acute coronary syndromes in India (CREATE): a prospective analysis of registry data. *Lancet* 2008 Apr 26;371(9622):1435–1442.

Zhao YT, Chen Q, Sun YX, Li XB, Zhang P, Xu Y, Guo JH. Prevention of sudden cardiac death with omega-3 fatty acids in patients with coronary heart disease: a meta-analysis of randomized controlled trials. *Ann Med* 2009;41(4):301–310.

Zhao JH, Sun SJ, Horiguchi H, Arao Y, Kanamori N, Kikuchi A, Oguma E, Kayama F. A soy diet accelerates renal damage in autoimmune MRL/Mp-lpr/lpr mice. *Int Immunopharmacol* 2005 Oct;5(11):1601–1610.

Zimmermann MB. The adverse effects of mild-to-moderate iodine deficiency during pregnancy and childhood: a review. *Thyroid* 2007 Sep;17(9):829–835.

Zimmermann MB. Iodine deficiency. *Endocr Rev* 2009 Jun;30(4):376–408.

5. Just Say No to the Milk Mustache

Adebamowo, C.A. Spiegelman D, Berkey CS, Danby FW, Rockett HH, Colditz GA, Willett WC, Holmes MD. Milk consumption and acne in adolescent girls. *Dermatol Online J* 12(4):1, 2006.

Adebamowo CA, Spiegelman D, Berkey CS, Danby FW, Rockett HH, Colditz GA, Willett WC, Holmes MD. Milk consumption and acne in teenaged boys. *J Am Acad Dermatol* 2008 May;58(5):787–793.

Adebamowo, C.A. Spiegelman D, Danby FW, Frazier AL, Willett WC, Holmes MD. High school dietary dairy intake and teenage acne. *J Am Acad Dermatol* 52(2):207–214, 2005.

Adly L, Hill D, Sherman ME, Sturgeon SR, Fears T, Mies C, Ziegler RG, Hoover RN, Schairer C. Serum concentrations of estrogens, sex hormone-binding globulin, and androgens and risk of breast cancer in postmenopausal women. *Int J Cancer* 2006 Nov 15;119(10):2402–2407.

Alcock N, Macintyre I. Inter-relation of calcium and magnesium absorption. *Clin Sci* 1962 Apr;22:185–193.

Arrar L, Hanachi N, Rouba K, Charef N, Khennouf S, Baghiani A. Anti-xanthine oxidase antibodies in sera and synovial fluid of patients with rheumatoid arthritis and other joint inflammations. *Saudi Med J* 2008 Jun;29(6):803–807.

Artaud-Wild S et al. Differences in coronary mortality can be explained by differences in cholesterol and saturated fat intake in 40 countries but not in France and Finland. *Circulation* 1993;88:2771–2779.

Appleby PN, Thorogood M, Mann JI, Key TJ. The Oxford Vegetarian Study: an overview. *Am J Clin Nutr* 1999 Sep;70(3 Suppl):525S–531S.

Bartley J, McGlashan SR. Does milk increase mucus production? *Med Hypotheses* 2010 Apr;74(4):732–734.

Bastian SE, Dunbar AJ, Priebe IK, Owens PC, Goddard C. Measurement of betacellulin levels in bovine serum, colostrum and milk. *J Endocrinol* 2001 Jan;168 (1):203–212.

Belvedere P, Gabai G, Dalla VL, et al. Occurrence of steroidogenic enzymes in the bovine mammary gland at different functional stages. *J Steroid Biochem Mol Biol* 1996;59:339–347.

Bischoff-Ferrari HA, Dawson-Hughes B, Baron JA, Kanis JA, Orav EJ, Staehelin HB, Kiel DP, Burckhardt P, Henschkowski J, Spiegelman D, Li R, Wong JB, Feskanich D, Willett WC.Milk intake and risk of hip fracture in men and women: A meta-analysis of prospective cohort studies. *J Bone Miner Res* 2010 Oct 14.

Bischoff-Ferrari HA. Optimal serum 25-hydroxyvitamin D levels for multiple health outcomes. *Adv Exp Med Biol* 2008;624:55–71.

Bischoff-Ferrari HA, Dawson-Hughes B, Baron JA, et al. Calcium intake and hip fracture risk in men and women: a meta-analysis of prospective cohort studies and randomized controlled trials. *Am J Clin Nutr* 2007;86:1780–1790.

Bischoff-Ferrari HA, Shao A, Dawson-Hughes B, Hathcock J, Giovannucci E, Willett WC. Benefit-risk assessment of vitamin D supplementation. *Osteoporos Int* 2010 Jul;21(7):1121–1132.

Bolland MJ, Avenell A, Baron JA, Grey A, MacLennan GS, Gamble GD, Reid IR. Effect of calcium supplements on risk of myocardial infarction and cardiovascular events: meta-analysis. *BMJ* 2010 Jul 29;341:c3691.

Briggs RD, Rubenberg ML, O'neal RM, Thomas WA, Hartroft WS. Myocardial infarction in patients treated with Sippy and other high-milk diets: an autopsy study of fifteen hospitals in the U.S.A. and Great Britain. *Circulation* 1960 Apr;21:538–542.

Bruder G. Jarasch ED, Heid HW. High concentrations of antibodies to xanthine oxidase in human and animal sera. *J Clin Invest* 1984;74:783–794.

Castillo-Duran C, Solomons NW. Studies on the bioavailability of zinc in humans. IX. Interaction of beef-zinc with iron, calcium and lactose. *Nutr Res* 1991;11:429–438.

Chen H, O'Reilly E, McCullough ML, Rodriguez C, Schwarzschild MA, Calle EE, Thun MJ, Ascherio A. Consumption of dairy products and risk of Parkinson's disease. *Am J Epidemiol* 2007 May 1;165(9):998–1006.

Clyne PS, Kulczycki A. Human breast milk contains bovine IgG. Relationship to Infant Colic? *Pediatrics* 1992; 87: 439–444.

Cordain L. Dietary implications for the development of acne: a shifting paradigm. In: *U.S. Dermatology Review II 2006*, Bedlow J (ed). London: Touch Briefings Publications, 2006.

Cordain L. Implications for the role of diet in acne. *Semin Cutan Med Surg* 2005 Jun;24(2):84–91.

Cordain L. The nutritional characteristics of a contemporary diet based upon Paleolithic food groups. *J Am Nutraceut Assoc* 2002; 5:15–24.

Cordain L, Eaton SB, Sebastian A, Mann N, Lindeberg S, Watkins BA, O'Keefe JH, Brand-Miller J. Origins and evolution of the Western diet: health implications for the 21st century. *Am J Clin Nutr* 2005 Feb;81(2):341–354.

Cordain L, Lindeberg S, Hurtado M, Hill K, Eaton SB, Brand-Miller J. Acne vulgaris: a disease of Western civilization. *Arch Dermatol* 2002 Dec;138(12):1584–1590.

Couet C, Jan P, Debry G. Lactose and cataract in humans: a review. *J Am Coll Nutr* 1991;10:79–86.

Davies DE, Chamberlin SG. Targeting the epidermal growth factor receptor for therapy of carcinomas. *Biochem Pharmacol* 1996 May 3;51(9):1101–1110.

Davies DF, Davies JR, Richards MA. Antibodies to reconstituted dried cow's milk protein in coronary heart disease. *J Atherocler Res* 1969;9:103–107.

Deeth HC. Homogenized milk and atherosclerotic disease: A review. *J. Dairy Sci* 1983;66:1419–1435.

de Rougemont A, Normand S, Nazare JA, Skilton MR, Sothier M, Vinoy S, Laville M. Beneficial effects of a 5-week low-glycaemic index regimen on weight control and cardiovascular risk factors in overweight non-diabetic subjects. *Br J Nutr* 2007 Dec;98(6):1288–1298.

Dietary Reference Intakes for Calcium and Vitamin D. Institute of Medicine of the National Academies, 2010 http://www.iom.edu/Reports/2010/Dietary-Reference-Intakes-for-Calcium-and-Vitamin-D.aspx.

Dunbar AJ, Priebe IK, Belford DA, Goddard C. Identification of betacellulin as a major peptide growth factor in milk: purification, characterization and molecular cloning of bovine betacellulin. *Biochem J* 1999 Dec 15;344 Pt 3:713–721.

Evans GH et al. Association of magnesium deficiency with the blood pressure lowering effects of calcium. *J Hypertension* 1990;8:327–337.

Evershed RP, Payne S, Sherratt AG, Copley MS, Coolidge J, Urem-Kotsu D, et al. Earliest date for milk use in the Near East and southeastern Europe linked to cattle herding. *Nature* 2008 Sep 25;455(7212):528–531.

Farlow DW, Xu X, Veenstra TD. Quantitative measurement of endogenous estrogen metabolites, risk-factors for development of breast cancer, in commercial milk products by LC-MS/MS. *J Chromatogr B Analyt Technol Biomed Life Sci* 2009;877(13):1327–1334.

Fields M, Lewis CG, Lure MD. Copper deficiency in rats: the effect of type of dietary protein. *J Am Coll Nutr* 1993;12:303–306.

Foster-Powell K, Holt SH, Brand-Miller JC. International table of glycemic index and glycemic load values: 2002. *Am J Clin Nutr* 2002 Jul;76(1):5–56.

Ganmaa D, Wang PY, Qin LQ, Hoshi K, Sato A. Is milk responsible for male reproductive disorders? *Med Hypotheses* 2001 Oct;57(4):510–514.

Ganmaa D, Sato A. The possible role of female sex hormones in milk from pregnant cows in the development of breast, ovarian and corpus uteri cancers. *Med Hypotheses* 2005;65(6):1028–1037.

Ganmaa D, Tezuka H, Enkhmaa D, Hoshi K, Sato A. Commercial cows' milk has uterotrophic activity on the uteri of young ovariectomized rats and immature rats. *Int J Cancer* 2006 May 1;118(9):2363–2365.

Gannon MC, Nuttall FQ, Krezowski PA, Billington CJ, Parker S. The serum insulin and plasma glucose responses to milk and fruit products in type 2 (non-insulin-dependent) diabetic patients. *Diabetologia* 1986 Nov;29(11):784–791.

Gao X, LaValley MP, Tucker KL. Prospective studies of dairy product and calcium intakes and prostate cancer risk: a meta-analysis. *J Natl Cancer Inst* 2005 Dec 7;97(23):1768–1777.

Genkinger JM, Hunter DJ, Spiegelman D, et al. Dairy products and ovarian cancer: a pooled analysis of 12 cohort studies. *Cancer Epidemiol Biomarkers Prev* 2006 Feb;15(2):364–372.

Gerrior S, Bente I. Nutrient Content of the U.S. Food Supply, 1909–99: A Summary Report. U.S.D.A, Center for Nutrition Policy and Promotion. Home Economics Research Report No. 55, 2002.

Gravis G, Bladou F, Salem N, Gonçalves A, Esterni B, Walz J, Bagattini S, Marcy M, Brunelle S, Viens P. Results from a monocentric phase II trial of erlotinib in patients with metastatic prostate cancer. *Ann Oncol.* 2008 Sep;19(9):1624–1628.

Gueux E, Cubizolles C, Bussière L, Mazur A, Rayssiguier Y., et al. Oxidative modification of triglyceride rich lipoprotein in hypertriglyceridemic rats following magnesium deficiency. *Lipids* 1993;28:573–575.

Hallberg L, Rossander-Hulten L, Brune M, Gleerup A. Calcium and iron absorption: mechanism of action and nutritional importance. *Eur J Clin Nutr* 1992 May;46(5):317–327.

Hankinson SE, Eliassen AH. Endogenous estrogen, testosterone and progesterone levels in relation to breast cancer risk. *J Steroid Biochem Mol Biol* 2007 Aug-Sep;106(1–5):24–30.

Harrison R. Milk xanthine oxidase: hazard or benefit. *J Nutr Environ Med* 2002;12:231–238.

Hartmann S, Lacorn M, Steinhart H. Natural occurrence of steroid hormones in food. *Food Chem* 1998;6:7–20.

Hartroft WS. The incidence of coronary artery disease in patients treated with Sippy diet. *Am J Clin Nutr* 1964 Oct;15:205–210.

Henson ES, Gibson SB. Surviving cell death through epidermal growth factor (EGF) signal transduction pathways: Implications for cancer therapy. *Cell Signal* 2006 Dec;18(12):2089–2097.

Holt SH Miller JC, Petocz P. An insulin index of foods: the insulin demand generated by 1000-kJ portions of common foods. *Am J Clin Nutr* 1997 Nov;66(5):1264–1276.

Hoppe C, Mølgaard C, Vaag A, Barkholt V, Michaelsen KF. High intakes of milk, but not meat increase s-insulin and insulin resistance in 8-year-old boys. *Eur J Clin Nutr* 2005 Mar;59(3):393–398.

Hormi K, Lehy T. Developmental expression of transforming growth factor-alpha and epidermal growth factor receptor proteins in the human pancreas and digestive tract. *Cell Tissue Res* 1994 Dec;278(3):439–450.

Horner SM et al. Efficacy of intravenous magnesium in acute myocardial infarction in reducing arrhythmias and mortality. Meta analysis of magnesium in acute myocardial infarction. *Circulation* 1992;86:774–779.

Høst A. Frequency of cow's milk allergy in childhood. *Ann Allergy Asthma Immunol* 2002 Dec;89(6 Suppl 1):33–37.

Hoyt G, Hickey MS, Cordain, L. Dissociation of the glycaemic and insulinaemic responses to whole and skimmed milk. *Br J Nutr* 2005 Feb;93(2):175–177.

Ingram CJ, Mulcare CA, Itan Y, Thomas MG, Swallow DM. Lactose digestion and the evolutionary genetics of lactase persistence. *Hum Genet* 2009 Jan;124(6):579–591.

Jakobsson I, Lindberg T. Cow's milk proteins cause infantile colic in breast-fed infants: a double-blind crossover study. *Pediatrics* 1983 Feb;71(2):268–271.

Kanis JA, Johansson H, Oden A, De Laet C, Johnell O, Eisman JA, Mc Closkey E, Mellstrom D, Pols H, Reeve J, Silman A, Tenenhouse A. A meta-analysis of milk intake and fracture risk: low utility for case finding. *Osteoporos Int* 2005 Jul;16(7):799–804.

Karas-Kuzelicki N, Pfeifer V, Lukac-Bajalo J. Synergistic effect of high lactase activity genotype and galactose-1-phosphate uridyl transferase (GALT) mutations on idiopathic presenile cataract formation. *Clin Biochem* 2008 Jul;41(10–11):869–874.

Koldovský, O (1995) Hormones in milk. In *Vitamins and Hormones 50*, Litwack G (ed). New Yorl: Academic Press, 77–149.

Koldovský, O. (1996) The potential physiological significance of milk-borne hormonally active substances for the neonate. *J Mammary Gland Biol Neoplasia* 1, 317–323.

Kostraba JN, Cruickshanks KJ, Lawler-Heavner J, Jobim LF, Rewers MJ, Gay EC, Chase HP, Klingensmith G, Hamman RF. Early exposure to cow's milk and solid foods in infancy, genetic predisposition, and risk of IDDM. *Diabetes* 1993 Feb;42(2): 288–295.

Kurahashi N, Inoue M, Iwasaki M, et al. Dairy product, saturated fatty acid, and calcium intake and prostate cancer in a prospective cohort of Japanese men. *Cancer Epidemiol Biomarkers Prev* 2008 Apr;17(4):930–937.

Larsson SC, Orsini N, Wolk A. Milk, milk products and lactose intake and ovarian cancer risk: a meta-analysis of epidemiological studies. *Int J Cancer* 2006 Jan 15;118(2):431–441.

Laugesen M, Elliott R. Ischaemic heart disease, Type 1 diabetes, and cow milk A1 beta-casein. *N Z Med J* 2003 Jan 24;116(1168):U295.

Liljeberg Elmstahl H, Bjorck I. Milk as a supplement to mixed meals may elevate postprandial insulinaemia. *Eur J Clin Nutr* 2001; 55:994–999.

Lothe L, Lindberg T. Cow's milk whey protein elicits symptoms of infantile colic in colicky formula-fed infants: a double-blind crossover study. *Pediatrics* 1989 Feb;83(2):262–266.

Luopajärvi K, Savilahti E, Virtanen SM, Ilonen J, Knip M, Akerblom HK, Vaarala O. Enhanced levels of cow's milk antibodies in infancy in children who develop type 1 diabetes later in childhood. *Pediatr Diabetes* 2008 Oct;9(5):434–441.

Lynch SM, Strain JJ. Effects of copper deficiency on hepatic and cardiac antioxidant enzyme activities in lactose and sucrose fed rats. *Brit J Nutr* 1989;61:345–354.

Marshall BJ. (1983). Unidentified curved bacillus on gastric epithelium in active chronic gastritis. *Lancet* 1 (8336): 1273–1275.

Marshall BJ, Warren JR. (1984). Unidentified curved bacilli in the stomach patients with gastritis and peptic ulceration. *Lancet* 1 (8390): 1311–1315.

McDermott CM, Beitz DC, Littledike ET, Horst RL. Effects of dietary vitamin D3 on concentrations of vitamin D and its metabolites in blood plasma and milk of dairy cows. *J Dairy Sci* 1985;68:1959–1967.

Meloni G, Ogana A, Mannazzu MC, Meloni T, Carta F, Carta A.High prevalence of lactose absorbers in patients with presenile cataract from northern Sardinia. *Br J Ophthalmol* 1995 Jul;79(7):709.

Moss M, Freed D. The cow and the coronary: epidemiology, biochemistry and immunology. *Int J Cardiol* 2003 Feb;87(2–3):203–216.

Munro JM, van der Walt JD, Munro CS, Chalmers JA, Cox EL. An immunolohistochemical analysis of human aortic fatty streaks. *Hum Pathol* 1987;18:375–380.

Muscari A, Volta U, Bonazzi C, Puddu GM, Bozzoli C, Gerratana C, Bianchi FB, Puddu P. Association of serum IgA antibodies to milk antigens with severe atherosclerosis. *Atherosclerosis* 1989;77:251–256.

Muslimov GF. Role of epidermal growth factor gene in the development of pancreatic cancer and efficiency of inhibitors of this gene in the treatment of pancreatic carcinoma. *Bull Exp Biol Med* 2008 Apr;145(4):535–538.

Nadler JL, Buchanan T, Natarajan R, Antonipillai I, Bergman R, Rude R. Magnesium deficiency produces insulin resistance and increased thromboxane synthesis. *Hypertension* 1993;21:1024–1029.

Nanda R. Targeting the human epidermal growth factor receptor 2 (HER2) in the treatment of breast cancer: recent advances and future directions. *Rev Recent Clin Trials* 2007 May;2(2):111–116.

Napoli C, Ambrosio G, Palumbo G, Elia PP, Chiariello M. Human low density lipoproteins are peroxidized by free radicals via chain reactions triggered by the superoxide radical. *Cardiologica* 1991;36:527–532.

National Institute of Allergy and Infectious Diseases (July 2004). "NIH Publication No. 04–5518: Food Allergy: An Overview.

Oski, FA. *Don't Drink Your Milk!: The Frightening New Medical Facts About the World's Most Overrated Nutrient.* New York: Wyden Books, 1977.

Ostman EM, Liljeberg Elmståhl HG, Björck IM. Inconsistency between glycemic and insulinemic responses to regular and fermented milk products. *Am J Clin Nutr* 2001;74:96–100.

Palayekar MJ, Herzog TJ. The emerging role of epidermal growth factor receptor inhibitors in ovarian cancer. *Int J Gynecol Cancer* 2008 Sep-Oct;18(5):879–890.

Park M, Ross GW, Petrovitch H, White LR, Masaki KH, Nelson JS, Tanner CM, Curb JD, Blanchette PL, Abbott RD. Consumption of milk and calcium in midlife and the future risk of Parkinson disease. *Neurology* 2005 Mar 22;64(6):1047–1051.

Playford RJ, Macdonald CE, Johnson WS. Colostrum and milk-derived peptide growth factors for the treatment of gastrointestinal disorders. *Am J Clin Nutr* 2000 Jul;72(1):5–14.

Precetti AS, Oria MP, Nielsen SS. Presence in bovine milk of two protease inhibitors of the plasmin system. J Dairy Sci 1997;80: 1490–1496.

Qin LQ, He K, Xu JY. Milk consumption and circulating insulin-like growth factor-I level: a systematic literature review. *Int J Food Sci Nutr* 2009;60 Suppl 7:330–340.

Qin LQ, Xu JY, Wang PY, Kaneko T, Hoshi K, Sato A. Milk consumption is a risk factor for prostate cancer: meta-analysis of case-control studies. *Nutr Cancer* 2004;48(1):22–7.

Qin LQ, Xu JY, Wang PY, Tong J, Hoshi K. Milk consumption is a risk factor for prostate cancer in Western countries: evidence from cohort studies. *Asia Pac J Clin Nutr* 2007;16(3):467–476.

Qin LQ, Wang PY, Kaneko T, Hoshi K, Sato A. Estrogen: one of the risk factors in milk for prostate cancer. *Med Hypotheses* 2004;62(1):133–142.

Rao RK, Baker RD, Baker SS. Bovine milk inhibits proteolytic degradation of epidermal growth factor in human gastric and duodenal lumen. *Peptides* 1998; 19(3):495–504.

Rasmussen HS et al. Influence of magnesium substitution therapy on blood lipid composition in patients with ischemic heart disease. *Arch Int Med* 1989;149:1050–1053.

Ratnakar KS. Interaction of galactose and dietary protein deficiency on rat lens. *Opthalmic Res* 1985;17:344–348.

Reid IR, Bolland MJ, Grey A. Does calcium supplementation increase cardiovascular risk? *Clin Endocrinol (Oxf)* 2010 Dec;73(6):689–695.

Renaud S, et al. Dietary lipids and their relation to ischaemic heart disease: from epidemiology to prevention. *J Int Med* 1989;225(supp 1):39–46.

Richter CP, Duke, JR. Cataracts produced in rats by yogurt. *Science* 1970;168: 1372–1374.

Rinaldi E, Albini L, Costagliola C, De Rosa G, Auricchio G, De Vizia B, Auricchio S. High frequency of lactose absorbers among adults with idiopathic senile and presenile cataract in a population with a high prevalence of primary adult lactose malabsorption. *Lancet* 1984 Feb 18;1(8373):355–357.

Rohrmann S, Platz EA, Kavanaugh CJ, et al. Meat and dairy consumption and subsequent risk of prostate cancer in a US cohort study. *Cancer Causes Control* 2007 Feb;18(1):41–50.

Rowlands MA, Gunnell D, Harris R, Vatten LJ, Holly JM, Martin RM. Circulating insulin-like growth factor peptides and prostate cancer risk: a systematic review and meta-analysis. *Int J Cancer* 2009 May 15;124(10):2416–2429.

Santayana G. *The Life of Reason or, The phases of Human Progress.* New York: C. Scribner's Sons, 1905.

Schairer C, Hill D, Sturgeon SR, Fears T, Mies C, Ziegler RG, Hoover RN, Sherman ME. Serum concentrations of estrogens, sex hormone binding globulin, and androgens and risk of breast hyperplasia in postmenopausal women. *Cancer Epidemiol Biomarkers Prev* 2005 Jul;14(7):1660–1665.

Segall JJ. Dietary lactose as a possible risk factor for ischemic heart disease: review of epidemiology. *Int J Cardiol* 1994;46:197–207.

Segall JJ. Plausibility of dietary lactose as a coronary risk factor. *J Nutr Environ Med* 2002:12:217–229.

Seiwert TY, Cohen E. The emerging role of EGFR and VEGF inhibition in the treatment of head and neck squamous cell carcinoma. *Angiogenesis Oncol* 2005;1:7–10.

Seelig MS. Increased need for magnesium with the use of combined oestrogen and calcium for osteoporosis treatment. *Magnes Res* 1990 Sep;3(3):197–215.

Séverin S, Wenshui X. Milk biologically active components as nutraceuticals: review. *Crit Rev Food Sci Nutr* 2005;45(7–8):645–656.

Sippy BW. Gastric and duodenal ulcer. Medical cure by an efficient removal of gastric juice corrosion. *JAMA* 1915;64:1625–630.

Smith RN, Mann NJ, Braue A, Mäkeläinen H, Varigos GA. A low-glycemic-load diet improves symptoms in acne vulgaris patients: a randomized controlled trial. *Am J Clin Nutr* 2007 Jul;86(1):107–115.

Soedamah-Muthu SS, Ding EL, Al-Delaimy WK, Hu FB, Engberink MF, Willett WC, Geleijnse JM. Milk and dairy consumption and incidence of cardiovascular diseases and all-cause mortality: dose-response meta-analysis of prospective cohort studies. *Am J Clin Nutr* 2011 Jan;93(1):158–171.

Sugumar A, Liu YC, Xia Q, Koh YS, Matsuo K. Insulin-like growth factor (IGF)-I and IGF-binding protein 3 and the risk of premenopausal breast cancer: a meta-analysis of literature. *Int J Cancer* 2004 Aug 20;111(2):293–297.

Swallow DM. Genetics of lactase persistence and lactose intolerance. *Annual Review of Genetics* 2003 37:197–219.

Thomas DE, Elliott EJ, Baur L. Low glycaemic index or low glycaemic load diets for overweight and obesity. *Cochrane Database Syst Rev* 2007 Jul 18;(3):CD005105.

Vaarala O, Knip M, Paronen J, et al. Cow's milk formula feeding induces primary immunization to insulin in infants at genetic risk for type 1 diabetes. *Diabetes* 1999;48:1389–1394.

Vaarala O, Paronen J, Otonkoski T, Akerblom HK. Cow milk feeding induces antibodies to insulin in children—a link between cow milk and insulin-dependent diabetes mellitus? *Scand J Immunol* 1998: 47: 131–135.

Varo P. Mineral element balance and coronary heart disease. *Internat J Vit Nutr Res* 1974;44:267–273.

Virtanen SM, Räsänen L, Ylönen K, Aro A, Clayton D, Langholz B, Pitkäniemi J, Savilahti E, Lounamaa R, Tuomilehto J, et al. Early introduction of dairy products associated with increased risk of IDDM in Finnish children. The Childhood in Diabetes in Finland Study Group. *Diabetes* 1993 Dec;42(12):1786–1790.

Wang TK, Bolland MJ, van Pelt NC, Horne AM, Mason BH, Ames RW, Grey AB, Ruygrok PN, Gamble GD, Reid IR. Relationships between vascular calcification, calcium metabolism, bone density, and fractures. *J Bone Miner Res* 2010 Dec;25(12):2501–2509.

Wilhelm KR, Yanamandra K, Gruden MA, Zamotin V, Malisauskas M, Casaite V, Darinskas A, Forsgren L, Morozova-Roche LA. Immune reactivity towards insulin, its amyloid and protein S100B in blood sera of Parkinson's disease patients. *Eur J Neurol* 2007 Mar;14(3):327–334.

Yudkin AM, Arnold CH. Cataracts produced in albino rats on a ration containing a high proportion of lactose or galactose. *Trans Am Opthalmol Soc* 1935;33:281–290.

Zhang J, Kesteloot H. Milk consumption in relation to incidence of prostate, breast, colon, and rectal cancers: is there an independent effect? *Nutr Cancer* 2005;53(1):65–72.

Zucker GM, Clayman CB. Landmark perspective: Bertram W. Sippy and ulcer disease therapy. *JAMA* 1983 Oct 28;250(16):2198–2202.

6. Grains Are Antinutritious

Alvarez JR, Torres-Pinedo R. Interactions of soybean lectin, soyasaponins, and glycinin with rabbit jejunal mucosa in vitro. *Pediatr Res* 1982 Sep;16(9):728–731.

Barratt SM, Leeds JS, Robinson K, Shah PJ, Lobo AJ, McAlindon ME, Sanders DS. Reflux and irritable bowel syndrome are negative predictors of quality of life in coeliac disease and inflammatory bowel disease. *J Gastroenterol Hepatol* 2011 Feb;23(2):159–165.

Barre A, Peumans WJ, Menu-Bouaouiche L, Van Damme EJ, May GD, Herrera AF, Van Leuven F, Rougé P. Purification and structural analysis of an abundant thaumatin-like protein from ripe banana fruit. *Planta* 2000 Nov;211(6):791–799.

Barsony J, Pike JW, DeLuca HF, Marx SJ. Immunocytology with microwave-fixed fibroblasts shows 1 alpha,25-dihydroxyvitamin D3-dependent rapid and estrogen-dependent slow reorganization of vitamin D receptors. *J Cell Biol* 1990 Dec;111(6 Pt 1):2385–2395.

Batchelor AJ, Watson G, Compston JE. Reduced plasma half-life of radio-labelled 25-hydroxyvitamin D3 in subjects receiving a high fiber diet. *Brit J Nutr* 1983;49:213–216.

Berlyne GM, Ben Ari J, Nord E, Shainkin R. Bedouin osteomalacia due to calcium deprivation caused by high phytic acid content of unleavened bread. *Am J Clin Nutr* 1973;26:910–911.

Bohn T, Davidsson L, Walczyk T, Hurrell RF. Phytic acid added to white-wheat bread inhibits fractional apparent magnesium absorption in humans. *Am J Clin Nutr* 2004 Mar;79(3):418–423.

Bomford R, Stapleton M, Winsor S, Beesley JE, Jessup EA, Price KR, Fenwick R. Adjuvanticity and ISCOM formation by structurally diverse saponins. *Vaccine* 1992;10(9):572–577.

Briani C, Samaroo D, Alaedini A. Celiac disease: from gluten to autoimmunity. *Autoimmun Rev* 2008 Sep;7(8):644–650.

Brooke OG, Brown IRF, Cleeve HJW. Observations of the vitamin D state of pregnant Asian women in London. *Brit J Obstet Gynaecol* 1981;88:18–26.

Cahill, J.P. 2003. Ethnobotany of chia, Salvia hispanica L. (Lamiaceae). *Economic Botany* 57(4):604–618.

Cascella NG, Kryszak D, Bhatti B, Gregory P, Kelly DL, Mc Evoy JP, Fasano A, Eaton WW. Prevalence of celiac disease and gluten sensitivity in the United States clinical antipsychotic trials of intervention effectiveness study population. *Schizophr Bull* 2011 Jan;37(1):94–100.

Clements MR, Johnson L, Fraser DR. A new mechanism for induced vitamin D deficiency in calcium deprivation. *Nature* 1987;325:62–65.

Cordain L. Cereal grains: humanity's double edged sword. *World Rev Nutr Diet* 1999; 84:19–73.

Cordain L, Eaton SB, Sebastian A, Mann N, Lindeberg S, Watkins BA, O'Keefe JH, Brand-Miller J. Origins and evolution of the Western diet: health implications for the 21st century. *Am J Clin Nutr* 2005 Feb;81(2):341–354.

Dalla Pellegrina C, Perbellini O, Scupoli MT, Tomelleri C, Zanetti C, Zoccatelli G, Fusi M, Peruffo A, Rizzi C, Chignola R. Effects of wheat germ agglutinin on human gastrointestinal epithelium: insights from an experimental model of immune/epithelial cell interaction. *Toxicol Appl Pharmacol* 2009 Jun 1;237(2):146–153.

Eigenmann PA. Mechanisms of food allergy. *Pediatr Allergy Immuol* 2009;20:5–11.

Estrada A, Li B, Laarveld B. Adjuvant action of *Chenopodium quinoa* saponins on the induction of antibody responses to intragastric and intranasal administered antigens in mice. *Comp Immunol Microbiol Infect Dis* 1998 Jul;21(3):225–236.

Ewer TK. Rachitogenicity of green oats. *Nature* 1950;166:732–733.

Fasano A, Berti I, Gerarduzzi T, Not T, Colletti RB, Drago S, Elitsur Y, Green PH, Guandalini S, Hill ID, Pietzak M, Ventura A, Thorpe M, Kryszak D, Fornaroli F, Wasserman SS, Murray JA, Horvath K. Prevalence of celiac disease in at-risk and not-at-risk groups in the United States: a large multicenter study. *Arch Intern Med* 2003 Feb 10;163(3):286–292.

Fernandez, S., M. Vidueiros, R. Ayerza, W. Coates and A. Pallaro. Impact of chia (Salvia hispanica L) on the immune system: preliminary study. *Proceedings of the Nutrition Society*, 2008 May;67(Issue OCE), E12.

Finlay DR, Newmeyer DD, Price TM, Forbes DJ. Inhibition of in vitro nuclear transport by a lectin that binds to nuclear pores. *J Cell Biol* 1987 Feb;104(2):189–200.

Ford JA, Colhoun EM, McIntosh WB, Dunnigan MG. Biochemical response of late rickets and osteomalacia to a chupatty-free diet. *Brit Med J* 1972;2:446–447.

Ford JA, McIntosh WB, Dunnigan MG. A possible relationship between high-extraction cereal and rickets and osteomalacia. *Adv Exp Med Biol* 1977;81:353–362.

Gee JM, Price KR, Ridout CL, Wortley GM, Hurrell RF, Johnson IT. Saponin of quinoa (Chenopodium quinoa): effects of processing on their abundance in quinoa products and their biological effects on intestinal mucosal tissue. *J Sci Food Agric* 1993;63:201–209.

Gélinas B, Seguin P. Oxalate in grain amaranth. *J Agric Food Chem* 2007 Jun 13;55(12): 4789–4794.

Gibson RS, Bindra GS, Nizan P, Draper HH. The vitamin D status of East Indian Punjabi immigrants to Canada. *Brit J Nutr* 1987;58:23–29.

Grammer JC, McGinnis J, Pubols MH. 1983. The rachitogenic effects of fractions of rye and certain polysaccharides. *Poultry Science* 62:103–109.

Guinez C, Morelle W, Michalski JC, Lefebvre T. O-GlcNAc glycosylation: a signal for the nuclear transport of cytosolic proteins? *Int J Biochem Cell Biol* 2005 Apr;37(4):765–774.

Hadjivassiliou M, Sanders DS, Grünewald RA, Woodroofe N, Boscolo S, Aeschlimann D. Gluten sensitivity: from gut to brain. *Lancet Neurol* 2010 Mar;9(3):318–330.

Halsted JA, Ronaghy HA, Abadi P, Haghshenass M, Amirhakemi GH, Barakat RM, Reinhold JG. Zinc deficiency in man, the Shiraz experiment. *Am J Med* 1972;53:277–284.

Harrison DC, Mellanby E. Phytic acid and the rickets-producing action of cereals. *Biochem J* 1939 Oct;33(10):1660–1680.

Hawkes K, Hill K, O'Connell JF. Why hunters gather: optimal foragingand the Ache of eastern Paraguay. *Am Ethnol* 1982;9:379–398.

Hidiroglou M, Ivan M, Proulx JG, Lessard JR. Effect of a single intramuscular dose of vitamin D on concentrations of liposoluble vitamins in the plasma of heifers winter-fed oat silage, grass silage or hay. *Can J Anim Sci* 1980;60:311–318.

Hunt SP, O'Riordan JLH, Windo J, Truswell AS. Vitamin D status in different subgroups of British Asians. *Br Med J* 1976;2:1351–54.

Ikeda K. Buckwheat: composition, chemistry, and processing. *Adv Food Nutr Res* 2002;44:395–434.

Ivarsson A, Persson LA, Juto P, Peltonen M, Suhr O, Hernell O. High prevalence of undiagnosed coeliac disease in adults: a Swedish population-based study. *J Intern Med* 1999 Jan;245(1):63–68.

Ixtainaa VY, Nolascoa SM, Tomás MC. Physical properties of chia (Salvia hispanica L.) seeds. *Industrial Crops and Products* 2008;28:286–293.

Johnson IT, Gee JM. Gastrointestinal adaptation in response to soluble non-available polysaccharides in the rat. *Br J Nutr* 1986 May;55(3):497–505.

Johnson IT, Gee JM, Price K, Curl C, Fenwick GR. Influence of saponins on gut permeability and active nutrient transport in vitro. *J Nutr* 1986 Nov;116(11):2270–2277.

Keukens EA, de Vrije T, van den Boom C, de Waard P, Plasman HH, Thiel F, Chupin V, Jongen WM, de Kruijff B. Molecular basis of glycoalkaloid induced membrane disruption. *Biochim Biophys Acta* 1995 Dec 13;1240(2):216–228.

Kozio MJ. Chemical composition and nutritional evaluation of quinoa (*Chenopodium quinoa Willd.*) *J Food Comp Anal* 1992;5:35–68.

Kumar V, Rajadhyaksha M, Wortsman J. Celiac disease-associated autoimmune endocrinopathies. *Clin Diagn Lab Immunol* 2001 Jul;8(4):678–685.

Kuzma JN, Cordain L. Ingestion of wheat germ in healthy subjects does not acutely elevate plasma wheat germ agglutinin concentrations. *FASEB J* 2010, 24:723.10.

Luo Z, Rouvinen J, Mäenpää PH. A peptide C-terminal to the second Zn finger of human vitamin D receptor is able to specify nuclear localization. *Eur J Biochem* 1994; 223:381–387.

MacAuliffe T, Pietraszek A, McGinnis J. Variable rachitogenic effects of grain and alleviation by extraction or supplementation with vitamin D, fat and antibiotics. *Poultry Sci* 1976;55:2142–2147.

Massey LK. Dietary influences on urinary oxalate and risk of kidney stones. *Front Biosci* 2003 May 1;8:s584–594.

Mellanby E. 1919. An experimental investigation of rickets. *Lancet* 1:407–412.

Monroy-Torres R, Mancilla-Escobar ML, Gallaga-Solorzano JC, Medina-Godoy S, Santiago-Garcia EJ. Protein digestibility of chia seed Salvia hispanica L. *Revista Salud Publica y Nutricion* 2008 Enero–Marzo;9(1). Monterey, Mexico.

Neuhausen SL, Steele L, Ryan S, Mousavi M, Pinto M, Osann KE, Flodman P, Zone JJ. Co-occurrence of celiac disease and other autoimmune diseases in celiacs and their first-degree relatives. *J Autoimmun* 2008 Sep;31(2):160–165.

Nieman, DC, Cayea, EJ, Austin, MD, Henson, DA, McAnulty SR, Jin F. Chia seed does not promote weight loss or alter disease risk factors in overweight adults. *Nutrition Research* 2009;(29):414–418.

Noma T, Yoshizawa I, Ogawa N, Ito M, Aoki K, Kawano Y. Fatal buckwheat dependent exercised-induced anaphylaxis. *Asian Pac J Allergy Immunol* 2001 Dec;19(4):283–286.

Oleszek W, Junkuszew M, Stochmal A. Determination and toxicity of saponins from Amaranthus cruentus seeds. *J Agric Food Chem* 1999 Sep;47(9):3685–3687.

Peiretti PB, Meineri G. Effects on growth performance, carcass characteristics, and the fat and meat fatty acid profile of rabbits fed diets with chia (Salvia hispanica L.) seed supplements. *Meat Science* 2008; (80):1116–1121.

Pusztai A, Ewen SW, Grant G, Brown DS, Stewart JC, Peumans WJ, Van Damme EJ, Bardocz S. Antinutritive effects of wheat-germ agglutinin and other N-acetylglucosamine-specific lectins. *Br J Nutr* 1993 Jul;70(1):313–321.

Ratner A. Interview of Dr. Alessio Fasano. *Gluten Free Living Magazine*, Dec 2010: 40–48, 54.

Reinhold JG. High phytate content of rural Iranian bread: a possible cause of human zinc deficiency. *Am J Clin Nutr* 1971;24:1204–1206.

Reinhold JG, Lahimgarzadeh A, Nasr K, Hedayati H. Effects of purified phytate and phytate rich bread upon metabolism of zinc, calcium, phosphorus and nitrogen in man. *Lancet* 1973;1:283–288.

Reynolds RD: Bioavailability of vitamin B-6 from plant foods. *Am J Clin Nutr* 1988;48:863–867.

Robertson I, Ford JA, McIntosh WB, Dunnigan MG. The role of cereals in the aetiology of nutritional rickets: the lesson of the Irish national nutritional survey 1943–8. *Brit J Nutr* 1981;45:17–22.

Rui T, Hongyu Z, Ruiqi W. Seven Chinese patients with buckwheat allergy. *Am J Med Sci* 2010 Jan;339(1):22–24.

Sander GR, Cummins AG, Henshall T, Powell BC. Rapid disruption of intestinal barrier function by gliadin involves altered expression of apical junctional proteins. *FEBS Lett* 2005 Aug 29;579(21):4851–4855.

Satoh R, Koyano S, Takagi K, Nakamura R, Teshima R, Sawada J. Immunological characterization and mutational analysis of the recombinant protein BWp16, a major allergen in buckwheat. *Biol Pharm Bull* 2008 Jun;31(6):1079–1085.

Shakeri R, Zamani F, Sotoudehmanesh R, Amiri A, Mohamadnejad M, Davatchi F, Karakani AM, Malekzadeh R, Shahram F. Gluten sensitivity enteropathy in patients with recurrent aphthous stomatitis. *BMC Gastroenterol* 2009 Jun 17;9:44.

Sheard C, Caylor HD, Schlotthauer C. Photosensitization of animals after the ingestion of buckwheat. *J Exp Med* 1928 May 31;47(6):1013–1028.

Simms SR. Behavioral Ecology and Hunter-Gatherer Foraging. An Example from the Great Basin. Oxford: BAR International Series 381, 1987: 47.

Sly MR, van der Walt WH, Du Bruyn DB, Pettifor JM, Marie PJ. Exacerbation of rickets and osteomalacia by maize: a study of bone histomorphometry and composition in young baboons. *Calcif Tissue Int* 1984;36:370–379.

Stephens WP, Berry JL, Klimiuk PS, Mawer EB: Annual high dose vitamin D prophylaxis in Asian immigrants. *Lancet* 1981;2:1199–1201.

Story JA, LePage SL, Petro MS, West LG, Cassidy MM, Lightfoot FG, Vahouny GV. Interactions of alfalfa plant and sprout saponins with cholesterol in vitro and in cholesterol-fed rats. *Am J Clin Nutr* 1984 Jun;39(6):917–929.

Thomas BH, Steenbock H. Cereals and rickets. The comparative rickets-producing properties of different cereals. *Biochemistry Journal* 1936;30:177–188.

Torre M, Rodriguez AR, Saura-Calixto F. Effects of dietary fiber and phytic acid on mineral availability. *Crit Rev Food Sci Nutr* 1991;1:1–22.

Vigers AJ, Roberts WK, Selitrennikoff CP. A new family of plant antifungal proteins. *Mol Plant Microbe Interact* 1991 Jul-Aug;4(4):315–323.

Wieslander G, Norbäck D, Wang Z, Zhang Z, Mi Y, Lin R. Buckwheat allergy and reports on asthma and atopic disorders in Taiyuan City, Northern China. *Asian Pac J Allergy Immunol* 2000 Sep;18(3):147–152.

Yu LG, Milton JD, Fernig DG, Rhodes JM. Opposite effects on human colon cancer cell proliferation of two dietary Thomsen-Friedenreich antigen-binding lectins. *J Cell Physiol* 2001 Feb;186(2):282–287.

Zhang R, Naughton DP. Vitamin D in health and disease: Current perspectives. *Nutr J* 2010 Dec 8;9:65.

Zoppi G, Gobio-Casali L, Deganello A, Astolfi R, Saccomani F, Cecchettin M. Potential complications in the use of wheat bran for constipation in infancy. *J Pediatr Gastroenterol Nutr* 1982;1(1):91–95.

7. The Trouble with Beans

Alvarez JR, Torres-Pinedo R. Interactions of soybean lectin, soyasaponins, and glycinin with rabbit jejunal mucosa in vitro. *Pediatr Res* 1982 Sep;16(9):728–731.

Banwell, JG, Howard R, Kabir I, Costerton JW. Bacterial overgrowth by indigenous microflora in the phytohemagglutinin-fed rat. *Canadian Journal of Microbiology* 1988; 34:1009–1013.

Baumann E, Stoya G, Völkner A, Richter W, Lemke C, Linss W. Hemolysis of human erythrocytes with saponin affects the membrane structure. *Acta Histochem* 2000 Feb;102(1):21–35.

Boufassa C, Lafont J, Rouanet JM, Besancon P. 1986 Thermal inactivation of lectins (PHA)isolated from Phaseolus vulgaris. *Food Chem* 1986;20:295–304.

Buera M P, Pilosof AMR, Bartholomai GB. 1984 Kinetics of trypsin inhibitory activity loss in heated flour from bean Phaseolus vulgaris. *J Food Sci* 1984;49:124–126.

Calloway DH, Carol A. Hickey CA, Murphy EL. Reduction of intestinal gas-forming properties of legumes by traditional and experimental processing methods. *J Food Sci* 1971;36: 251–255.

Cappellini MD, Fiorelli G. Glucose-6-phosphate dehydrogenase deficiency. *Lancet* 2008;371(9606): 64–74.

Carmalt J, Rosel K, Burns T, Janzen E. Suspected white kidney bean (Phaseolus vulgaris) toxicity in horses and cattle. *Aust Vet J* 2003 Nov;81(11):674–676.

Caron M, Steve, AP. *Lectins and Pathology*. London: Taylor & Francis, 2000.

Chrispeels MJ, Raikel NV. Lectins, lectin genes, and their role in plant defense. *Plant Cell* 1991;3:1–9.

Collins JL, Beaty BF. Heat inactivation of trypsin inhibitor in fresh green soybeans and physiological responses of rats fed the beans. *J Food Sci* 1980; 45: 542–546.

Cordain L, Toohey L, Smith MJ, Hickey MS. Modulation of immune function by dietary lectins in rheumatoid arthritis. *Br J Nutr* 2000 Mar;83(3):207–217.

Couzy F, Mansourian R, Labate A, Guinchard S, Montagne DH, Dirren H. Effect of dietary phytic acid on zinc absorption in the healthy elderly, as assessed by serum concentration curve tests. *Br J Nutr* 1998 Aug;80(2):177–182.

FAO/WHO Expert Consultation. Protein Quality Evaluation. Food and Agricultural Organization of the United Nations, FAO Food and Nutrition Paper 51, Rome.

Firestein GS, Alvaro-Gracia JM, Maki R. Quantitative analysis of cytokine gene expression in rheumatoid arthritis. *Journal of Immunology* 1990;144: 33347–33353.

Francis G, Kerem Z, Makkar HP, Becker K. The biological action of saponins in animal systems: a review. *Br J Nutr* 2002 Dec;88(6):587–605.

Gee JM, Johnson IT. Interactions between hemolytic saponins, bile salts and small intestinal mucosa in the rat. *J Nutr* 1988 Nov;118(11):1391–1397.

Gee JM, Wal JM, Miller K, Atkinson H, Grigoriadou F, Wijnands MV, Penninks AH, Wortley G, Johnson IT. Effect of saponin on the transmucosal passage of beta-lactoglobulin across the proximal small intestine of normal and beta-lactoglobulin-sensitised rats. *Toxicology* 1997 Feb 28;117(2–3):219–228.

Gibson RS, Bailey KB, Gibbs M, Ferguson EL. A review of phytate, iron, zinc, and calcium concentrations in plant-based complementary foods used in low-income countries and implications for bioavailability. *Food Nutr Bull* 2010 Jun;31(2 Suppl):S134–146.

Gilani GS, Cockell KA, Sepehr E. Effects of antinutritional factors on protein digestibility and amino acid availability in foods. *J AOAC Int* 2005 May–Jun;88(3):967–987.

Grant G. Anti-nutritional effects of soyabean: a review. *Prog Food Nutr Sci* 1989;13 (3–4):317–348.

Grant G, More LJ, McKenzie NH, Pusztai A. The effect of heating on the haemagglutinating activity and nutritional properties of bean (Phaseolus vulgaris) seeds. *J Sci Food Agric* 1982;33: 1324–1326.

Grant G, More LJ, McKenzie NH, Stewart JC, Pusztai A. A survey of the nutritional and haemagglutination properties of legume seeds generally available in the UK. *Br J Nutr* 1983 Sep;50(2):207–214.

Greer F, Pusztai A. (1985). Toxicity of kidney bean (Phaseolus vulgaris) in rats: changes in intestinal permeability. *Digestion* 1985 32: 42–46.

Gupta YP. Anti-nutritional and toxic factors in food legumes: a review. *Plant Foods Hum Nutr* 1987;37:201–228.

Hallberg L, Hulthén L. Prediction of dietary iron absorption: an algorithm for calculating absorption and bioavailability of dietary iron. *Am J Clin Nutr* 2000 May;71(5):1147–1160.

Hintz HF, Hogue DE, Krook L. Toxicity of red kidney beans (Phaseolus vulgaris) in the rat. *J Nutr* 1967 Sep;93(1):77–86.

Hooper L, Ryder JJ, Kurzer MS, Lampe JW, Messina MJ, Phipps WR, Cassidy A. Effects of soy protein and isoflavones on circulating hormone concentrations in pre- and post-menopausal women: a systematic review and meta-analysis. *Hum Reprod Update* 2009 Jul–Aug;15(4):423–440.

Hughes JS, Acevedo E, Bressani R, Swanson BG. Effects of dietary fiber and tannins on protein utilization in dry beans (Phaseolus vulgaris). *Food Res Int* 1996;29:331–338.

Hurrell RF, Juillerat MA, Reddy MB, Lynch SR, Dassenko SA, Cook JD. Soy protein, phytate, and iron absorption in humans. *Am J Clin Nutr* 1992 Sep;56(3):573–578.

Ishizuki Y, Hirooka Y, Murata Y, Togashi K. The effects on the thyroid gland of soybeans administered experimentally in healthy subjects. *Nippon Naibunpi Gakkai Zasshi* 1991 May 20;67(5):622–629.

Johnson IT, Gee JM, Price K, Curl C, Fenwick GR. Influence of saponins on gut permeability and active nutrient transport in vitro. *J Nutr* 1986 Nov;116(11):2270–2277.

Keukens EA, de Vrije T, van den Boom C, de Waard P, Plasman HH, Thiel F, Chupin V, Jongen WM, de Kruijff B. Molecular basis of glycoalkaloid induced membrane disruption. Biochim Biophys Acta 1995 Dec 13;1240(2):216–228.

Kilpatrick DC, Pusztai A, Grant G, Graham C, Ewen SW. Tomato lectin resists digestion in the mammalian alimentary canal and binds to intestinal villi without deleterious effects. *FEBS Lett* 1985;185:299–305.

Knudsen D, Jutfelt F, Sundh H, Sundell K, Koppe W, Frøkiaer H. Dietary soya saponins increase gut permeability and play a key role in the onset of soyabean-induced enteritis in Atlantic salmon (Salmo salar L.). *Br J Nutr* 2008 Jul;100(1):120–129.

Kritchevsky D et al. Influence of native and randomized peanut oil on lipid metabolism and aortic sudanophilia in the vervet monkey. *Atherosclerosis* 1982;42:53–58.

Kritchevsky D, Tepper SA, Klurfeld DM. Lectin may contribute to the atherogenicity of peanut oil. *Lipids* 1998 Aug;33(8):821–823.

Liener IE. Nutritional significance of lectins in the diet. In *The Lectins: Properties, Functions, and Applications in Biology and Medicine*, Liener IE, Sharon N, Goldstein IJ (eds). Orlando: Academic Press, 1986: 527–552.

Liener IE. Implications of antinutritional components in soybean foods. *Crit Rev Food Sci Nutr* 1994;34:31–67.

Lochner N, Pittner F, Wirth M, Gabor F. Wheat germ agglutinin binds to the epidermal growth factor receptor of artificial Caco-2 membranes as detected by silver nanoparticle enhanced fluorescence. *Pharm Res* 2003 May;20(5):833–839.

Losso JN. The biochemical and functional food properties of the Bowman-Birk inhibitor. *Crit Rev Food Sci Nutr* 2008 Jan;48(1):94–118.

Noah ND, Bender AE, Reaidi GB, Gilbert RJ. Food poisoning from raw red kidney beans. *Br Med J* 1980 Jul 19;281 (6234):236–237.

Muraille E, Pajak B, Urbain J, Leo O. Carbohydrate-bearing cell surface receptors involved in innate immunity: interleukin-12 induction by mitogenic and nonmitogenic lectins. *Cell Immunol* 1999 Jan 10;191(1):1–9.

Pusztai A. Dietary lectins are metabolic signals for the gut and modulate immune and hormone functions. *European Journal of Clinical Nutrition* 1993;47: 691–699.

Pusztai A, Clarke EM, Grant G, King TP. The toxicity of Phaseolus vulgaris lectins. Nitrogen balance and immunochemical studies. *J Sci Food Agric* 1981 Oct;32(10):1037–1046.

Pusztai A, Ewen SW, Grant G, Brown DS, Stewart JC, Peumans WJ, Van Damme EJ, Bardocz S. Antinutritive effects of wheat-germ agglutinin and other N-acetylglucosamine-specific lectins. *Br J Nutr* 1993 Jul;70(1):313–321.

Pusztai A, Ewen SWB, Grant G, Peumans WJ, Van Damme EJM, Rubio LA, Bardocz S. Plant (food) lectins as signal molecules: effects on the morphology and bacterial ecology of the small intestine. In *Lectin Reviews*, Volume I, pp. 1–15, Kilpatrick, DC, Van Driessche E, Bog-Hansen TC (eds). St. Louis: Sigma, 1991.

Pusztai A, Grant G. Assessment of lectin inactivation by heat and digestion. In: *Methods in Molecular Medicine: Vol. 9: Lectin methods and protocols*, Rhodes JM, Milton JD (eds). Totowa, NJ: Humana Press Inc., 1998.

Pusztai A, Grant G, Spencer RJ, Duguid TJ, Brown DS, Ewen, SWB, Peumans WJ, Van Damme EJM, Bardocz S. Kidney bean lectin-induced Escherichia coli overgrowth in the small intestine is blocked by GNA, a mannose-specific lectin. *Journal of Applied Bacteriology* 1993;75: 360–368.

Pusztai A, Greer F, Grant G. Specific uptake of dietary lectins into the systemic circulation of rats. *Biochemical Society Transactions* 1989;17, 527–528.

Rattray EAS, Palmer R, Pusztai A. Toxicity of kidney beans (Phaseolus vulgaris L.) to conventional and gnotobiotic rats. *Journal of the Science of Food and Agriculture* 1974;25:1035–1040.

Rodhouse JC, Haugh CA, Roberts D, Gilbert RJ. Red kidney bean poisoning in the UK: an analysis of 50 suspected incidents between 1976 and 1989. *Epidemiol Infect* 1990 Dec;105(3):485–491.

Róka R, Demaude J, Cenac N, Ferrier L, Salvador-Cartier C, Garcia-Villar R, Fioramonti J, Bueno L. Colonic luminal proteases activate colonocyte proteinase-activated receptor-2 and regulate paracellular permeability in mice. *Neurogastroenterol Motil* 2007 Jan;19(1):57–65.

Román GC. Autism: transient in utero hypothyroxinemia related to maternal flavonoid ingestion during pregnancy and to other environmental antithyroid agents. *J Neurol Sci* 2007 Nov 15;262(1–2):15–26.

Ruiz RG, Price KR, Arthur AE, Rose ME, Rhodes MJ, Fenwick RG. Effect of soaking and cooking on saponin content and composition of chickpeas (*Cicer arietinum*) and lentils (*Lens culinaris*). *J Agric Food Chem* 1996;44:1526–1530.

Ryder SD, Smith JA, Rhodes JM. Peanut lectin: a mitogen for normal human colonic epithelium and human HT29 colorectal cancer cells. *Journal of the National Cancer Institute* 1992;84:1410–16.

Sandberg AS. Bioavailability of minerals in legumes. *Br J Nutr* 2002 Dec;88 Suppl 3:S281–5.

Sanford GL, Harris-Hooker S. Stimulation of vascular proliferation by beta-galactoside specific lectins. *FASEB J* 1990;4:2912–2918.

Singleton VL. Naturally occurring food toxicants: phenolic substances of plant origin. *Adv Food Res* 1981;27:149–242.

Tuxen MK, Nielsen HV, Birgens H. [Poisoning by kidney beans (Phaseolus vulgaris)]. *Ugeskr Laeger* 1991 Dec 16;153(51):3628–3629.

U.S.D.A. My Pyramid. http://www.mypyramid.gov/index.html.

van den Bourne BE, Kijkmans BA, de Rooij HH, le Cessie S, Verweij CL. Chloroquine and hydroxychloroquine equally affect tumor necrosis factor-alpha, interleukin 6, and interferon-gamma production by peripheral blood mononuclear cells. *Journal of Rheumatology* 1997;24: 55–60.

Venter FS, Thiel PG. Red kidney beans—to eat or not to eat? *S Afr Med J* 1995 Apr;85(4):250–252.

Wang Q, Yu LG, Campbell BJ, Milton JD, Rhodes JM. Identification of intact peanut lectin in peripheral venous blood. *Lancet* 1998;352:1831–1832.

Wilson AB, King TP, Clarke EMW, Pusztai A. Kidney bean (Phaseolus vulgaris) lectin-induced lesions in the small intestine. II. Microbiological studies. *Journal of Comparative Pathology* 1980; 90:597–602.

8. Potatoes Should Stay below Ground

Cani PD, Amar J, Iglesias MA, Poggi M, Knauf C, Bastelica D et al. Metabolic endotoxemia initiates obesity and insulin resistance. *Diabetes* 2007 Jul;56(7):1761–1772.

Cordain L, Eades MR, Eades MD. Hyperinsulinemic diseases of civilization: more than just Syndrome X. *Comp Biochem Physiol A Mol Integr Physiol* 2003 Sep;136(1):95–112.

Cordain L, Toohey L, Smith MJ, Hickey MS. Modulation of immune function by dietary lectins in rheumatoid arthritis. *Br J Nutr* 2000 Mar;83(3):207–217.

De Swert LF, Cadot P, Ceuppens JL. Diagnosis and natural course of allergy to cooked potatoes in children. *Allergy* 2007 Jul;62(7):750–757.

El-Tawil AM. Prevalence of inflammatory bowel diseases in the Western nations: high consumption of potatoes may be contributing. *Int J Colorectal Dis* 2008 Oct;23(10):1017–1018.

Fasano A. Surprises from celiac disease. *Sci Am* 2009 Aug;301(2):54–61.

Fernandes G, Velangi A, Wolever TM. Glycemic index of potatoes commonly consumed in North America. *J Am Diet Assoc* 2005 Apr;105(4):557–562.

Foster-Powell K, Holt SH, Brand-Miller JC. International table of glycemic index and glycemic load values: 2002. *Am J Clin Nutr* 2002 Jul;76(1):5–56.

Francis G, Kerem Z, Makkar HP, Becker K. The biological action of saponins in animal systems: a review. *Br J Nutr* 2002 Dec;88(6):587–605.

Friedman M. Potato glycoalkaloids and metabolites: roles in the plant and in the diet. *J Agric Food Chem* 2006 Nov 15;54(23):8655–8681.

Gabor F, Stangl M, Wirth M. Lectin-mediated bioadhesion: binding characteristics of plant lectins on the enterocyte-like cell lines Caco-2, HT-29 and HCT-8. *J Control Release* 1998 Nov 13;55(2–3):131–142.

Härtig W, Reichenbach A, Voigt C, Boltze J, Bulavina L, Schuhmann MU, Seeger J, Schusser GF, Freytag C, Grosche J. Triple fluorescence labelling of neuronal, glial and vascular markers revealing pathological alterations in various animal models. *J Chem Neuroanat* 2009 Mar;37(2):128–138.

Hellenäs KE, Nyman A, Slanina P, Lööf L, Gabrielsson J. Determination of potato glycoalkaloids and their aglycone in blood serum by high-performance liquid chromatography. Application to pharmacokinetic studies in humans. *J Chromatogr* 1992 Jan 3;573(1):69–78.

Henry CJ, Lightowler HJ, Strik CM, Storey M. Glycaemic index values for commercially available potatoes in Great Britain. *Br J Nutr* 2005 Dec;94(6):917–921.

Higashihara M, Ozaki Y, Ohashi T, Kume S. Interaction of Solanum tuberosum agglutinin with human platelets. *Biochem Biophys Res Commun* 1984 May 31;121(1):27–33.

Iablokov V, Sydora BC, Foshaug R, Meddings J, Driedger D, Churchill T, Fedorak RN. Naturally occurring glycoalkaloids in potatoes aggravate intestinal inflammation in two mouse models of inflammatory bowel disease. *Dig Dis Sci* 2010 Nov;55(11):3078–3085.

Morris SC, Lee TH. The toxicity and teratogenicity of Solanaceae glycoalkaloids, particularly those of the potato (*Solanum tuberosum*): a review. *Food Technol Aust* 36 (no. 3) (1984): 118–124.

Kallio P, Kolehmainen M, Laaksonen DE, Pulkkinen L, Atalay M, Mykkänen H, Uusitupa M, Poutanen K, Niskanen L. Inflammation markers are modulated by responses to diets differing in postprandial insulin responses in individuals with the metabolic syndrome. *Am J Clin Nutr* 2008 May;87(5):1497–1503.

Keukens EA, de Vrije T, van den Boom C, de Waard P, Plasman HH, Thiel F, Chupin V, Jongen WM, de Kruijff B. Molecular basis of glycoalkaloid induced membrane disruption. *Biochim Biophys Acta* 1995 Dec 13;1240(2):216–228.

Keukens EA, de Vrije T, Jansen LA, de Boer H, Janssen M, de Kroon AI, Jongen WM, de Kruijff B. Glycoalkaloids selectively permeabilize cholesterol containing biomembranes. *Biochim Biophys Acta* 1996 Mar 13;1279(2):243–250.

Leeman M, Ostman E, Björck I. Glycaemic and satiating properties of potato products. *Eur J Clin Nutr* 2008 Jan;62(1):87–95

Manning PJ, Sutherland WH, McGrath MM, de Jong SA, Walker RJ, Williams MJ. Postprandial Cytokine Concentrations and Meal Composition in Obese and Lean Women. *Obesity (Silver Spring)* 2008 Jun 26.

Mensinga TT, Sips AJ, Rompelberg CJ, van Twillert K, Meulenbelt J, van den Top HJ, van Egmond HP. Potato glycoalkaloids and adverse effects in humans: an ascending dose study. *Regul Toxicol Pharmacol* 2005 Feb;41(1):66–72.

Morris SC, Lee TH. The toxicity and teratogenicity of Solanaceae glycoalkaloids, particularly those of the potato (*Solanum tuberosum*): a review. *Food Technol Aust* 1984;36:118–124.

Morrow-Brown H. Clinical experience with allergy and intolerance to potato (Solanum tuberosum). *Immunol Allergy Practice* 1993;15:41–47.

Naruszewicz M, Zapolska-Downar D, Kośmider A, Nowicka G, Kozłowska-Wojciechowska M, Vikström AS, Törnqvist M. Chronic intake of potato chips in humans increases the production of reactive oxygen radicals by leukocytes and increases plasma C-reactive protein: a pilot study. *Am J Clin Nutr* 2009 Mar;89(3):773–777.

Patel B, Schutte R, Sporns P, Doyle J, Jewel L, Fedorak RN. Potato glycoalkaloids adversely affect intestinal permeability and aggravate inflammatory bowel disease. *Inflamm Bowel Dis* 2002 Sep;8(5):340–346.

Pramod SN, Venkatesh YP, Mahesh PA. Potato lectin activates basophils and mast cells of atopic subjects by its interaction with core chitobiose of cell-bound non-specific immunoglobulin E. *Clin Exp Immunol* 2007 Jun;148(3):391–401.

Qaddoumi M, Lee VH. Lectins as endocytic ligands: an assessment of lectin binding and uptake to rabbit conjunctival epithelial cells. *Pharm Res* 2004 Jul;21(7):1160–1166.

Rauchhaus M, Coats AJ, Anker SD. The endotoxin-lipoprotein hypothesis. *Lancet* 2000 Sep 9;356(9233):930–933.

Root and Tuber Source: http://www.uga.edu/rootandtubercrops/English/.

Smith DB, Roddick JG, Jones JL. Potato glycoalkaloids: some unanswered questions. *Trends Food Sci Technol* 1996;7:126–131.

Stoll LL, Denning GM, Weintraub NL. Endotoxin, TLR4 signaling and vascular inflammation: potential therapeutic targets in cardiovascular disease. *Curr Pharm Des* 2006;12(32):4229–4245.

Sweet MJ, Hume DA. Endotoxin signal transduction in macrophages. *J Leukoc Biol* 1996;60: 8–26.

Ryan CA, Hass GM. Structural, evolutionary and nutritional properties of proteinase inhibitors from potatoes. 1981. In: *Antinutrients and natural toxicants in foods*, Ory RL (ed). Westport, CT: Food and Nutrition Press Inc., 1981.

United States Department of Agriculture. Economic Research Service. Sugar and Sweeteners Yearbook Tables http://www.ers.usda.gov/Briefing/Sugar/Data.htm.

Vetter J. Plant cyanogenic glycosides. *Toxicon* 2000;38:11–36.

9. The Food-Autoimmune Disease Connection

Ansaldi N, Palmas T, Corrias A, Barbato M, D'Altiglia MR, Campanozzi A, Baldassarre M, Rea F, Pluvio R, Bonamico M, Lazzari R, Corrao G. Autoimmune thyroid disease and celiac disease in children. *J Pediatr Gastroenterol Nutr* 2003 Jul;37(1):63–66.

Albert LJ, Inman RD. (1999) Molecular mimicry and autoimmunity. *N Engl J Med* 341, 2068–2074.

Alvarez JR, Torres-Pinedo R. Interactions of soybean lectin, soyasaponins, and glycinin with rabbit jejunal mucosa in vitro. *Pediatr Res* 1982;16:728–731.

Arrieta MC, Bistritz L, Meddings JB. Alterations in intestinal permeability. *Gut* 2006 Oct;55(10):1512–1520.

Benko S, Magyarics Z, Szabó A, Rajnavölgyi E. Dendritic cell subtypes as primary targets of vaccines: the emerging role and cross-talk of pattern recognition receptors. *Biol Chem* 2008 May;389(5):469–485.

Bies C, Lehr CM, Woodley JF. Lectin-mediated drug targeting: history and applications. *Adv Drug Deliv Rev* 2004 Mar 3;56(4):425–35.

Ch'ng CL, Jones MK, Kingham JG. Celiac disease and autoimmune thyroid disease. *Clin Med Res* 2007 Oct;5(3):184–192.

Blank M, Barzilai O, Shoenfeld Y. Molecular mimicry and auto-immunity. *Clin Rev Allergy Immunol* 2007;32:111–118.

Bosland PW. Chiles: history, cultivation, and uses. In: *Spices, Herbs and Edible Fungi (Herbs)*, Charalambous G (ed). Amsterdam: Elsevier Science Publishers, 1994: 347–366.

Cani PD, Amar J, Iglesias MA, Poggi M, Knauf C, Bastelica D, et al. Metabolic endotoxemia initiates obesity and insulin resistance. *Diabetes* 2007 Jul;56(7):1761–1772.

Carreno-Gómez B, Woodley JF, Florence AT. Studies on the uptake of tomato lectin nanoparticles in everted gut sacs. *Int J Pharm* 1999 Jun 10;183(1):7–11.

Childers NF. *Arthritis—Childer's Diet to Stop It. Nightshades, Aging and Ill Health*, 4th ed. *Gainesville*, FL: Horticultural Publications, 1993.

Cordain L, Toohey L, Smith MJ, Hickey MS. Modulation of immune function by dietary lectins in rheumatoid arthritis. *Br J Nutr* 2000 Mar;83(3):207–217.

Elfström P, Montgomery SM, Kämpe O, Ekbom A, Ludvigsson JF. Risk of thyroid disease in individuals with celiac disease. *J Clin Endocrinol Metab* 2008 Oct;93(10):3915–3921.

Fairweather D, Frisancho-Kiss S, Rose NR. Viruses as adjuvants for autoimmunity: evidence from Coxsackievirus-induced myocarditis. *Rev Med Virol* 2005 Jan–Feb;15(1):17–27.

Fairweather D, Kaya Z, Shellam GR, Lawson CM, Rose NR. From infection to autoimmunity. *J Autoimmun* 2001 May;16(3):175–186.

Fairweather D, Rose NR. Women and autoimmune disease. *Emerg Infect Dis* 2004; 10:2005–2011.

Fasano A. Physiological, pathological, and therapeutic implications of zonulin-mediated intestinal barrier modulation: living life on the edge of the wall. *Am J Pathol* 2008 Nov;173(5):1243–1252.

Fasano A. Surprises from celiac disease. *Sci Am* 2009 Aug;301(2):54–61.

Fogh K, Kragballe K. New vitamin D analogs in psoriasis. *Curr Drug Targets Inflamm Allergy* 2004 Jun;3(2):199–204.

Francis G, Kerem Z, Makkar HP, Becker K. The biological action of saponins in animal systems: a review. *Br J Nutr* 2002 Dec;88(6):587–605.

Friedman M, Levin CE. Alpha tomatine content in tomato and tomato products determined by HPLC with pulsed amperometric detection. *J Agric Food Chem* 1995;43:1507–1511.

Gabor F, Bogner E, Weissenboeck A, Wirth M. The lectin-cell interaction and its implications to intestinal lectin-mediated drug delivery. *Adv Drug Deliv Rev* 2004 Mar 3;56(4):459–480.

Gee JM, Wortley GM, Johnson IT, Price KR, Rutten AA, Houben GF, Penninks, AJ. Effects of saponins and glycoalkaloids on the permeability and viability of mammalian intestinal cells and on the integrity of tissue preparations. *Toxicol in Vitro* 1996;10:117–128.

Govindarajan VS, Sathyanarayana MN. Capsicum—production, technology, chemistry, and quality. Part V. Impact on physiology, pharmacology, nutrition, and metabolism; structure, pungency, pain, and desensitization sequences. *Crit Rev Food Sci Nutr* 1991;29(6):435–474.

Greer F, Pusztai A. Toxicity of kidney bean (Phaseolus vulgaris) in rats: changes in intestinal permeability. *Digestion* 1985;32, 42–46.

Han J, Isoda H, Maekawa T. Analysis of the mechanism of the tight-junctional permeability increase by capsaicin treatment on the intestinal Caco-2 cells. *Cytotechnology* 2002 Nov;40(1–3):93–98.

Han JK, Akutsu M, Talorete TP, Maekawa T, Tanaka T, Isoda H. Capsaicin-enhanced Ribosomal Protein P2 Expression in Human Intestinal Caco-2 Cells. *Cytotechnology* 2005 Jan;47(1–3):89–96.

Heiser CB. *Nightshades, the Paradoxical Plants*. San Francisco: W.H. Freeman and Company, 1969.

Hoorfar J, Buschard K, Dagnaes-Hansen F. Prophylactic nutritional modification of the incidence of diabetes in autoimmune non-obese diabetic (NOD) mice. *Br J Nutr* 1993 Mar;69(2):597–607.

Hormi K, Lehy T. Developmental expression of transforming growth factor-alpha and epidermal growth factor receptor proteins in the human pancreas and digestive tract. *Cell Tissue Res* 1994 Dec;278(3):439–450.

Humbert P, Bidet A, Treffel P, Drobacheff C, Agache P. Intestinal permeability in patients with psoriasis. *J Dermatol Sci* 1991;2:324–326.

Hyppönen E, Läärä E, Reunanen A, Järvelin MR, Virtanen SM. Intake of vitamin D and risk of type 1 diabetes: a birth-cohort study. *Lancet* 2001 Nov 3;358(9292):1500–1503.

Isoda H, Han J, Tominaga M, Maekawa T. Effects of capsaicin on human intestinal cell line Caco-2. *Cytotechnology* 2001 Jul;36(1–3):155–161.

Iuorio R, Mercuri V, Barbarulo F, D'Amico T, Mecca N, Bassotti G, Pietrobono D, Gargiulo P, Picarelli A. Prevalence of celiac disease in patients with autoimmune thyroiditis. *Minerva Endocrinol* 2007 Dec;32(4):239–243.

Jensen-Jarolim E, Gajdzik L, Haberl I, Kraft D, Scheiner O, Graf J. Hot spices influence permeability of human intestinal epithelial monolayers. *J Nutr* 1998 Mar;128(3):577–581.

Johnson IT, Gee JM, Price K, Curl C, Fenwick GR. Influence of saponins on gut permeability and active nutrient transport in vitro. *J Nutr* 1986 Nov;116(11):2270–2277.

Kavanaghi R, Workman E, Nash P, Smith M, Hazleman BL, Hunter JO. The effects of elemental diet and subsequent food reintroduction on rheumatoid arthritis. *British Journal of Rheumatology* 1995;34: 70–273.

Katz KD, Hollander D. Intestinal mucosal permeability and rheumatological diseases. *Baillières Clinical Rheumatology* 1989;3:271–284.

Kagnoff MF. Celiac disease: pathogenesis of a model immunogenetic disease. *J Clin Invest* 2007 Jan;117(1):41–49.

Keukens EA, de Vrije T, van den Boom C, de Waard P, Plasman HH, Thiel F, Chupin V, Jongen WM, de Kruijff B. Molecular basis of glycoalkaloid induced membrane disruption. *Biochim Biophys Acta* 1995;1240: 216–228.

Kilpatrick DC, Pusztai A, Grant G, Graham C, Ewen SW. Tomato lectin resists digestion in the mammalian alimentary canal and binds to intestinal villi without deleterious effects. *FEBS Lett* 1985 Jun 17;185(2):299–305.

Komori Y, Aiba T, Nakai C, Sugiyama R, Kawasaki H, Kurosaki Y. Capsaicin-induced increase of intestinal cefazolin absorption in rats. *Drug Metab Pharmacokinet* 2007 Dec;22(6):445–449.

Kozukue N, Han JS, Kozukue E, Lee SJ, Kim JA, Lee KR, Levin CE, Friedman M. Analysis of eight capsaicinoids in peppers and pepper-containing foods by high-performance liquid chromatography and liquid chromatography-mass spectrometry. *J Agric Food Chem* 2005 Nov 16;53(23):9172–9181.

Lee S, Levin MC. Molecular mimicry in neurological disease: what is the evidence? *Cell Mol Life Sci* 2008 Apr;65(7–8):1161–1175.

Lidén M, Kristjánsson G, Valtýsdóttir S, Hällgren R. Gluten sensitivity in patients with primary Sjögren's syndrome. *Scand J Gastroenterol* 2007 Aug;42(8):962–967.

Lochner N, Pittner F, Wirth M, Gabor F. Wheat germ agglutinin binds to the epidermal growth factor receptor of artificial Caco-2 membranes as detected by silver nanoparticle enhanced fluorescence. *Pharm Res* 2003 May;20(5):833–839.

Michaelsson G, Ahs S, Hammarstrom I, Lundin IP, Hagforsen E. Gluten-free diet in psoriasis patients with antibodies to gliadin results in decreased expression of tissue transglutaminase and fewer Ki67+ cells in the dermis. *Acta Derm Venereol* 2003;83(6):425–429.

Michaëlsson G, Gerdén B, Hagforsen E, Nilsson B, Pihl-Lundin I, Kraaz W, Hjelmquist G, Lööf L. Psoriasis patients with antibodies to gliadin can be improved by a gluten-free diet. *Br J Dermatol* 2000 Jan;142(1):44–51.

Michaëlsson G, Gerdén B, Ottosson M, Parra A, Sjöberg O, Hjelmquist G, Lööf L. Patients with psoriasis often have increased serum levels of IgA antibodies to gliadin. *Br J Dermatol* 1993 Dec;129(6):667–673.

Mielants H. Reflections on the link between intestinal permeability and inflammatory joint disease. *Clinical and Experimental Rheumatology* 1990;8:523–524.

Maclaurin BP, Matthews N, Kilpatrick JA. Coeliac disease associated with auto-immune thyroiditis, Sjogren's syndrome, and a lymphocytotoxic serum factor. *Aust N Z J Med* 1972 Nov;2(4):405–411.

McGough N, Cummings JH. Coeliac disease: a diverse clinical syndrome caused by intolerance of wheat, barley and rye. *Proc Nutr Soc* 2005 Nov;64(4):434–450.

Morrow WJ, Yang YW, Sheikh NA. Immunobiology of the Tomatine adjuvant. *Vaccine* 2004 Jun 23;22(19):2380–2384.

Mowat AM. Dendritic cells and immune responses to orally administered antigens. *Vaccine* 2005;23:1797–1799.

Nachbar MS, Oppenheim JD, Thomas JO. Lectins in the U.S. Diet. Isolation and characterization of a lectin from the tomato (Lycopersicon esculentum). *J Biol Chem* 1980 Mar 10;255(95):2056–2061.

Naisbett B, Woodley J. The potential use of tomato lectin for oral drug delivery: 4. Immunological consequences. *Int J Pharm* 1995;120:247–254.

Norris JM, Yin X, Lamb MM, Barriga K, Seifert J, Hoffman M, Orton HD, Barón AE, Clare-Salzler M, Chase HP, Szabo NJ, Erlich H, Eisenbarth GS, Rewers M. Omega-3 polyunsaturated fatty acid intake and islet autoimmunity in children at increased risk for type 1 diabetes. *JAMA* 2007 Sep 26;298(12):1420–1428.

O'Hara AM, Shanahan F. The gut flora as a forgotten organ. *EMBO Rep* 2006 Jul;7(7):688–693.

Paimela L, Kurki P, Leirisalo-Repo M, Piirainen H. Gliadin immune reactivity in patients with rheumatoid arthritis. *Clin Exp Rheumatol* 1995 Sep–Oct;13(5):603–607.

Pengiran Tengah CD, Lock RJ, Unsworth DJ, Wills AJ. Multiple sclerosis and occult gluten sensitivity. *Neurology* 2004 Jun 22;62(12):2326–2327.

Pittman Fe, Holub Da. Sjögren's Syndrome and Adult Celiac Disease. *Gastroenterology* 1965 Jun;48:869–876.

Prinz JC. Psoriasis vulgaris—a sterile antibacterial skin reaction mediated by cross-reactive T cells? An immunological view of the pathophysiology of psoriasis. *Clin Exp Dermatol* 2001;26:326–332.

Progress in Autoimmune Disease Research. The Autoimmune Disease Coordinating Committee Report to Congress. U.S. Department of Health and Human Services, National Institutes of Health, National Institute of Allergy and Infectious Diseases. Bethesda (MD), 2005.

Pruthi JS. Spices and Condiments. In: *Advances in Food Research*, Chichester EM, Stewart GF (eds). New York: Academic Press, 1980: 13.

Pusztai A. Dietary lectins are metabolic signals for the gut and modulate immune and hormone functions. *European Journal of Clinical Nutrition* 1993; 47: 691–699.

Pusztai A, Ewen SW, Grant G, Peumans WJ, van Damme EJ, Rubio L, Bardocz S. Relationship between survival and binding of plant lectins during small intestinal passage and their effectiveness as growth factors. *Digestion* 1990;46 Suppl 2:308–316.

Pusztai A, Greer F, Grant G. Specific uptake of dietary lectins into the systemic circulation of rats. *Biochemical Society Transactions* 1989;17:527–528.

Rauchhaus M, Coats AJ, Anker SD. The endotoxin-lipoprotein hypothesis. *Lancet* 2000 Sep 9;356(9233):930–933.

Rose NR, Mackay IR. *The Auto-Immune Diseases*. New York: Academic Press, 2006.

Schmid S, Koczwara K, Schwinghammer S, Lampasona V, Ziegler AG, Bonifacio E. Delayed exposure to wheat and barley proteins reduces diabetes incidence in non-obese diabetic mice. *Clin Immunol* 2004 Apr;111(1):108–118.

Scott FW. Food-induced type 1 diabetes in the BB rat. *Diabetes Metab Rev* 1996;12:341–359.

Shatin R. Preliminary report of the treatment of rheumatoid arthritis with high protein gluten free diet and supplementation. *Medical Journal of Australia* 1964;2:169–172.

Sjolander A, Magnusson KE, Latkovic S. The effect of concanavalin A and wheat germ agglutinin on the ultrastructure and permeability of rat intestine. *Int Arch Allergy Appl Immunol* 1984;75:230–236.

Smith MD, Gibson RA, Brooks PM. Abnormal bowel permeability in ankylosing spondylitis and rheumatoid arthritis. *Journal of Rheumatology* 1985;12:299–305.

Spadaccino AC, Basso D, Chiarelli S, Albergoni MP, D'Odorico A, Plebani M, Pedini B, Lazzarotto F, Betterle C. Celiac disease in North Italian patients with autoimmune thyroid diseases. *Autoimmunity* 2008 Feb;41(1):116–121.

Stoll LL, Denning GM, Weintraub NL. Endotoxin, TLR4 signaling and vascular inflammation: potential therapeutic targets in cardiovascular disease. *Curr Pharm Des* 2006;12(32):4229–4245.

Strobel S, Mowat MA. Oral tolerance and allergic responses to food proteins. *Curr Opin Allergy Clin Immunol* 2006 Jun;6(3):207–213.

Surh YJ, Lee SS. Capsaicin in hot chili pepper: carcinogen, co-carcinogen or anticarcinogen? *Fd Chem Toxic* 1996;34:313–316.

Szodoray P, Barta Z, Lakos G, Szakáll S, Zeher M. Coeliac disease in Sjögren's syndrome—a study of 111 Hungarian patients. *Rheumatol Int* 2004 Sep;24(5):278–282.

Teppo AM, Maury CP. Antibodies to gliadin, gluten and reticulin glycoprotein in rheumatic diseases: elevated levels in Sjögren's syndrome. *Clin Exp Immunol* 1984 Jul;57(1):73–78.

Thapa B, Skalko-Basnet N, Takano A, Masuda K, Basnet P. High-performance liquid chromatography analysis of capsaicin content in 16 Capsicum fruits from Nepal. *J Med Food* 2009;12:908–913.

Toumi D, Mankai A, Belhadj R, Ghedira-Besbes L, Jeddi M, Ghedira I. Thyroid-related autoantibodies in Tunisian patients with coeliac disease. *Clin Chem Lab Med* 2008;46(3):350–353.

Tsukura Y, Mori M, Hirotani Y, Ikeda K, Amano F, Kato R, Ijiri Y, Tanaka K. Effects of capsaicin on cellular damage and monolayer permeability in human intestinal Caco-2 cells. *Biol Pharm Bull* 2007 Oct;30(10):1982–1986.

Vasconcelos IM, Oliveira JT. Antinutritional properties of plant lectins. *Toxicon* 2004 Sep 15;44(4):385–403.

Walsh SJ, Rau LM. Autoimmune diseases: a leading cause of death among young and middle-aged women in the United States. *Am J Public Health* 2000 Sep;90(9):1463–1466.

Wang Q, Yu LG, Campbell BJ, Milton JD, Rhodes JM. Identification of intact peanut lectin in peripheral venous blood. *Lancet* 1998 Dec 5;352(9143):1831–1832.

Yang YW, Wu CA, Morrow WJ. The apoptotic and necrotic effects of tomatine adjuvant. *Vaccine* 2004 Jun 2;22(17–18):2316–2327.

10. The Paleo Answer 7-Day Diet Plan

Agren MS. Studies on zinc in wound healing. *Acta Derm Venereol Suppl (Stockh)* 1990;154:1–36.

Agren MS, Ostenfeld U, Kallehave F, Gong Y, Raffn K, Crawford ME, Kiss K, Friis-Møller A, Gluud C, Jorgensen LN. A randomized, double-blind, placebo-controlled multicenter trial evaluating topical zinc oxide for acute open wounds following pilonidal disease excision. *Wound Repair Regen* 2006 Sep–Oct;14(5):526–535.

Basford JR, Oh JK, Allison TG, Sheffield CG, Manahan BG, Hodge DO, Tajik AJ, Rodeheffer RJ, Tei C. Safety, acceptance, and physiologic effects of sauna bathing in people with chronic heart failure: a pilot report. *Arch Phys Med Rehabil* 2009 Jan;90(1):173–177.

Billhult A, Lindholm C, Gunnarsson R, Stener-Victorin E. The effect of massage on immune function and stress in women with breast cancer—a randomized controlled trial. *Auton Neurosci* 2009 Oct 5;150(1–2):111–115

Cordain L. *The Paleo Diet.* John Wiley & Sons, New York, 2010.

Cordain L, Friel J. *The Paleo Diet for Athletes.* Emmaus, PA: Rodale Press, 2006.

Cordain L, Gotshall RW, Eaton SB. Evolutionary aspects of exercise. *World Rev Nutr Diet* 1997;81:49–60.

Cordain L, Gotshall RW, Eaton SB, Eaton SB 3rd. Physical activity, energy expenditure and fitness: an evolutionary perspective. *Int J Sports Med* 1998 Jul;19(5):328–335.

Cordain L, Stephenson N, Cordain L. *The Paleo Diet Cookbook.* John Wiley & Sons, New York, 2010.

Cotterman ML, Darby LA, Skelly WA. Comparison of muscle force production using the Smith machine and free weights for bench press and squat exercises. *J Strength Cond Res* 2005;19: 169–176.

DeVoe D, Israel RG, Lipsey T, Voyles W. A long-duration (118-day) backpacking trip (2669 km) normalizes lipids without medication: A case study. *Wilderness & Environmental Medicine* 2009, 20(4): 347–352.

Elli M, Cattivelli D, Soldi S, Bonatti M, Morelli L. Evaluation of prebiotic potential of refined psyllium (Plantago ovata) fiber in healthy women. *J Clin Gastroenterol* 2008 Sep;42 Suppl 3 Pt 2:S174–176.

Fujimori S, Tatsuguchi A, Gudis K, Kishida T, Mitsui K, Ehara A, Kobayashi T, Sekita Y, Seo T, Sakamoto CJ. High dose probiotic and prebiotic cotherapy for remission induction of active Crohn's disease. *Gastroenterol Hepatol* 2007 Aug;22(8):1199–1204.

Hansen D, Dendale P, van Loon LJ, Meeusen R. The impact of training modalities on the clinical benefits of exercise intervention in patients with cardiovascular disease risk or type 2 diabetes mellitus. *Sports Med* 2010 Nov 1;40(11):921–940.

Harvey R, Hannan SA, Badia L, Scadding G. Nasal saline irrigations for the symptoms of chronic rhinosinusitis. *Cochrane Database Syst Rev* 2007 Jul 18;(3):CD006394.

Jungers, W. L. Biomechanics: Barefoot running strikes back. *Nature* 2010; 463(7280), 433–434.

Kihara T, Biro S, Imamura M, Yoshifuku S, Takasaki K, Ikeda Y, Otuji Y, Minagoe S, Toyama Y, Tei C. Repeated sauna treatment improves vascular endothelial and cardiac function in patients with chronic heart failure. *J Am Coll Cardiol* 2002 Mar 6;39(5):754–759.

Kukkonen-Harjula K, Kauppinen K. Health effects and risks of sauna bathing. *Int J Circumpolar Health* 2006 Jun;65(3):195–205.

Labrique-Walusis F, Keister KJ, Russell AC. Massage therapy for stress management: implications for nursing practice. *Orthop Nurs* 2010 Jul–Aug;29(4):254–257.

Lansdown AB, Mirastschijski U, Stubbs N, Scanlon E, Agren MS. Zinc in wound healing: theoretical, experimental, and clinical aspects. *Wound Repair Regen* 2007 Jan–Feb;15(1):2–16.

Lieberman DE, Venkadesan M, Werbel WA, Daoud AI, D'Andrea S, Davis IS, et al. Foot strike patterns and collision forces in habitually barefoot versus shod runners. *Nature* 2010; 463(7280), 531–535.

Lyons TS, McLester JR, Arnett SW, Thoma MJ. Specificity of training modalities on upper-body one repetition maximum performance: free weights vs. hammer strength equipment. *J Strength Cond Res* 2010 Nov;24(11):2984–2988.

Miller MM. Low sodium chloride intake in the treatment of insomnia and tension states. *JAMA* 1945;129:262–266.

Mizushima T. HSP-dependent protection against gastrointestinal diseases. *Curr Pharm Des* 2010;16(10):1190–1196.

Nerbass FB, Feltrim MI, Souza SA, Ykeda DS, Lorenzi-Filho G.Effects of massage therapy on sleep quality after coronary artery bypass graft surgery. *Clinics (Sao Paulo)* 2010;65(11):1105–1110.

O'Keefe JH, Vogel R, Lavie CJ, Cordain L. Achieving hunter-gatherer fitness in the 21(st) century: back to the future. *Am J Med* 2010 Dec;123(12):1082–1086.

O'Keefe JH, Vogel R, Lavie CJ, Cordain L. Organic fitness: physical activity consistent with our hunter-gatherer heritage. *Phys Sportsmed* 2010 Dec;38(4):11–8.

Pinhasi R, Gasparian B, Areshian G, Zardaryan D, Smith A, Bar-Oz G, Higham T. First direct evidence of Chalcolithic footwear from the near eastern highlands. *PLoS One* 2010 Jun 9;5(6):e10984.

Rabago D, Guerard E, Bukstein D. Nasal irrigation for chronic sinus symptoms in patients with allergic rhinitis, asthma, and nasal polyposis: a hypothesis generating study. *WMJ* 2008 Apr;107(2):69–75.

Ratel S. High-intensity and resistance training and elite young athletes. *Med Sport Sci* 2011;56:84–96.

Rodríguez-Cabezas ME, Gálvez J, Camuesco D, Lorente MD, Concha A, Martinez-Augustin O, Redondo L, Zarzuelo A. Intestinal anti-inflammatory activity of dietary fiber (Plantago ovata seeds) in HLA-B27 transgenic rats. *Clin Nutr* 2003 Oct;22(5):463–471.

Simpson, SR, Rozeneck, R, Garhammer, J, Lacourse, M, and Storer, T. Comparison of one repetition maximums between free weight and universal machine exercises. *J Strength Cond Res* 1997; 11: 103–106.

Squadrone R, Gallozzi C. Biomechanical and physiological comparison of barefoot and two shod conditions in experienced barefoot runners. *J Sports Med Phys Fitness* 2009;49(1): 6–13.

Stein MD, Friedmann PD. Disturbed sleep and its relationship to alcohol use. *Subst Abus* 2005 Mar;26(1):1–13.

Stetler RA, Gan Y, Zhang W, Liou AK, Gao Y, Cao G, Chen J. Heat shock proteins: cellular and molecular mechanisms in the central nervous system. *Prog Neurobiol* 2010 Oct;92(2):184–211.

Takács T, Rakonczay Z Jr, Varga IS, Iványi B, Mándi Y, Boros I, Lonovics J. Comparative effects of water immersion pretreatment on three different acute pancreatitis models in rats. *Biochem Cell Biol* 2002;80(2):241–251.

Tolson JK, Roberts SM. Manipulating heat shock protein expression in laboratory animals. *Methods* 2005 Feb;35(2):149–157.

Trinkaus, E. Anatomical evidence for the antiquity of human footwear use. *J Archaeol Sci* 2005;32(10):1515–1526.

Trinkaus E, Shang H. Anatomical evidence for the antiquity of human footwear: Tianyuan and Sunghir. *J Archaeol Sci* 2008; 35(7), 1928–1933.

Willardson, JM and Bressel, E. Predicting a 10 repetition maximum for the free weight parallel squat using the 45* angled leg press. *J Strength Cond Res* 2004;18:567–561.

11. Paleo Supplements and Sunshine

Adams M, Lucock M, Stuart J, Fardell S, Baker K, Ng X. Preliminary evidence for involvement of the folate gene polymorphism 19bp deletion-DHFR in occurrence of autism. *Neurosci Lett* 2007 Jul 5;422(1):24–29.

Alcock N, Macintyre I. Inter-relation of calcium and magnesium absorption. *Clin Sci* 1962 Apr;22:185–193.

Autier P. Sunscreen abuse for intentional sun exposure. *Br J Dermatol* 2009 Nov;161 Suppl 3:40–45.

Autier P, Boniol M, Doré JF. Sunscreen use and increased duration of intentional sun exposure: still a burning issue. *Int J Cancer* 2007 Jul 1;121(1):1–5.

Autier P, Doré JF, Eggermont AM, Coebergh JW. Epidemiological evidence that UVA radiation is involved in the genesis of cutaneous melanoma. *Curr Opin Oncol* 2011 Mar;23(2):189–196.

ATBC Cancer Prevention Study Group. The effect of vitamin E and beta carotene on the incidence of lung cancer and other cancers in male smokers. The Alpha-Tocopherol, Beta Carotene Cancer Prevention Study Group. *N Engl J Med* 1994 Apr 14;330(15):1029–1035.

Autism and Developmental Disabilities Monitoring Network Surveillance Year 2006 Principal Investigators; Centers for Disease Control and Prevention (CDC). Prevalence of autism spectrum disorders—Autism and Developmental Disabilities Monitoring Network, United States, 2006. *MMWR Surveill Summ* 2009 Dec 18;58(10):1–20.

Beard CM, Panser LA, Katusic SK. Is excess folic acid supplementation a risk factor for autism? *Med Hypotheses* 2011 Jul;77(1):15–17.

Beaudet AL, Goin-Kochel RP. Some, but not complete, reassurance on the safety of folic acid fortification. *Am J Clin Nutr* 2010 Dec;92(6):1287–1288.

Berwick M. The good, the bad, and the ugly of sunscreens. *Clin Pharmacol Ther* 2011 Jan;89(1):31–33.

Binkley N, Novotny R, Krueger D, Kawahara T, Daida YG, Lensmeyer G, Hollis BW, Drezner MK. Low vitamin D status despite abundant sun exposure. *J Clin Endocrinol Metab* 2007 Jun;92(6):2130–2135.

Bjelakovic G, Gluud C. Surviving antioxidant supplements. *J Natl Cancer Inst* 2007 May 16;99(10):742–743.

Bjelakovic G, Nikolova D, Gluud LL, Simonetti RG, Gluud C. Antioxidant supplements for prevention of mortality in healthy participants and patients with various diseases. *Cochrane Database Syst Rev* 2008 Apr 16;(2):CD007176.

Bjelakovic G, Nikolova D, Gluud LL, Simonetti RG, Gluud C. Mortality in randomized trials of antioxidant supplements for primary and secondary prevention: systematic review and meta-analysis. *JAMA* 2007 Feb 28;297(8):842–857. Review. Erratum in: *JAMA* 2008 Feb 20;299(7):765–766.

Bjelakovic G, Nikolova D, Simonetti RG, Gluud C. Systematic review: primary and secondary prevention of gastrointestinal cancers with antioxidant supplements. *Aliment Pharmacol Ther* 2008 Sep 15;28(6):689–703.

Bleys J, Miller ER 3rd, Pastor-Barriuso R, Appel LJ, Guallar E. Vitamin-mineral supplementation and the progression of atherosclerosis: a meta-analysis of randomized controlled trials. *Am J Clin Nutr* 2006 Oct;84(4):880–887.

Bolland MJ, Avenell A, Baron JA, Grey A, MacLennan GS, Gamble GD, Reid IR. Effect of calcium supplements on risk of myocardial infarction and cardiovascular events: meta-analysis. *BMJ* 2010 Jul 29;341:c3691. doi: 10.1136/bmj.c3691.

Boulet SL, Gambrell D, Shin M, et al. Racial/ethnic differences in the birth prevalence of spina bifida-United States, 1995–2005. *MMWR* 2009;57:1409–1413.

Burnett ME, Wang SQ. Current sunscreen controversies: a critical review. *Photodermatol Photoimmunol Photomed* 2011 Apr;27(2):58–67.

Chiaffarino F, Ascone GB, Bortolus R, Mastroia-Covo P, Ricci E, Cipriani S, Parazzini F. [Effects of folic acid supplementation on pregnancy outcomes: a review of randomized clinical trials]. *Minerva Ginecol* 2010 Aug;62(4):293–301.

Chiang EC, Shen S, Kengeri SS, Xu H, Combs GF, Morris JS, Bostwick DG, Waters DJ. Defining the optimal selenium dose for prostate cancer risk reduction: insights from the U-shaped relationship between selenium status, DNA damage, and apoptosis. *Dose Response* 2009 Dec 21;8(3):285–300.

Cho E, Hunter DJ, Spiegelman D, Albanes D, Beeson WL, van den Brandt PA, Colditz GA, et al. Intakes of vitamins A, C and E and folate and multivitamins and lung cancer: a pooled analysis of 8 prospective studies. *Int J Cancer* 2006 Feb 15;118(4):970–978.

Clarke R, Halsey J, Lewington S, Lonn E, Armitage J, Manson JE, et al. Effects of lowering homocysteine levels with B vitamins on cardiovascular disease, cancer, and cause-specific mortality: Meta-analysis of 8 randomized trials involving 37 485 individuals. *Arch Intern Med* 2010 Oct 11;170(18):1622–1631.

Close, G. L., Ashton, T., Cable, T., Doran, D., Holloway, C., McArdle, F., et al. (2006). Ascorbic acid supplementation does not attenuate post-exercise muscle soreness following muscle-damaging exercise but may delay the recovery process. *Brit J Nutr* 2006; 95:976–981.

Cole BF, Baron JA, Sandler RS, Haile RW et al. Folic acid for the prevention of colorectal adenomas: a randomized clinical trial. *JAMA* 2007 Jun 6;297(21):2351–2359.

Collin SM, Metcalfe C, Refsum H, Lewis SJ, Smith GD et al. Associations of folate, vitamin B12, homocysteine, and folate-pathway polymorphisms with prostate-specific antigen velocity in men with localized prostate cancer. *Cancer Epidemiol Biomarkers Prev* 2010 Nov;19(11):2833–2838.

Collin SM, Metcalfe C, Refsum H, Lewis SJ, et al.Circulating folate, vitamin B12, homocysteine, vitamin B12 transport proteins, and risk of prostate cancer: a case-control study, systematic review, and meta-analysis. *Cancer Epidemiol Biomarkers Prev* 2010 Jun;19(6):1632–1642.

Dobnig H, Pilz S, Scharnagl H, Renner W, Seelhorst U, Wellnitz B, Kinkeldei J, Boehm BO, Weihrauch G, Maerz W. Independent association of low serum 25-hydroxyvitamin d and 1,25-dihydroxyvitamin d levels with all-cause and cardiovascular mortality. *Arch Intern Med* 2008 Jun 23;168(12):1340–1349.

Ebbing M, Bønaa KH, Nygård O, Arnesen E, Ueland PM, et al. Cancer incidence and mortality after treatment with folic acid and vitamin B12. *JAMA* 2009 Nov 18;302(19):2119–2126.

Field S, Newton-Bishop JA. Melanoma and vitamin D. *Mol Oncol* 2011 Feb 3. Epub ahead of print.

Figueiredo JC, Grau MV, Haile RW, Sandler RS, Summers RW, Bresalier RS, Burke CA, McKeown-Eyssen GE, Baron JA. Folic acid and risk of prostate cancer: results from a randomized clinical trial. *J Natl Cancer Inst* 2009 Mar 18;101(6):432–435.

Forouhi NG, Luan J, Cooper A, Boucher BJ, Wareham NJ. Baseline serum 25-hydroxy vitamin D is predictive of future glycaemic status and insulin resistance: The MRC Ely prospective study 1990–2000. *Diabetes* 2008 Oct;57(10):2619–2125.

Garland CF, Garland FC, Gorham ED. Epidemiologic evidence for different roles of ultraviolet A and B radiation in melanoma mortality rates. *Ann Epidemiol* 2003 Jul;13(6):395–404.

Gaziano JM, Glynn RJ, Christen WG, Kurth T, Belanger C, MacFadyen J, Bubes V, Manson JE, Sesso HD, Buring JE. Vitamins E and C in the prevention of prostate and total cancer in men: the Physicians' Health Study II randomized controlled trial. *JAMA* 2009 Jan 7;301(1):52–62. Epub 2008 Dec 9.

Gomez-Cabrera, M-C, Domenech E, Romagnoli M, Arduini A, Borras C, Pallardo FV, et al. Oral administration of vitamin C decreases muscle mitochondrial biogenesis and hampers training-induced adaptations in endurance performance. *Am J Clin Nutr* 2008; 87(1), 142–149.

Gore F, Fawell J, Bartram J. Too much or too little? A review of the conundrum of selenium.*J Water Health* 2010 Sep;8(3):405–416.

Gorham ED, Mohr SB, Garland CF, Chaplin G, Garland FC. Do sunscreens increase risk of melanoma in populations residing at higher latitudes? *Ann Epidemiol* 2007 Dec;17(12):956–963.

Greenough A, Shaheen SO, Shennan A, Seed PT, Poston L. Respiratory outcomes in early childhood following antenatal vitamin C and E supplementation. *Thorax* 2010 Nov;65(11):998–1003.

Herbert K, Fletcher S, Chauhan D, Ladapo A, Nirwan J, Munson S, et al. (2006). Dietary supplementation with different vitamin C doses: no effect on oxidative DNA damage in healthy people. *Eur J Nutr* 2006;45(2): 97–104.

Herbert V. Staging vitamin B-12 (cobalamin) status in vegetarians. *Am J Clin Nutr* 1994 May;59(5 Suppl):1213S–1222S.

Holick MF. Optimal vitamin d status for the prevention and treatment of osteoporosis. *Drugs Aging* 2007; 24(12):1017–1029.

Holick MF. Vitamin D and sunlight: strategies for cancer prevention and other health benefits. *Clin J Am Soc Nephrol* 2008;3:1548–1554.

Holick MF, Chen TC. Vitamin D deficiency: a worldwide problem with health consequences. *Am J Clin Nutr* 2008 Apr;87(4):1080S–1086S.

Hollis BW. Circulating 25-hydroxyvitamin D levels indicative of vitamin D sufficiency: implications for establishing a new effective dietary intake recommendation for vitamin D. *J Nutr* 2005 Feb;135(2):317–322.

Honein MA, Paulozzi LJ, Mathews TJ, Erickson JD, Wong LY. Impact of folic acid fortification of the US food supply on the occurrence of neural tube defects. *JAMA* 2001 Jun 20;285(23):2981–2986.

Johnson FO, Gilbreath ET, Ogden L, Graham TC, Gorham S. Reproductive and developmental toxicities of zinc supplemented rats. *Reprod Toxicol* 2011 Feb;31(2):134–143.

Khan AT, Graham TC, Ogden L, Ali S, Salwa, Thompson SJ, Shireen KF, Mahboob M. A two-generational reproductive toxicity study of zinc in rats. *J Environ Sci Health B* 2007 May;42(4):403–415.

King CR. A novel embryological theory of autism causation involving endogenous biochemicals capable of initiating cellular gene transcription: A possible link between twelve autism risk factors and the autism 'epidemic.' *Med Hypotheses* 2011 Mar 7. Epub ahead of print.

Kull I, Bergström A, Melén E, Lilja G, van Hage M, Pershagen G, Wickman M. Early-life supplementation of vitamins A and D, in water-soluble form or in peanut oil, and allergic diseases during childhood. *J Allergy Clin Immunol* 2006 Dec;118(6):1299–1304.

Kumar J, Muntner P, Kaskel FJ, Hailpern SM, Melamed ML. Prevalence and associations of 25-hydroxyvitamin D deficiency in US children: NHANES 2001–2004. *Pediatrics* 2009 Sep;124(3):e362–370.

Ledesma MC, Jung-Hynes B, Schmit TL, Kumar R, Mukhtar H, Ahmad N. Selenium and vitamin E for prostate cancer: post-SELECT (Selenium and Vitamin E Cancer Prevention Trial) status. *Mol Med* 2011 Jan-Feb;17(1–2):134–143.

Leeming RJ, Lucock M. Autism: Is there a folate connection? *J Inherit Metab Dis* 2009 Jun;32(3):400–402.

Levine AJ, Figueiredo JC, Lee W, Conti DV, Kennedy K, Duggan DJ, Poynter JN, Campbell PT, Newcomb P, Martinez ME, Hopper JL, Le Marchand L, Baron JA, Limburg PJ, Ulrich CM, Haile RW. A candidate gene study of folate-associated one carbon metabolism genes and colorectal cancer risk. *Cancer Epidemiol Biomarkers Prev* 2010 Jul;19(7):1812–1821.

Lichtenstein AH, Russell RM. Essential nutrients: food or supplements? Where should the emphasis be? *JAMA* 2005 Jul 20;294(3):351–358.

Lin J, Lee IM, Cook NR, Selhub J, Manson JE, Buring JE, Zhang SM. Plasma folate, vitamin B-6, vitamin B-12, and risk of breast cancer in women. *Am J Clin Nutr* 2008 Mar;87(3):734–743.

Lindzon GM, Medline A, Sohn KJ, Depeint F, Croxford R, Kim YI. Effect of folic acid supplementation on the progression of colorectal aberrant crypt foci. *Carcinogenesis* 2009 Sep;30(9):1536–1543.

Løland KH, Bleie O, Blix AJ, Strand E, Ueland PM, Refsum H, Ebbing M, Nordrehaug JE, Nygård O. Effect of homocysteine-lowering B vitamin treatment on angiographic progression of coronary artery disease: a Western Norway B Vitamin Intervention Trial (WENBIT) substudy. *Am J Cardiol* 2010 Jun 1;105(11):1577–1584.

Main PA, Angley MT, Thomas P, O'Doherty CE, Fenech M. Folate and methionine metabolism in autism: a systematic review. *Am J Clin Nutr* 2010 Jun;91(6):1598–1620.

McCance DR, Holmes VA, Maresh MJ, Patterson CC, Walker JD, Pearson DW, Young IS, Diabetes and Pre-eclampsia Intervention Trial (DAPIT) Study Group. Vitamins C and E for prevention of pre-eclampsia in women with type 1 diabetes (DAPIT): a randomised placebo-controlled trial. *Lancet* 2010 Jul 24;376(9737):259–266.

Melamed ML, Kumar J. Low levels of 25-hydroxyvitamin D in the pediatric populations: prevalence and clinical outcomes. *Ped Health* 2010 Feb;4(1):89–97.

Millen AE, Dodd KW, Subar AF. Use of vitamin, mineral, nonvitamin, and nonmineral supplements in the United States: the 1987, 1992, and 2000 National Health Interview Survey results. *J Am Diet Assoc* 2004;104:942–950.

Miller ER 3rd, Pastor-Barriuso R, Dalal D, Riemersma RA, Appel LJ, Guallar E. Meta-analysis: high-dosage vitamin E supplementation may increase all-cause mortality. *Ann Intern Med* 2005 Jan 4;142(1):37–46.

Milner JD, Stein DM, McCarter R, Moon RY. Early infant multivitamin supplementation is associated with increased risk for food allergy and asthma. *Pediatrics* 2004 Jul;114(1):27–32.

Mohr SB, Garland CF, Gorham ED, Grant WB, Garland FC. Relationship between low ultraviolet B irradiance and higher breast cancer risk in 107 countries. *Breast J* 2008 May–Jun;14(3):255–260.

Moyal DD, Fourtanier AM. Broad-spectrum sunscreens provide better protection from solar ultraviolet-simulated radiation and natural sunlight-induced immunosuppression in human beings. *J Am Acad Dermatol* 2008 May;58(5 Suppl 2):S149–154.

Mozaffarian D, Ludwig DS. Dietary guidelines in the 21st century—a time for food. *JAMA* 2010 Aug 11;304(6):681–682.

Omenn GS, Goodman GE, Thornquist MD, Balmes J, Cullen MR, Glass A, Keogh JP, Meyskens FL, Valanis B, Williams JH, Barnhart S, Hammar S. Effects of a combination of beta carotene and vitamin A on lung cancer and cardiovascular disease. *N Engl J Med* 1996 May 2;334(18):1150–1155.

Plum LA, DeLuca HF. Vitamin D, disease and therapeutic opportunities. *Nat Rev Drug Discov* 2010 Dec;9(12):941–955.

Refsum H, Smith AD. Are we ready for mandatory fortification with vitamin B-12? *Am J Clin Nutr* 2008 Aug;88(2):253–254.

Rice C, Nicholas J, Baio J, Pettygrove S, Lee LC et al. Changes in autism spectrum disorder prevalence in 4 areas of the United States. *Disabil Health J* 2010 Jul;3(3):186–201.

Ristow M, Zarse K, Oberbach A, KlÃting N, Birringer M, Kiehntopf M, et al. Antioxidants prevent health-promoting effects of physical exercise in humans. *Proc Natl Acad Sci* 2009;106(21):8665–8670.

Rogers EJ. Has enhanced folate status during pregnancy altered natural selection and possibly Autism prevalence? A closer look at a possible link. *Med Hypotheses* 2008 Sep;71(3):406–410.

Rosenberg IH. Science-based micronutrient fortification: which nutrients, how much, and how to know? *Am J Clin Nutr* 2005 Aug;82(2):279–280.

Sauer J, Mason JB, Choi SW. Too much folate: a risk factor for cancer and cardiovascular disease? *Curr Opin Clin Nutr Metab Care* 2009 Jan;12(1):30–36.

Schürks M, Glynn RJ, Rist PM, Tzourio C, Kurth T. Effects of vitamin E on stroke subtypes: meta-analysis of randomised controlled trials. *BMJ* 2010 Nov 4;341:c5702. doi: 10.1136/bmj.c5702.

Seelig MS. Increased need for magnesium with the use of combined oestrogen and calcium for osteoporosis treatment. *Magnes Res* 1990 Sep;3(3):197–215.

Sharief S, Jariwala S, Kumar J, Muntner P, Melamed ML. Vitamin D levels and food and environmental allergies in the United States: results from the National Health and Nutrition Examination Survey 2005–2006. *J Allergy Clin Immunol* 2011 Feb 15.

Smith AD, Kim YI, Refsum H. Is folic acid good for everyone? *Am J Clin Nutr* 2008 Mar;87(3):517–533.

Smulders YM, Blom HJ. The homocysteine controversy. *J Inherit Metab Dis* 2011 Feb;34(1):93–99.

Soni MG, Thurmond TS, Miller ER 3rd, Spriggs T, Bendich A, Omaye ST. Safety of vitamins and minerals: controversies and perspective. *Toxicol Sci* 2010 Dec;118(2):348–355.

Stevens VL, McCullough ML, Sun J, Gapstur SM. Folate and other one-carbon metabolism-related nutrients and risk of postmenopausal breast cancer in the Cancer Prevention Study II Nutrition Cohort. *Am J Clin Nutr* 2010 Jun;91(6):1708–1715.

Stolzenberg-Solomon RZ, Chang SC, Leitzmann MF, Johnson KA, Johnson C, Buys SS, Hoover RN, Ziegler RG. Folate intake, alcohol use, and postmenopausal breast cancer risk in the Prostate, Lung, Colorectal, and Ovarian Cancer Screening Trial. *Am J Clin Nutr* 2006 Apr;83(4):895–904.

Ulrich CM, Potter JD. Folate and cancer—timing is everything. *JAMA* 2007 Jun 6;297(21):2408–2409.

Vieth R. Why the optimal requirement for vitamin D3 is probably much higher than what is officially recommended for adults. *J Steroid Biochem Mol Biol* 2004; 89–90:575–579.

Walter PB, Knutson MD, Paler-Martinez A, Lee S, Xu Y, Viteri FE, Ames BN. Iron deficiency and iron excess damage mitochondria and mitochondrial DNA in rats. *Proc Natl Acad Sci USA* 2002 Feb 19;99(4):2264–2269.

Wu J, Lyons GH, Graham RD, Fenech MF. The effect of selenium, as selenomethionine, on genome stability and cytotoxicity in human lymphocytes measured using the cytokinesis-block micronucleus cytome assay. *Mutagenesis* 2009 May;24(3):225–232.

12. Paleo Water

Amiridou D, Voutsa D. Alkylphenols and phthalates in bottled waters. *J Hazard Mater* 2011 Jan 15;185(1):281–286.

Barbier O, Arreola-Mendoza L, Del Razo LM. Molecular mechanisms of fluoride toxicity. *Chem Biol Interact* 2010 Nov 5;188(2):319–333.

Biedermann S, Tschudin P, Grob K. Transfer of bisphenol A from thermal printer paper to the skin. *Anal Bioanal Chem* 2010 Sep;398(1):571–576.

Brewer GJ. The risks of copper toxicity contributing to cognitive decline in the aging population and to Alzheimer's disease. *J Am Coll Nutr* 2009 Jun;28(3):238–342.

Cao XL, Corriveau J, Popovic S. Sources of low concentrations of bisphenol A in canned beverage products. *J Food Prot* 2010 Aug;73(8):1548–1551.

Chandrajith R, Dissanayake CB, Ariyarathna T, Herath HM, Padmasiri JP. Dose-dependent Na and Ca in fluoride-rich drinking water—another major cause of chronic renal failure in tropical arid regions. *Sci Total Environ* 2011 Jan 15;409(4):671–675.

Chinoy NJ, Rao MV, Narayana MV, Neelakanta E. Microdose vasal injection of sodium fluoride in the rat. *Reprod Toxicol* 1991;5(6):505–512.

Crinnion WJ. Toxic effects of the easily avoidable phthalates and parabens. *Altern Med Rev* 2010 Sep;15(3):190–196.

Danielson C, Lyon JL, Egger M, Goodenough GK. Hip fractures and fluoridation in Utah's elderly population. *JAMA* 1992 Aug 12;268(6):746–748.

Do LG, Spencer AJ. Risk-benefit balance in the use of fluoride among young children. *J Dent Res* 2007 Aug;86(8):723–728.

Durand ML, Dietrich AM. Contributions of silane cross-linked PEX pipe to chemical/solvent odours in drinking water. *Water Sci Technol* 2007;55(5):153–160.

Freni SC. Exposure to high fluoride concentrations in drinking water is associated with decreased birth rates. *J Toxicol Environ Health* 1994 May;42(1):109–121.

Gazzano E, Bergandi L, Riganti C, Aldieri E, Doublier S, Costamagna C, Bosia A, Ghigo D. Fluoride effects: the two faces of janus. *Curr Med Chem* 2010;17(22):2431–2441.

Guart A, Bono-Blay F, Borrell A, Lacorte S. Migration of plasticizersphthalates, bisphenol A and alkylphenols from plastic containers and evaluation of risk. *Food Addit Contam Part A Chem Anal Control Expo Risk Assess* 2011 Mar 11:1–10.

Gutowska I, Baranowska-Bosiacka I, Baśkiewicz M, Milo B, Siennicka A, Marchlewicz M, Wiszniewska B, Machaliński B, Stachowska E. Fluoride as a pro-inflammatory factor and inhibitor of ATP bioavailability in differentiated human THP1 monocytic cells. *Toxicol Lett* 2010 Jul 1;196(2):74–79.

Hedlund LR, Gallagher JC. Increased incidence of hip fracture in osteoporotic women treated with sodium fluoride. *J Bone Miner Res* 1989 Apr;4(2):223–225.

Hua G, Reckhow DA. Comparison of disinfection byproduct formation from chlorine and alternative disinfectants. *Water Res* 2007 Apr;41(8):1667–1678.

Inkielewicz-Stepniak I, Czarnowski W. Oxidative stress parameters in rats exposed to fluoride and caffeine. *Food Chem Toxicol* 2010 Jun;48(6):1607–1611.

Joyce SJ, Cook A, Newnham J, Brenters M, Ferguson C, Weinstein P. Water disinfection by-products and pre-labor rupture of membranes. *Am J Epidemiol* 2008 Sep 1;168(5):514–521. Epub 2008 Jul 16.

Kimber I, Dearman RJ. An assessment of the ability of phthalates to influence immune and allergic responses. *Toxicology* 2010 May 27;271(3):73–82.

Kitazawa M, Cheng D, Laferla FM. Chronic copper exposure exacerbates both amyloid and tau pathology and selectively dysregulates cdk5 in a mouse model of AD. *J Neurochem* 2009 Mar;108(6):1550–1560.

Krasner SW. The formation and control of emerging disinfection by-products of health concern. *Philos Transact A Math Phys Eng Sci* 2009 Oct 13;367(1904):4077–4095.

Krasner SW, Weinberg HS, Richardson SD, Pastor SJ, Chinn R, Sclimenti MJ, Onstad GD, Thruston AD Jr. Occurrence of a new generation of disinfection byproducts. *Environ Sci Technol* 2006 Dec 1;40(23):7175–7185.

Kristiana I, Gallard H, Joll C, Croué JP. The formation of halogen-specific TOX from chlorination and chloramination of natural organic matter isolates. *Water Res* 2009 Sep;43(17):4177–4186.

Künzel W, Fischer T, Lorenz R, Brühmann S. Decline of caries prevalence after the cessation of water fluoridation in the former East Germany. *Community Dent Oral Epidemiol* 2000 Oct;28(5):382–389.

Lang IA, Galloway TS, Scarlett A, Henley WE, Depledge M, Wallace RB, Melzer D. Association of urinary bisphenol A concentration with medical disorders and laboratory abnormalities in adults. *JAMA* 2008 Sep 17;300(11):1303–1310.

Loganathan SN, Kannan K. Occurrence of Bisphenol A in indoor dust from two locations in the Eastern United States and implications for human exposures. *Arch Environ Contam Toxicol* 2011 Jan 8;61(1): 68–73.

McDonald TA, Komulainen H. Carcinogenicity of the chlorination disinfection by-product MX. *J Environ Sci Health C Environ Carcinog Ecotoxicol Rev* 2005;23(2):163–214.

Morris RD, Audet AM, Angelillo IF, Chalmers TC, Mosteller F. Chlorination, chlorination by-products, and cancer: a meta-analysis. *Am J Public Health* 1992 Jul;82(7):955–963.

Mullenix PJ, Denbesten PK, Schunior A, Kernan WJ. Neurotoxicity of sodium fluoride in rats. *Neurotoxicol Teratol* 1995 Mar–Apr;17(2):169–177.

Pizzo G, Piscopo MR, Pizzo I, Giuliana G. Community water fluoridation and caries prevention: a critical review. *Clin Oral Investig* 2007 Sep;11(3):189–193.

Prystupa J. Fluorine—a current literature review. An NRC and ATSDR based review of safety standards for exposure to fluorine and fluorides. *Toxicol Mech Methods* 2011 Feb;21(2):103–170.

Rahman MB, Driscoll T, Cowie C, Armstrong BK. Disinfection by-products in drinking water and colorectal cancer: a meta-analysis. *Int J Epidemiol* 2010 Jun;39(3):733–745.

Raj SD. Bottled water: how safe is it? *Water Environ Res* 2005 Nov–Dec;77(7):3013–3018.

Richardson SD, Plewa MJ, Wagner ED, Schoeny R, Demarini DM. Occurrence, genotoxicity, and carcinogenicity of regulated and emerging disinfection by-products in drinking water: a review and roadmap for research. *Mutat Res* 2007 Nov–Dec;636 (1–3):178–242.

Schecter A, Malik N, Haffner D, Smith S, Harris TR, Paepke O, Birnbaum L. Bisphenol A (BPA) in U.S. food. *Environ Sci Technol* 2010 Dec 15;44(24):9425–9430.

Schettler T. Human exposure to phthalates via consumer products. *Int J Androl* 2006 Feb;29(1):134–139; discussion 181–185.

Sedman RM, Beaumont J, McDonald TA, Reynolds S, Krowech G, Howd R. Review of the evidence regarding the carcinogenicity of hexavalent chromium in drinking water. *J Environ Sci Health C Environ Carcinog Ecotoxicol Rev* 2006 Apr;24(1):155–182.

Soto AM, Sonnenschein C. Environmental causes of cancer: endocrine disruptors as carcinogens. *Nat Rev Endocrinol* 2010 Jul;6(7):363–370.

Sparks DL, Friedland R, Petanceska S, Schreurs BG, Shi J, Perry G, Smith MA, Sharma A, Derosa S, Ziolkowski C, Stankovic G. Trace copper levels in the drinking water, but not zinc or aluminum influence CNS Alzheimer-like pathology. *J Nutr Health Aging* 2006 Jul-Aug;10(4):247–254.

Streltsov VA, Titmuss SJ, Epa VC, Barnham KJ, Masters CL, Varghese JN. The structure of the amyloid-beta peptide high-affinity copper II binding site in Alzheimer disease. *Biophys J* 2008 Oct;95(7):3447–3456.

Swan SH, Waller K, Hopkins B, Windham G, Fenster L, Schaefer C, Neutra RR. A prospective study of spontaneous abortion: relation to amount and source of drinking water consumed in early pregnancy. *Epidemiology* 1998 Mar;9(2):126–133.

Tang QQ, Du J, Ma HH, Jiang SJ, Zhou XJ. Fluoride and children's intelligence: a meta-analysis. *Biol Trace Elem Res* 2008 Winter;126(1–3):115–120.

Varner JA, Jensen KF, Horvath W, Isaacson RL. Chronic administration of aluminum-fluoride or sodium-fluoride to rats in drinking water: alterations in neuronal and cerebrovascular integrity. *Brain Res* 1998 Feb 16;784(1–2):284–298.

Villanueva CM, Fernández F, Malats N, Grimalt JO, Kogevinas M. Meta-analysis of studies on individual consumption of chlorinated drinking water and bladder cancer. *J Epidemiol Community Health* 2003 Mar;57(3):166–173.

Wagner M, Oehlmann J. Endocrine disruptors in bottled mineral water: estrogenic activity in the E-Screen. *J Steroid Biochem Mol Biol* 2010 Nov 2. Epub ahead of print.

Wagner M, Oehlmann J. Endocrine disruptors in bottled mineral water: total estrogenic burden and migration from plastic bottles. *Environ Sci Pollut Res Int* 2009 May;16(3):278–286.

Waller K, Swan SH, DeLorenze G, Hopkins B. Trihalomethanes in drinking water and spontaneous abortion. *Epidemiology* 1998 Mar;9(2):134–140.

Ward MH, Mark SD, Cantor KP, Weisenburger DD, Correa-Villasenor A, Zahm SH. Drinking water nitrate and the risk of non-Hodgkin's lymphoma. *Epidemiology* 1996 Sep;7(5):465–471.

Wiesenthal KE, McGuire MJ, Suffet IH. Characteristics of salt taste and free chlorine or chloramine in drinking water. *Water Sci Technol* 2007;55(5):293–300.

Windham GC, Waller K, Anderson M, Fenster L, Mendola P, Swan S. Chlorination by-products in drinking water and menstrual cycle function. *Environ Health Perspect* 2003 Jun;111(7):935–941.

Wormuth M, Scheringer M, Vollenweider M, Hungerbühler K. What are the sources of exposure to eight frequently used phthalic acid esters in Europeans? *Risk Anal* 2006 Jun;26(3):803–824.

Wrensch M, Swan SH, Lipscomb J, Epstein DM, Neutra RR, Fenster L. Spontaneous abortions and birth defects related to tap and bottled water use, San Jose, California, 1980–1985. *Epidemiology* 1992 Mar;3(2):98–103.

13. The Paleo Diet for Women and 14. The Paleo Diet for Children

Abrams SA, Griffin IJ. Microminerals and Bone Health. In: Holick MF, Dawson-Hughes B, *Nutrition and Bone Health*. Totowa, NJ: Humana Press, 2004: 377–387.

American Heart Association, 2010 Heart & Stroke Statistical Update http://www.americanheart.org/presenter.jhtml?identifier=3000090.

Barclay AW, Petocz P, McMillan-Price J, Flood VM, Prvan T, Mitchell P, Brand-Miller JC. Glycemic index, glycemic load, and chronic disease risk—a meta-analysis of observational studies. *Am J Clin Nutr* 2008 Mar;87(3):627–637.

Barzel US. The skeleton as an ion exchange system: implications for the role of acid-base imbalance in the genesis of osteoporosis. *J Bone Miner Res* 1995; 10:1431–1436.

Borer KT. Physical activity in the prevention and amelioration of osteoporosis in women: interaction of mechanical, hormonal and dietary factors. *Sports Med* 2005;35(9):779–830.

Bulkley JL. Cancer among primitive tribes. *Cancer* 1927;4:289–295.

Bürk K, Farecki ML, Lamprecht G, Roth G, Decker P, Weller M, Rammensee HG, Oertel W. Neurological symptoms in patients with biopsy proven celiac disease. *Mov Disord* 2009 Dec 15;24(16):2358–2362.

Capaso LL. Antiquity of cancer. *Int J Cancer* 2005;113:2–13.

Chen Y, Quick WW, Yang W, Zhang Y, Baldwin A, Moran J, Moore V, Sahai N, Dall TM. Cost of gestational diabetes mellitus in the United States in 2007. *Popul Health Manag* 2009 Jun;12(3):165–174.

Clifton P. High protein diets and weight control. *Nutr Metab Cardiovasc Dis* 2009 Jul;19(6):379–382.

Cockayne S, Adamson J, Lanham-New S, Shearer MJ, Gilbody S, Torgerson DJ. Vitamin K and the prevention of fractures: systematic review and meta-analysis of randomized controlled trials. *Arch Intern Med* 2006 Jun 26;166(12):1256–1261.

Coletta JM, Bell SJ, Roman AS. Omega-3 Fatty acids and pregnancy. *Rev Obstet Gynecol* 2010 Fall;3(4):163–171.

Cordain L. The nutritional characteristics of a contemporary diet based upon Paleolithic food groups. *J Am Nutraceut Assoc* 2002; 5:15–24.

Cordain L, Eades MR, Eades MD. Hyperinsulinemic diseases of civilization: more than just syndrome X. *Comp Biochem Physiol Part A* 2003;136:95–112.

Cordain L, Miller JB, Eaton SB, Mann N, Holt SH, Speth JD. Plant-animal subsistence ratios and macronutrient energy estimations in worldwide hunter-gatherer diets. *Am J Clin Nutr* 2000 Mar;71(3):682–692.

Cussons AJ, Watts GF, Mori TA, Stuckey BG. Omega-3 fatty acid supplementation decreases liver fat content in polycystic ovary syndrome: a randomized controlled trial employing proton magnetic resonance spectroscopy. *J Clin Endocrinol Metab* 2009 Oct;94(10):3842–3848.

David AR, Zimmerman MR. Cancer: an old disease, a new disease or something in between? *Nat Rev Cancer* 2010 Oct;10(10):728–733.

Dawson-Hughes B. Protein intake and calcium absorption—Potential role of the calcium sensor receptor. In Burckhardt P, Heaney R, Dawson-Hughes B. *Proceedings of the International Symposium on Nutritional Aspects of Osteoporosis, 4–6 May 2006, Lausanne, Switzerland*. Elsevier, 2007: 217–227.

DeFronzo RA, Cooke CR, Andres R, Faloona GR, Davis PJ. The effect of insulin on renal handling of sodium, potassium, calcium, and phosphate in man. *J Clin Invest* 1975;55:845–855.

Department of Health and Human Services. Centers for Disease Control and Prevention. United States Cancer Statistics http://apps.nccd.cdc.gov/uscs/.

Dohan FC. Genetic hypothesis of idiopathic schizophrenia: its exorphin connection. *Schizophr Bull* 1988;14(4):489–494.

Dohan FC. Hypothesis: genes and neuroactive peptides from food as cause of schizophrenia. *Adv Biochem Psychopharmacol* 1980;22:535–548.

Dohan FC, Harper EH, Clark MH, Rodrigue RB, Zigas V. Is schizophrenia rare if grain is rare? *Biol Psychiatry* 1984 Mar;19(3):385–399.

Dong JY, Qin LQ. Dietary glycemic index, glycemic load, and risk of breast cancer: meta-analysis of prospective cohort studies. *Breast Cancer Res Treat* 2011 Apr;126(2):287–294.

Eaton SB et al. Women's reproductive cancers in evolutionary context. *Quart Rev Biol* 1994;69:353–367.

Ford RP. The gluten syndrome: a neurological disease. *Med Hypotheses* 2009 Sep; 73(3):438–440.

Frassetto LA, Morris RC Jr, Sebastian A. Dietary sodium chloride intake independently predicts the degree of hyperchloremic metabolic acidosis in healthy humans consuming a net acid-producing diet. *Am J Physiol Renal Physiol* 2007 Aug;293(2):F521–525.

Frassetto LA, Morris Jr RC, Sebastian A. A practical approach to the balance between acid production and renal acid excretion in humans. *J Nephrol* 2006 Mar–Apr;19 Suppl 9:S33–40.

Frassetto L. Diet, evolution and aging—the pathophysiologic effects of the post-agricultural inversion of the potassium-to-sodium and base-to-chloride ratios in the human diet. *Eur J Nutr* 2001 Oct;40(5):200–213.

Friborg JT, Melbye M. Cancer patterns in Inuit populations. *Lancet Oncol* 2008 Sep;9(9):892–900.

Gandini S, Merzenich H, Robertson C, Boyle P. Meta-analysis of studies on breast cancer risk and diet: the role of fruit and vegetable consumption and the intake of associated micronutrients. *Eur J Cancer* 2000 Mar;36(5):636–646.

Gannon MC, Nuttall FQ, Krezowski PA, Billington CJ, Parker S. The serum insulin and plasma glucose responses to milk and fruit products in type 2 (non-insulin-dependent) diabetic patients. *Diabetologia* 1986 Nov;29(11):784–791.

Halperin EC. Pale-oncology the role of ancient remains in the study of cancer. *Perspect Biol Med* 2004;47:1–14.

Hearsey H. The rarity of cancer among the aborigines of British Central Africa. *Brit Med J* 1906 Dec 1:1562–1563.

Henson, WW. Cancer in Kafirs: suggested cause. *Guy's Hospital Gazette* 1904 Mar 26:131–133.

Herrick K, Phillips DIW, Haselden S, Shiell AW, Campbell-Brown M, Godfrey KM. Maternal consumption of a high-meat, low-carbohydrate diet in late pregnancy: relation to adult cortisol concentrations in the offspring. *J Clin Endocrinol Metab* 2003;88(8):3554–3560.

Hildes JA, Schaefer O. The changing picture of neoplastic disease in the western and central Canadian Arctic (1950–1980). *Can Med Assoc J* 1984;130:25–32.

Holick MF, Chen TC. Vitamin D deficiency: a worldwide problem with health consequences. *Am J Clin Nutr* 2008 Apr;87(4):1080S–1086S.

Holt SH, et al. An insulin index of foods: the insulin demand generated by 1000-kJ portions of common foods. *Am J Clin Nutr* 1997 Nov;66(5):1264–1276.

Hoyt G, Hickey MS, Cordain L. Dissociation of the glycaemic and insulinaemic responses to whole and skimmed milk. *Br J Nutr* 2005 Feb;93(2):175–177.

Kalhan, S. Protein metabolism in pregnancy. *Am J Clin Nutr* 2000;71 (suppl): 1249S–1255S.

Kelly J, Lanier A, Santos M, Healey S, Louchini R, Friborg J, Young K, Ng C. Cancer among the circumpolar Inuit, 1989–2003. I. Background and methods. *Int J Circumpolar Health* 2008 Dec;67(5):396–407.

Kerstetter JE, Gaffney ED, O'Brien O, et al. Dietary Protein increases intestinal calcium absorption and improves bone balance : an hypothesis. In Burckhardt P, Heaney R, Dawson-Hughes B. *Proceedings of the International Symposium on Nutritional Aspects of Osteoporosis, 4–6 May 2006, Lausanne, Switzerland.* Elsevier, 2007: 204–216.

Lanier AP, Bender TR, Blot WJ, Fraumeni JF Jr. Cancer in Alaskan Natives: 1974–78. *Natl Cancer Inst Monogr* 1982;62:79–81.

Larsen TM, Dalskov SM, van Baak M, Jebb SA, Papadaki A, Pfeiffer AF, Martinez JA, Handjieva-Darlenska T, Kunešová M, Pihlsgård M, Stender S, Holst C, Saris WH, Astrup A. Diet, Obesity, and Genes (Diogenes) Project. Diets with high or low protein content and glycemic index for weight-loss maintenance. *N Engl J Med* 2010 Nov 25;363(22):2102–2113.

Liljeberg Elmstahl H, Bjorck I. Milk as a supplement to mixed meals may elevate postprandial insulinaemia. *Eur J Clin Nutr* 2001; 55:994–999.

Lissowska J, Gaudet MM, Brinton LA, Peplonska B, Sherman M, Szeszenia-Dabrowska N, Zatonski W, Garcia-Closas M. Intake of fruits, and vegetables in relation to breast cancer risk by hormone receptor status. *Breast Cancer Res Treat* 2008;107:113–117.

Lorenz K. Cereals and schizophrenia. *Adv Cereal Sci Technol* 1990;10:435–469.

Louie JC, Brand-Miller JC, Markovic TP, Ross GP, Moses RG. Glycemic index and pregnancy: a systematic literature review. *J Nutr Metab* 2010;2010:282464.

Marsh KA, Steinbeck KS, Atkinson FS, Petocz P, Brand-Miller JC. Effect of a low glycemic index compared with a conventional healthy diet on polycystic ovary syndrome. *Am J Clin Nutr* 2010 Jul;92(1):83–92.

McDowell M, Briefel R, Alaimo K, et al. Energy and macronutrientintakes of persons ages 2 months and over in the United States: Third National Health and Nutrition Examination Survey, Phase 1, 1988–91. Washington, DC: US Government Printing Office, Vital and Health Statistics; 1994. CDC publication No. 255.

Niederhofer H, Pittschieler K. A preliminary investigation of ADHD symptoms in persons with celiac disease. *J Atten Disord* 2006 Nov;10(2):200–2004.

Noli D, Avery G. Protein poisoning and coastal subsistence. *J Archaeological Sci* 1988;15:395–401.

Ostman EM, et al. Inconsistency between glycemic and insulinemic responses to regular and fermented milk products. *Am J Clin Nutr* 2001;74:96–100.

Papadaki A, Linardakis M, Larsen TM, van Baak MA, Lindroos AK, Pfeiffer AF, Martinez JA, Handjieva-Darlenska T, Kunesová M, Holst C, Astrup A, Saris WH, Kafatos A, DiOGenes Study Group. The effect of protein and glycemic index on children's body composition: the DiOGenes randomized study. *Pediatrics* 2010 Nov;126(5):e1143–1152.

Phelan N, O'Connor A, Kyaw Tun T, Correia N, Boran G, Roche HM, Gibney J. Hormonal and metabolic effects of polyunsaturated fatty acids in young women with polycystic ovary syndrome: results from a cross-sectional analysis and a randomized, placebo-controlled, crossover trial. *Am J Clin Nutr* 2011 Mar;93(3):652–662.

Pols H, Yazdanpanah N, van Meurs J. Homocysteine, the vitamin B complex family and bone. In Burckhardt P, Heaney R, Dawson-Hughes B. *Proceedings of the International Symposium on Nutritional Aspects of Osteoporosis, 4–6 May 2006, Lausanne, Switzerland.* Elsevier, 2007, pp 151–157.

Pynnönen PA, Isometsä ET, Aronen ET, Verkasalo MA, Savilahti E, Aalberg VA. Mental disorders in adolescents with celiac disease. *Psychosomatics* 2004 Jul–Aug;45(4):325–335.

Pynnönen PA, Isometsä ET, Verkasalo MA, Kähkönen SA, Sipilä I, Savilahti E, Aalberg VA. Gluten-free diet may alleviate depressive and behavioural symptoms in adolescents with coeliac disease: a prospective follow-up case-series study. *BMC Psychiatry* 2005 Mar 17;5:14.

Rabinowitch IM. Clinical and other observations on Canadian Eskimos in the Eastern Arctic. *Can Med Assoc J* 1936;34:487–501.

Reichelt KL, Seim AR, Reichelt WH. Could schizophrenia be reasonably explained by Dohan's hypothesis on genetic interaction with a dietary peptide overload? *Prog Neuropsychopharmacol Biol Psychiatry* 1996 Oct;20(7):1083–1114.

Remer T, Manz F. Potential renal acid load of foods and its influence on urine pH. *J Am Diet Assoc* 1995;95:791–797.

Renner W. The spread of cancer among the descendants of the liberated Africans or Creoles of Sierre Leone. *Brit Med J* 1910 Sept 3;587–589.

Rhodes ET, Pawlak DB, Takoudes TC, Ebbeling CB, Feldman HA, Lovesky MM, Cooke EA, Leidig MM, Ludwig DS. Effects of a low-glycemic load diet in overweight and obese pregnant women: a pilot randomized controlled trial. *Am J Clin Nutr* 2010 Dec;92(6):1306–1315.

Riboli E, Norat T. Epidemiologic evidence of the protective effect of fruit and vegetables on cancer risk. *Am J Clin Nutr* 2003 Sep;78(3 Suppl):559S–569S.

Riveros M. First observation of cancer among the Pampidos (Chulupi) Indians of the Paraguayan Chaco. *Int Surg* 1970;53:51–55.

Rudman D, DiFulco TJ, Galambos JT, Smith RB 3rd, Salam AA, Warren WD. Maximal rates of excretion and synthesis of urea in normal and cirrhotic subjects. *J Clin Invest* 1973 Sep;52(9):2241–2249.

Ruuskanen A, Kaukinen K, Collin P, Huhtala H, Valve R, Mäki M, Luostarinen L. Positive serum antigliadin antibodies without celiac disease in the elderly population: does it matter? *Scand J Gastroenterol.* 2010 Oct;45(10):1197–1202.

Saadatian-Elahi M, Norat T, Goudable J, Riboli E. Biomarkers of dietary fatty acid intake and the risk of breast cancer: a meta-analysis. *Int J Cancer* 2004 Sep 10;111(4):584–591.

Sebastian A. Dietary protein content and the diet's net acid load: opposing effects on bone health. *Am J Clin Nutr* 2005 Nov;82(5):921–922.

Simonelli C, et al. (July 2006). *ICSI Health Care Guideline: Diagnosis and Treatment of Osteoporosis, 5th edition (PDF).* Institute for Clinical Systems Improvement.

Speth JD. Early hominid hunting and scavenging: the role of meat as an energy source. *J Hum Evol* 1989;18:329–343.

Speth JD. Protein selection and avoidance strategies of contemporary and ancestral foragers: unresolved issues. *Philos Trans R Soc Lond B Biol Sci* 1991 Nov 29;334 (1270):265–269; discussion 269–270.

Speth JD, Spielmann KA. Energy source, protein metabolism, and hunter-gatherer subsistence strategies. *J Anthropological Archaeology* 1983;2:1–31.

Sojka JE, Weaver CM. Magnesium supplementation and osteoporosis. *Nutr Rev* 1995 Mar;53(3):71–74.

Stefansson V. *Cancer: Disease of Civilization?* New York: Hill and Wang, 1960.

St Jeor ST, Howard BV, Prewitt TE, Bovee V, Bazzarre T, Eckel RH, et al. Dietary protein and weight reduction: a statement for healthcare professionals from the Nutrition Committee of the Council on Nutrition, Physical Activity, and Metabolism of the American Heart Association. *Circulation* 2001 Oct 9;104(15):1869–1874.

Urquhart JA. The most northerly practice in Canada. *Can Med Assoc J* 1935;33:193–196.

Vojdani A, O'Bryan T, Green JA, Mccandless J, Woeller KN, Vojdani E, Nourian AA, Cooper EL. Immune response to dietary proteins, gliadin and cerebellar peptides in children with autism. *Nutr Neurosci* 2004 Jun;7(3):151–161.

Vojdani A, Pangborn JB, Vojdani E, Cooper EL. Infections, toxic chemicals and dietary peptides binding to lymphocyte receptors and tissue enzymes are major instigators of autoimmunity in autism. *Int J Immunopathol Pharmacol* 2003 Sep–Dec;16(3):189–199.

Watkins BA, Li Y, Seifert MF. Dietary ratio of n-6/n-3 PUFAs and docosahexaenoic acid: actions on bone mineral and serum biomarkers in ovariectomized rats. *J Nutr Biochem* 2006; 17(4):282–289, 2006.

Weiss La, Barrett-Connor E, Von Muhlen D. Ratio of omega-6 to omega-3 fatty acids and bone mineral density in older adults: the Rancho Bernardo Study. *Am J Clin Nutr* 2005;81(4):934–938.

Wright JD, J Kennedy-Stephenson J, Wang CY, McDowell MA, Johnson CL, National Center for Health Statistics, CDC. Trends in intake of energy and macronutrients—United States, 1971–2000. *JAMA* 2004;291:1193–1194.

Yee LD, Lester JL, Cole RM, Richardson JR, Hsu JC, Li Y, Lehman A, Belury MA, Clinton SK. Omega-3 fatty acid supplements in women at high risk of breast cancer have dose-dependent effects on breast adipose tissue fatty acid composition. *Am J Clin Nutr* 2010 May;91(5):1185–1194.

Zhang CX, Ho SC, Chen YM, Fu JH, Cheng SZ, Lin FY. Greater vegetable and fruit intake is associated with a lower risk of breast cancer among Chinese women. *Int J Cancer* 2009 Jul 1;125(1):181–188.

Index